Access your Clinics anywhere you go with our new App!

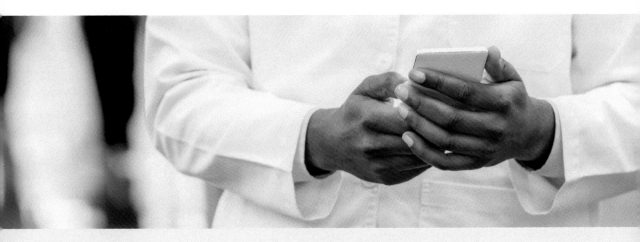

The new and improved Clinics Review Articles mobile app offers subscribers rapid access to recently published content from all Clinics Review Articles titles.

KEY FEATURES OF THE CLINICS APP:

- **Download full issues** while reading – no need to wait!
- **Access articles quickly and conveniently** with new, improved layouts and navigation.
- **Interact with figures, tables, videos**, and other supplementary content.
- **Personalize your experience** by creating reading lists and adding your own notes to articles.
- **Share your favorite articles** on social media and email useful content to colleagues.

DOWNLOAD THE CLINICS APP TODAY!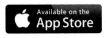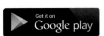

Clinics Review Articles

Imaging of the Pelvis and Lower Extremity

Editors

KURT F. SCHERER
LAURA W. BANCROFT

RADIOLOGIC CLINICS OF NORTH AMERICA

www.radiologic.theclinics.com

Consulting Editor
FRANK H. MILLER

November 2018 • Volume 56 • Number 6

ELSEVIER

1600 John F. Kennedy Boulevard • Suite 1800 • Philadelphia, Pennsylvania, 19103-2899

http://www.theclinics.com

RADIOLOGIC CLINICS OF NORTH AMERICA Volume 56, Number 6
November 2018 ISSN 0033-8389, ISBN 13: 978-0-323-64155-5

Editor: John Vassallo (j.vassallo@elsevier.com)
Developmental Editor: Donald Mumford

Radiologic Clinics of North America (ISSN 0033-8389) is published bimonthly by Elsevier Inc., 360 Park Avenue South, New York, NY 10010-1710. Months of issue are January, March, May, July, September, and November. Periodicals postage paid at New York, NY and additional mailing offices. Subscription prices are USD 493 per year for US individuals, USD 889 per year for US institutions, USD 100 per year for US students and residents, USD 573 per year for Canadian individuals, USD 1136 per year for Canadian institutions, USD 680 per year for international individuals, USD 1136 per year for international institutions, and USD 315 per year for Canadian and international students/residents. To receive student and resident rate, orders must be accompanied by name of affiliated institution, date of term and the signature of program/residency coordinatior on institution letterhead. Orders will be billed at individual rate until proof of status is received. Foreign air speed delivery is included in all *Clinics* subscription prices. All prices are subject to change without notice. **POSTMASTER:** Send address changes to *Radiologic Clinics of North America*, Elsevier Health Sciences Division, Subscription Customer Service, 3251 Riverport Lane, Maryland Heights, MO63043. **Customer Service: Telephone: 1-800-654-2452** (U.S. and Canada); **1-314-447-8871** (outside U.S. and Canada). **Fax: 1-314-447-8029. E-mail: journalscustomerservice-usa@ elsevier.com (for print support); journalsonlinesupport-usa@elsevier.com (for online support).**

Reprints. For copies of 100 or more of articles in this publication, please contact the Commercial Reprints Department, Elsevier Inc., 360 Park Avenue South, New York, New York 10010-1710. Tel.: +1-212-633-3874; Fax: +1-212-633-3820; E-mail: reprints@elsevier.com.

Radiologic Clinics of North America also published in Greek Paschalidis Medical Publications, Athens, Greece.

Radiologic Clinics of North America is covered in *MEDLINE/PubMed (Index Medicus), EMBASE/Excerpta Medica, Current Contents/Life Sciences, Current Contents/Clinical Medicine, RSNA Index to Imaging Literature, BIOSIS, Science Citation Index,* and *ISI/BIOMED*.

Printed in the United States of America.

Contributors

CONSULTING EDITOR

FRANK H. MILLER, MD, FACR
Lee F. Rogers MD Professor of Medical
Education, Chief, Body Imaging Section and
Fellowship Program, Medical Director, MRI,
Department of Radiology, Northwestern
Memorial Hospital, Northwestern University
Feinberg School of Medicine, Chicago, Illinois

EDITORS

KURT F. SCHERER, MD
Program Director, Diagnostic Radiology
Residency Program, Florida Hospital Orlando,
Clinical Assistant Professor of Radiology,
Florida State University College of Medicine,
Adjunct Assistant Professor, University of
Central Florida College of Medicine, Orlando,
Florida

LAURA W. BANCROFT, MD, FACR
Chief of Musculoskeletal Imaging, Florida
Hospital Orlando, Clinical Professor of
Radiology, Florida State University College of
Medicine, Department Chair of Radiology and
Adjunct Professor, University of Central Florida
College of Medicine, Orlando, Florida

AUTHORS

BEHRANG AMINI, MD, PhD
Associate Professor, Department of Diagnostic
Radiology, The University of Texas MD
Anderson Cancer Center, Houston, Texas

TOLU ASHIMOLOWO, MD
Department of Radiology, University of
Washington, Seattle, Washington

JENNY T. BENCARDINO, MD
Department of Radiology, NYU Langone
Medical Center, New York, New York

BRIAN Y. CHAN, MD
Musculoskeletal Imaging and Intervention
Fellow, Department of Radiology, University of
Wisconsin-Madison School of Medicine and
Public Health, Madison, Wisconsin

RUSSELL CHAPIN, MD
Associate Professor, Department of Radiology,
Medical University of South Carolina,
Charleston, South Carolina

IVAN DAVIS, MD
Assistant Professor, Department of Radiology,
College of Medicine, University of Florida,
Gainesville, Florida

ALEJANDRA DUARTE, MD
Department of Radiology, NYU
Langone Medical Center, New York,
New York

GREGOR DUNHAM, MD
Department of Radiology, University of
Washington, Seattle, Washington

ANGELA M. FAST, MD
Department of Radiology, Stanford University,
Stanford, California

ELISABETH R. GARWOOD, MD
Department of Radiology, NYU
Langone Orthopedic Hospital, New York,
New York

ARIA GHAFFARI, MD
Resident Physician, Department of Radiology,
College of Medicine, University of Florida,
Gainesville, Florida

AARON HODES, MD
Resident, Department of Radiology, Jacobi
Medical Center, Bronx, New York

OMAR KHAN, MD
Department of Radiology, House Officer,
University of Michigan Health System,
Ann Arbor, Michigan

KENNETH S. LEE, MD
Associate Professor, Department of Radiology,
University of Wisconsin-Madison School of
Medicine and Public Health, Madison,
Wisconsin

GARY M. LIMARZI, MD
Clinical Lecturer, Department of Radiology,
MSK Division, University of Michigan Health
System, Ann Arbor, Michigan

WILLIAM C. MEYERS, MD
Vincera Institute, Philadelphia, Pennsylvania

DANIEL J. MIZRAHI, MD
Division of Musculoskeletal Radiology, Thomas
Jefferson University, Philadelphia,
Pennsylvania

MICHAEL MOSER, MD
Associate Professor, Department of
Orthopaedics and Rehabilitation, UF
Orthopaedics and Sports Medicine Institute,
University of Florida, Gainesville, Florida

HYOJEONG MULCAHY, MD
Associate Professor, Department of Radiology,
University of Washington, Seattle, Washington

NAOKI O. MURAI, MD
Resident, Department of Diagnostic and
Interventional Imaging, The University of Texas
Health Science Center, Houston, Texas

ALEX E. POOR, MD
Vincera Institute, Philadelphia, Pennsylvania

JACK PORRINO, MD
Radiology and Biomedical Imaging, Yale
School of Medicine, New Haven, Connecticut

GEOFFREY RILEY, MD
Department of Radiology, Stanford University,
Stanford, California

JOHANNES B. ROEDL, MD, PhD
Division of Musculoskeletal Radiology, Thomas
Jefferson University, Philadelphia,
Pennsylvania

YASHESH SHAH, MD
Department of Radiology, House Officer,
University of Michigan Health System,
Ann Arbor, Michigan

JAKE W. SHARP, MD
Department of Radiology, University of
Washington, Seattle, Washington

TROY STOREY, MD
Associate Professor, Department of Radiology,
College of Medicine, University of Florida,
Gainesville, Florida

PREETI ARUN SUKERKAR, MD, PhD
Department of Radiology, Stanford University,
Stanford, California

OLUWADAMILOLA TENIOLA, MD
Resident, Department of Radiology,
Baylor College of Medicine, Houston,
Texas

HILARY UMANS, MD
Professor, Department of Radiology,
Albert Einstein College of Medicine, Bronx,
New York; Musculoskeletal Radiologist,
Department of Radiology, Lenox Hill Radiology
& Imaging Associates, P.C., New York,
New York

WEI-LIEN WANG, MD, MPH
Assistant Professor, Department of Pathology,
The University of Texas MD Anderson Cancer
Center, Houston, Texas

CORRIE M. YABLON, MD
Associate Professor, Department of Radiology,
MSK Division, University of Michigan Health
System, Ann Arbor, Michigan

ADAM C. ZOGA, MD
Division of Musculoskeletal Radiology, Thomas
Jefferson University, Philadelphia,
Pennsylvania

Contents

The foot and ankle delicately balance the need for support of the weight of the human body, with the need for flexibility. Palpable masses about the foot and ankle, therefore, are most commonly related to trauma or mechanical instability. Non-neoplastic causes, such as ganglion cysts and callus, therefore, predominate. However, the radiologist must be aware of the imaging appearance of less common benign and malignant neoplasms that can involve the foot and ankle.

The posterolateral corner (PLC) of the knee is composed of numerous ligamentous and tendinous structures that provide restraint and stability. This anatomy is complex, and at times controversial. We present a comprehensive review of the normal anatomy and pathology of the PLC. We highlight potential pitfalls of image interpretation and detail what the referring physician needs to know.

In the postmeniscectomy or meniscal repair setting, there is overlap between expected postoperative change and findings of a re-torn meniscus, particularly increased T1-weighted or proton density signal contacting the articular surface. Protocol selection and accurate diagnosis requires knowledge of meniscal tear treatment, the expected postoperative appearance, and criteria for re-tear. Criteria for meniscal re-tear on MR imaging are high T2-weighted signal reaching the articular surface, abnormal meniscal morphology not explained by the surgery, or a displaced fragment. When MR arthrography is performed, a meniscal tear may or may not exhibit signal intensity as high as that of the intraarticular contrast.

Femoroacetabular impingement (FAI) is a prevalent clinical syndrome and likely a primary contributor to idiopathic hip osteoarthritis. It is characterized by osseous pathomorphology in the hip that alters normal biomechanics, causing accelerated joint degeneration and characteristic patterns of chondral and labral injuries. Early intervention in well-selected patients can provide symptomatic relief and delay progression to osteoarthritis. Because imaging findings of FAI are subtle, a checklist approach based on current concepts is necessary to efficiently generate imaging reports that advance clinical decision-making. This article details an approach to the imaging assessment of FAI.

Pelvic pain can result from gastrointestinal, gynecologic, urologic, neurologic, and musculoskeletal sources. This article focuses on the musculoskeletal lesions that contribute to acute and chronic pain throughout the musculoskeletal core. Armed with an understanding of musculoskeletal core anatomy and biomechanics, imagers play an integral role in the accurate diagnosis and treatment planning for patients with pain and dysfunction from pelvic sources. MR imaging is the primary imaging modality used, but focused sonographic and radiographic techniques have a role. Ultimately, radiologists can help guide patients to the most appropriate subspecialty clinicians based on the underlying source of symptoms.

Entrapment neuropathies of the lower extremity are commonly encountered and present a diagnostic challenge. Historical diagnostic workhorses—the physical examination combined with electrodiagnostic studies—are now frequently supplemented by MR neurography. MR neurography is a high-resolution, noninvasive, and operator-independent imaging modality that has proven useful in diagnosis, disease severity assessment, and informing treatment decisions in the management of lower extremity entrapment neuropathies. Currently, the assessment of the peripheral nerves relies heavily on reader identification of morphologic nerve changes; however, emerging innovative MR sequences and PET/MR imaging hold the potential to provide noninvasive means of functional assessment.

Extreme sports are growing in popularity, and physicians are becoming increasingly aware of injuries related to these activities. Imaging plays a key role in diagnosing and determining clinical management of many of these injuries. This article describes general imaging techniques and findings in various injuries specific to multiple extreme sports.

Musculoskeletal (MSK) conditions are growing in prevalence. Ultrasound (US) is increasingly used for managing MSK conditions due to its low cost and ability to provide real-time image guidance during therapeutic interventions. As MSK US becomes more widespread, familiarity and comfort with US-guided interventions will become increasingly important. This article focuses on general concepts regarding therapeutic US-guided injections of corticosteroids and platelet-rich plasma and highlights several of the US-guided procedures commonly performed, involving the pelvis and lower extremity.

PROGRAM OBJECTIVE

The objective of the *Radiologic Clinics of North America* is to keep practicing radiologists and radiology residents up to date with current clinical practice in radiology by providing timely articles reviewing the state of the art in patient care.

TARGET AUDIENCE

Practicing radiologists, radiology residents, and other healthcare professionals who provide patient care utilizing radiologic findings.

LEARNING OBJECTIVES

Upon completion of this activity, participants will be able to:
1. Review imaging manifestations of ankle impingement syndromes
2. Discuss current concepts in the diagnosis and treatment of Femoroacetabular Impingement
3. Recognize uncommon sources of pelvic pain through imaging of the pelvis and lower extremity

ACCREDITATION

The Elsevier Office of Continuing Medical Education (EOCME) is accredited by the Accreditation Council for Continuing Medical Education (ACCME) to provide continuing medical education for physicians.

The EOCME designates this enduring material for a maximum of 15 *AMA PRA Category 1 Credit*(s)™. Physicians should claim only the credit commensurate with the extent of their participation in the activity.

All other healthcare professionals requesting continuing education credit for this enduring material will be issued a certificate of participation.

DISCLOSURE OF CONFLICTS OF INTEREST

The EOCME assesses conflict of interest with its instructors, faculty, planners, and other individuals who are in a position to control the content of CME activities. All relevant conflicts of interest that are identified are thoroughly vetted by EOCME for fair balance, scientific objectivity, and patient care recommendations. EOCME is committed to providing its learners with CME activities that promote improvements or quality in healthcare and not a specific proprietary business or a commercial interest.

The planning committee, staff, authors and editors listed below have identified no financial relationships or relationships to products or devices they or their spouse/life partner have with commercial interest related to the content of this CME activity:

Behrang Amini, MD, PhD; Tolu Ashimolowo, MD; Jenny T. Bencardino, MD; Brian Y. Chan, MD; Russell Chapin, MD; Ivan Davis, MD; Alejandra Duarte, MD; Gregor Dunham, MD; Angela M. Fast, MD; Elisabeth R. Garwood, MD; Aria Ghaffari, MD; Aaron Hodes, MD; Alison Kemp; Omar Khan, MD; Pradeep Kuttysankaran; Gary M. LiMarzi, MD; William C. Meyers, MD; Frank H. Miller, MD, FACR; Daniel J. Mizrahi, MD; Michael Moser, MD; Hyojeong Mulcahy, MD; Naoki O. Murai, MD; Alex E. Poor, MD; Jack Porrino, MD; Geoffrey Riley, MD; Johannes B. Roedl, MD, PhD; Yashesh Shah, MD; Jake W. Sharp, MD; Troy Storey, MD; Preeti Arun Sukerkar, MD, PhD; Oluwadamilola Teniola, MD; Hilary Umans, MD; John Vassallo; Wei-Lien Wang, MD, MPH; Corrie M. Yablon, MD; Adam C. Zoga, MD.

The planning committee, staff, authors and editors listed below have identified financial relationships or relationships to products or devices they or their spouse/life partner have with commercial interest related to the content of this CME activity:

Kenneth S. Lee, MD: receives research support from General Electric Company and DePuy Synthesis; is a consultant/advisor for Echometrix, LLC; and receives royalties from Elsevier.

UNAPPROVED/OFF-LABEL USE DISCLOSURE

The EOCME requires CME faculty to disclose to the participants:
1. When products or procedures being discussed are off-label, unlabelled, experimental, and/or investigational (not US Food and Drug Administration [FDA] approved); and
2. Any limitations on the information presented, such as data that are preliminary or that represent ongoing research, interim analyses, and/or unsupported opinions. Faculty may discuss information about pharmaceutical agents that is outside of FDA-approved labelling. This information is intended solely for CME and is not intended to promote off-label use of these medications. If you have any questions, contact the medical affairs department of the manufacturer for the most recent prescribing information.

TO ENROLL

To enroll in the *Radiologic Clinics of North America* Continuing Medical Education program, call customer service at 1-800-654-2452 or sign up online at http://www.theclinics.com/home/cme. The CME program is available to subscribers for an additional annual fee of USD 327.60.

METHOD OF PARTICIPATION

In order to claim credit, participants must complete the following:

1. Complete enrolment as indicated above.
2. Read the activity.
3. Complete the CME Test and Evaluation. Participants must achieve a score of 70% on the test. All CME Tests and Evaluations must be completed online.

CME INQUIRIES/SPECIAL NEEDS

For all CME inquiries or special needs, please contact elsevierCME@elsevier.com.

RADIOLOGIC CLINICS OF NORTH AMERICA

RELATED SERIES

Magnetic Resonance Imaging Clinics
Neuroimaging Clinics
PET Clinics

THE CLINICS ARE AVAILABLE ONLINE!
Access your subscription at:
www.theclinics.com

Preface
Imaging of the Pelvis and Lower Extremity

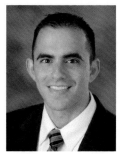
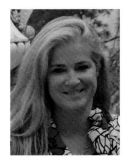

Kurt F. Scherer, MD   Laura W. Bancroft, MD, FACR

Editors

This issue of the *Radiologic Clinics of North America* serves as a centralized, practical resource for radiologists who interpret musculoskeletal imaging of the pelvis and lower extremity. This collection of articles reviews the relevant clinical and multimodality imaging features found in posttraumatic and sports-related injuries of the foot/ankle, knee, and pelvis. In addition, various experts have compiled focused articles on ankle impingement, postoperative meniscus, bone and soft tissue tumors about the foot and ankle, ultrasound-guided interventions of the lower extremity and pelvis, and lower-extremity entrapment neuropathy.

We would like to extend our gratitude to all of the authors who have contributed to this issue. We appreciate their willingness to share their expertise and provide the most relevant and updated references from the literature.

Kurt F. Scherer, MD
Department of Radiology
Florida Hospital
601 E Rollins
Orlando, FL 32803, USA

Laura W. Bancroft, MD, FACR
Department of Radiology
Florida Hospital
601 E Rollins
Orlando, FL 32803, USA

E-mail addresses:
Kurt.scherer.md@flhosp.org (K.F. Scherer)
Laura.bancroft.md@flhosp.org (L.W. Bancroft)

Radiol Clin N Am 56 (2018) xi
https://doi.org/10.1016/j.rcl.2018.08.015
0033-8389/18/© 2018 Published by Elsevier Inc.

Turf Toe
An Update and Comprehensive Review

Tolu Ashimolowo, MD[a], Gregor Dunham, MD[a],
Jake W. Sharp, MD[a], Jack Porrino, MD[b],*

KEYWORDS

- Turf toe • Metatarsophalangeal joint • Plantar plate • Accessory sesamoid ligament
- Intersesamoid ligament • Metatarsal-sesamoidal ligament • Sesamoid-phalangeal ligament
- Deep transverse intermetatarsal ligament

KEY POINTS

- Turf toe was originally believed to involve injury only to the central plantar plate; however, numerous other structures may be involved.
- The injury may be severely debilitating and can result in premature end to an athlete's career.
- Understanding the anatomy and accurately identifying the pathology to the structures involved is critical to arriving at the appropriate diagnosis and management strategy.
- MR imaging is routinely used in conjunction with radiographs, ultrasound, and computed tomography, to fully diagnose the extent of the turf toe injury.
- Turf toe is typically managed conservatively; however, surgical intervention is used if less invasive measures fail.

INTRODUCTION

The term *turf toe* was initially used to describe a classic sports-related injury pattern involving the first metatarsophalangeal joint (MTP) in collegiate level football players wearing flexible cleats on artificial turf.[1] The traditional definition was a sprain of the plantar capsule-ligament caused by hyperextension of the first MTP joint on forced contact.[1] It has since evolved to include a more detailed description of injuries that encompass the small structures surrounding the first MTP joint, and has also been reported in professional football, soccer, tennis, and basketball players.[2–4]

The mechanism of injury involves an axial loading force on the posterior aspect of the leg, a fixed-planted foot, and resultant forced hyperextension (dorsiflexion) of the first MTP joint. In extreme cases, the player develops severe pain and inability to bear weight. Additional mechanisms of injury have also been reported. The most common variant involves a valgus-directed force to the first MTP joint with injury to the medial plantar complex and medial sesamoid.[4,5] This specific variant has been linked to the development of a traumatic hallux valgus deformity.[4] An alternative pattern of injury to the first MTP joint originally described in 1978 by Coker and colleagues[5] consists of forced hyperflexion of the joint, and should be differentiated from turf toe. Frey and colleagues[6] coined the term "sand toe" to describe this injury due to the preponderance of this pathology in beach volleyball players. Although also affecting the first MTP joint, it should

Disclosures: The authors report no commercial or financial conflicts of interest, nor any funding sources.
[a] Department of Radiology, University of Washington, 1959 Northeast Pacific Street, Seattle, WA 98195-7117, USA; [b] Radiology and Biomedical Imaging, Yale School of Medicine, 20 York Street, New Haven, CT 06510, USA
* Corresponding author.
E-mail address: rhees27@yahoo.com

Radiol Clin N Am 56 (2018) 847–858
https://doi.org/10.1016/j.rcl.2018.06.002

not be considered analogous to turf toe because it involves injury to a different set of structures, particularly the extensor mechanism.[4]

Specific predisposing causes for the development of a turf toe injury have been a topic of controversy for decades. Nonetheless, it is widely accepted that the use of an artificial playing surface and softer, more flexible cleats serve as risk factors in football-related injuries of the first MTP joint.[7] Improved imaging techniques have contributed immensely to the detection and characterization of turf toe–related injuries.

NORMAL ANATOMY

The first MTP joint plays an essential role in walking, running, jumping, and weight bearing. The joint is surrounded by ligaments and tendons, which provide extrinsic and intrinsic support (**Fig. 1**). The rounded first metatarsal head forms a hinge joint with the concave end of the first proximal phalanx. The paired sesamoids are located at the plantar surface of the first metatarsal head, separated by a bony protuberance on the undersurface of the first metatarsal head called the crista. The sesamoids are bridged by the intersesamoid (IS) ligament, essentially a proximal thickening of the plantar plate. There is limited range of motion at the first

MTP joint, with approximately 30° of flexion and 50° of extension.[8] Although the hallux sesamoids are a set of small bones at the joint, they play a critical role in its stabilization. Injury to the sesamoids or absence (congenital or postsurgical) may contribute to joint pathology (**Fig. 2**).[9]

The IS ligament is situated deep to the flexor hallucis longus tendon. The paired medial and lateral heads of the flexor hallucis brevis (FHB) tendons surround and attach to the medial/tibial and lateral/fibular sesamoid bones (**Fig. 3**).[8,10] The plantar plate is a strand of fibrocartilaginous tissue that originates at the first metatarsal head/neck, wraps around the hallux sesamoids, and attaches distally to the base of the first proximal phalanx.[3,11] The central portion is relatively thin compared with the thick, lateral margins that encapsulate the sesamoids (**Fig. 4**). The distal attachment is fixed, taut, and more stable compared with the weaker proximal attachment.[11]

The accessory sesamoid ligaments originate from the first metatarsal head and terminate at the margins of the medial and lateral sesamoids. Paired with the accessory sesamoid ligaments on either side of the joint are the main collateral ligaments, which extend obliquely from the first metatarsal head to the base of the first proximal phalanx. Together, the accessory sesamoid ligaments and main collateral ligaments form the

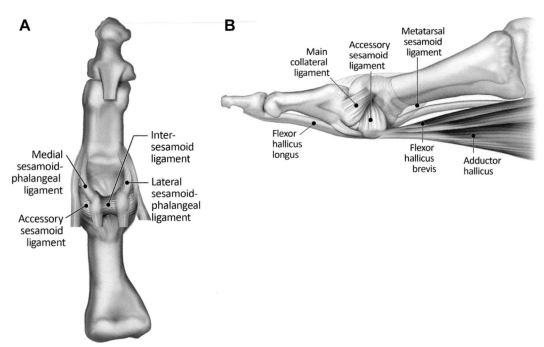

Fig. 1. Anatomy of the first metatarsophalangeal joint. Plantar (*A*) and lateral (*B*) schematic views of the first metatarsophalangeal joint.

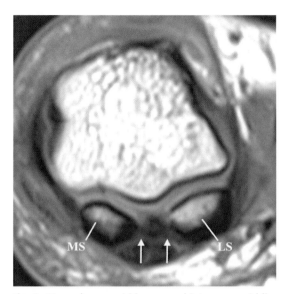

Fig. 2. Normal sesamoid bones and intersesamoid ligament in a 31-year-old woman. Short-axis T1-weighted image through the first metatarsal head shows the medial sesamoid (MS) and lateral sesamoid (LS), bridged by the intersesamoid ligament (*arrows*).

collateral ligament complex (**Fig. 5**).[12] The paired medial and lateral metatarsal-sesamoidal (MS), and sesamoid-phalangeal (SP) ligaments provide peripheral stabilization along the more plantar aspect of the joint in conjunction with the collateral ligament complex (**Fig. 6**).[3,11] Further intrinsic support is provided by the tendons of the abductor hallucis and adductor hallucis attaching to the medial and lateral sesamoids, respectively, along the outer periphery of the FHB (see **Fig. 3**).[3]

The capsuloligamentous-sesamoid complex is collectively composed of the deep transverse intermetatarsal ligament (DTIL), tendons of the FHB, abductor hallucis, adductor hallucis, and the plantar plate. Together, these structures serve as the principal volar support unit of the joint. The DTIL acts as a bridge between the plantar plates of the first and second MTP joints (**Fig. 7**).[13] Some investigators have also referenced a fibrocartilaginous complex, which includes the plantar plate, SP, and IS ligaments.[13]

A detailed review of the neurovascular supply of the MTP joint is beyond the scope of this review; nonetheless, it should be considered and well understood before operative management. The medial plantar nerve runs adjacent to the flexor hallucis longus tendon. Paired hallucal nerves are located on the plantar surface of the medial and lateral sesamoids.[14] The plantar arch gives off multiple small branches that terminate as the sesamoid arteries and supply each sesamoid bone. These vessels enter the tibial sesamoid on its medial aspect and the fibular sesamoid on its lateral margin.[14]

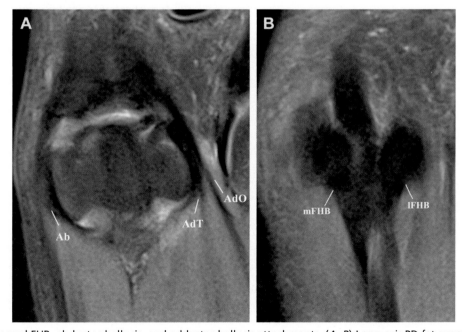

Fig. 3. Normal FHB, abductor hallucis, and adductor hallucis attachments. (*A, B*) Long-axis PD fat-suppressed images demonstrate the normal attachments of the medial (mFHB) and lateral (lFHB) heads of the FHB tendon, abductor hallucis (Ab) tendon, and the oblique (AdO) and transverse (AdT) heads of the adductor hallucis tendon.

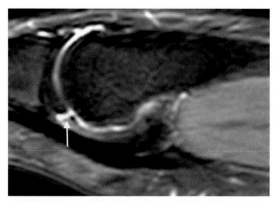

Fig. 4. Normal central plantar plate with normal recess. Sagittal STIR image shows the central plantar plate with normal well-demarcated distal recess (*arrow*).

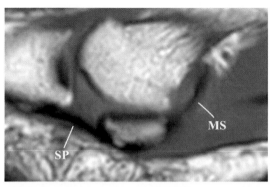

Fig. 6. Normal metatarsal-sesamoidal and sesamoid-phalangeal ligaments. Sagittal T1-weighted image shows the medial metatarsal-sesamoidal (MS) and sesamoid-phalangeal (SP) ligaments.

IMAGING TECHNIQUE AND PROTOCOLS

Several imaging modalities can be used to assess the first MTP joint for radiologic signs of turf toe injury, with radiographs considered first line in the evaluation process. Computed tomography (CT) can be used as an adjunct to radiography. Ultrasound is easily obtainable, safe, relatively cost-effective, and useful in assessing the plantar plate; however, other intrinsic structures may be difficult to visualize and the overall utility is highly operator dependent. Feuerstein and colleagues[15]

advocated the use of dynamic ultrasound over static images acquired by the sonographer for the diagnosis of plantar plate pathology. When performed correctly, ultrasound has demonstrated a high sensitivity (96%) and low specificity for detecting plantar plate injury.

Magnetic resonance (MR) imaging remains the most useful modality for the evaluation of the ligamentous structures, tendons, and sesamoids involved in turf toe injury.[3] For optimal visualization of the joint, a focused extremity coil should be used in conjunction with immobilization and adequate positioning.[16] Specific imaging parameters will vary based on institution; however, on a 1.5-T magnet, thin slices (<3 mm), a small field of view (10–14 mm), and short slice spacing (0.25–0.3 mm) are paramount for assessing the small structures of the first MTP joint.[16] Notably, at our institution, we perform all turf toe studies on a 3-T magnet. The standard MR protocol for evaluation of turf toe injury includes a combination of 3 planes of fat-sensitive T1-weighted (T1W) imaging and fluid-sensitive sequences (**Table 1**).[3] Anatomic survey for pathology of the ligaments, tendons, and bony structures is

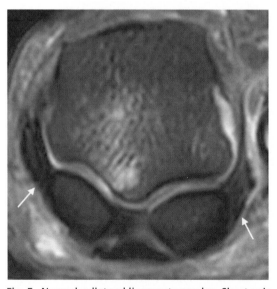

Fig. 5. Normal collateral ligament complex. Short-axis PD fat-suppressed image shows the attachments of the accessory sesamoid ligaments (*arrows*), which combine with the main collateral ligaments to form the collateral ligament complex.

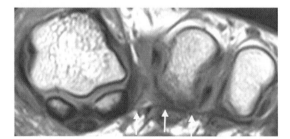

Fig. 7. Normal deep transverse intermetatarsal ligament. Short-axis T1-weighted image shows the normal deep transverse intermetatarsal ligament (*arrows*) bridging the plantar plates of the MTP joints.

Table 1
First metatarsophalangeal joint/turf toe MR imaging protocol for 3-T magnet

Pulse Sequences	Field of View, mm; Frequency × Phase	Slice Thickness, mm	Slice Gap, mm	Acquisition Matrix, Frequency × Phase	Parallel Imaging Factor	TR/TE	Echo Train Length	Bandwidth, Hz/Pixel
Axial proton-density fat suppressed	120 × 70	2	0	344 × 171	1.5	1800/30	9	293
Axial T2 fat suppressed	120 × 70	2	0	220 × 119	1.7	2742/80	17	248
Coronal proton-density fat suppressed	70 × 70	3	0.3	200 × 174	1.5	1879/30	9	286
Sagittal proton-density fat suppressed	120 × 70	2	0	344 × 171	1.5	1800/30	9	293
Sagittal T1	120 × 70	2	0	268 × 143	0	685/20	5	211

Abbreviations: TE, echo time; TR, repetition time.

best achieved with non–fat-suppressed T1W or proton-density (PD) sequences. Fat-suppressed PD and short tau inversion recovery (STIR) imaging are helpful for evaluation of abnormal soft tissue and marrow edema. T1W images are useful for further characterizing bone marrow abnormalities, whereas PD sequences are ideal for evaluating the articular cartilage.[3] A recent study by Lepage-Saucier and colleagues[17] demonstrated the utility of toe traction and MR arthrography in the assessment of the plantar plate, and other structures of the first MTP joint.

IMAGING FINDINGS/PATHOLOGY
Radiographic Findings

A routine 3-view (dorsoplantar, lateral, and oblique) conventional weight-bearing radiograph series of the foot can be used to assess for anatomic derangement of the bony structures. Osteocartilaginous injuries may occur due to impaction of the metatarsal head on the proximal phalanx during forced dorsiflexion, and are often identifiable on radiographs.[18] The presence of an intra-articular fragment at the first MTP joint potentially arising from the sesamoids or proximal phalanx may portend capsular avulsion or disruption.[19] Additionally, the presence of a bipartite sesamoid bone and accompanying traumatic diastasis may be seen on routine radiograph views.[18]

Additional, more specialized views can be obtained in the assessment of a turf toe injury. The functional integrity of the plantar plate may be indirectly evaluated using a lateral stress test view at 45° of MTP joint hyperextension.[10] Standing bilateral AP views may be helpful to assess for asymmetry in the position of the sesamoid bones.[4] Injury to the plantar complex may be inferred by assessing the distance between the sesamoids and the first proximal phalanx.[4] Evidence of proximal migration is suggested, and plantar plate injury is inferred, when the distance from the distal tip of the medial sesamoid to the proximal phalangeal base is greater than 10.4 mm, and 13.3 mm for the lateral sesamoid.[4] Compared with the uninjured side, an increased interval of 3 mm between the affected sesamoid and the base of the proximal phalanx is indicative of proximal migration.[10] Waldrop and colleagues[10] found that the presence of proximal migration of a sesamoid was associated with injury to at least 3 of the following 4 ligaments: medial collateral ligament, lateral collateral ligament, medial SP ligament, and lateral SP ligament. Although not routinely used in the evaluation of the MTP joint, fluoroscopy can be performed to identify abnormal motion of the sesamoids during dorsiflexion.[19]

MR Imaging Findings

As with most other ligaments, the normal plantar plate displays homogeneously low signal on all pulse sequences. The presence of increased intrasubstance signal or surrounding fluid should raise the suspicion for injury.[3] MR evidence of synovitis, which is noted by the presence of intermediate signal throughout the MTP joint, is seen in relation to plantar plate injury.[20] An indistinct appearance of the plantar plate associated with either thickening or thinning, denotes the presence of a partial-thickness tear.[3] Frank discontinuity, retraction, and the presence of a fluid gap, are indicative of a full-thickness plantar plate tear (**Fig. 8**).[3]

In the context of turf toe, the SP ligaments are frequently injured; this may occur on the medial, lateral, or both aspects. Partial or complete tear of the SP ligament may be seen with proximal migration of the affected sesamoid, most often present in cases of complete ligament rupture (**Fig. 9**).[16] Injury to the paired MS ligaments also can be seen; however, sesamoid migration is not routinely noted (**Fig. 10**). The sagittal and short-axis planes offer the best view of both the SP and MS ligaments.

Injuries to the collateral ligament complexes are often most conspicuous in the short-axis and long-axis planes. The collateral ligaments

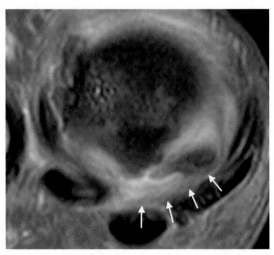

Fig. 8. Plantar plate tear in a 32-year-old man with chronic first MTP pain. Short-axis PD fat-suppressed image shows diffuse hyperintensity (*arrows*) in the expected location of the central plantar plate and medial sesamoid-phalangeal ligament, compatible with full-thickness tear.

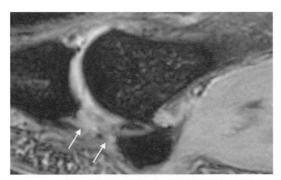

Fig. 9. Full-thickness sesamoid-phalangeal ligament tear in an 18-year-old man with sports-related injury. Sagittal fast field echo image shows disruption of the medial sesamoid-phalangeal ligament (*arrows*) with associated proximal migration of the medial sesamoid.

are more likely to tear at the less flexible proximal metatarsal attachment point, rather than at the phalangeal attachment.[16] Abnormal increased intrasubstance signal at the proximal attachment to the metatarsal head/neck is typically seen with this injury (**Fig. 11**). Complete tear of the IS ligament leads to widening of the intersesamoid interval. Visualization of this structure is best achieved on short-axis and long-axis views. Partial or complete rupture of the IS ligament is associated with abnormal increased intrasubstance signal, variable degrees of fiber discontinuity, and with adjacent soft tissue edema and hemorrhage around the sesamoids (**Fig. 12**).

Partial tear of the abductor or adductor hallucis tendons results in abnormal increased intrasubstance signal. Full-thickness tears and avulsion injury involving the abductor or adductor hallucis from the sesamoid can also

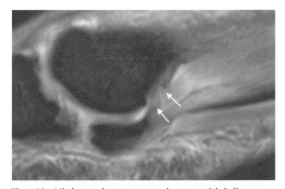

Fig. 10. High-grade metatarsal-sesamoidal ligament tear in an 18-year-old woman with sports-related injury. Sagittal T2 fat-suppressed image shows abnormal increased signal along the course of the medial metatarsal-sesamoidal ligament (*arrows*).

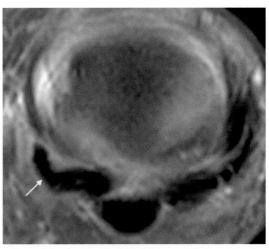

Fig. 11. Full-thickness accessory sesamoid ligament tear in a 39-year-old man with chronic first MTP pain. Short-axis PD fat-suppressed image shows dorsal disruption of the lateral accessory sesamoid ligament of the collateral ligament complex, with a wavy appearance of residual inferior ligament fibers (*arrow*).

occur. The abductor hallucis is more frequently injured during hyperextension and valgus-directed trauma to the first MTP joint. This results in capsular and/or tendinous avulsion with resultant edema at the site of injury. The lateral sesamoid and adductor hallucis will be intact and can serve as a normal comparison. Short-axis and long-axis images are most useful in detecting these muscle and tendon abnormalities (**Fig.13**).[13] Variable degrees of injury to the paired FHB muscles and tendons also may occur (**Fig. 14**).

In the acute or chronic phase, MR imaging provides great utility for detecting osteochondral defects at the first MTP joint. A focal defect in the articular cartilage and adjacent bone marrow edema are unequivocal findings.[12] Regional soft tissue edema and swelling are routinely noted and best seen on fat-suppressed, fluid-sensitive sequences in the acute injury phase. These findings are absent with chronic injuries.[12]

DIAGNOSIS AND CLASSIFICATION

The diagnosis of turf toe relies on a thorough clinical history, physical examination, and imaging findings. The typical patient is a collegiate/professional athlete who has experienced an axially loaded force to the posterior leg with resultant forced hyperextension of the first MTP joint. Pain, of varying degrees, may serve as a prognostic

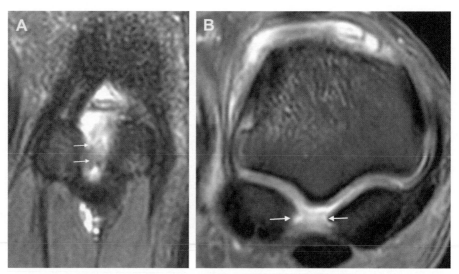

Fig. 12. Full-thickness intersesamoid ligament tear. Long-axis T2 fat-suppressed image (*A*) and short-axis PD fat-suppressed image (*B*) of a 32-year-old man with chronic first metatarsophalangeal joint pain. There is disruption/absence of the intersesamoid ligament with abnormal hyperintense signal within the intersesamoid interval (*arrows*).

indicator of injury severity. On physical examination, patients may exhibit an inability to bear weight on the affected side and limited range of motion at the first MTP joint.

A well-recognized and straightforward clinical classification system of turf toe injury was first devised by Clanton and Ford.[21] Several revisions of this classification system have been performed.

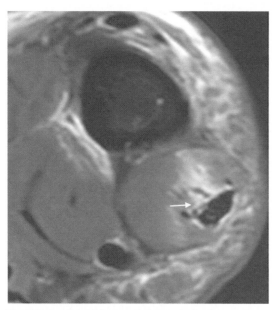

Fig. 13. Partial-thickness abductor hallucis tear in an 18-year-old woman with sports-related injury. Short-axis T2 fat-suppressed image shows edema present at the abductor hallucis myotendinous junction (*arrow*).

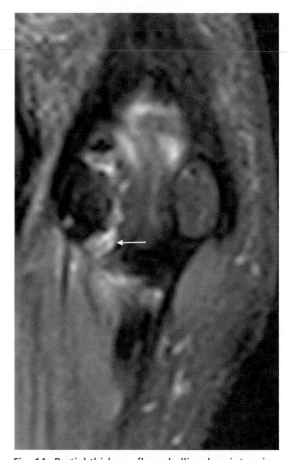

Fig. 14. Partial-thickness flexor hallucis brevis tear in a 21-year-old woman with a sports-related injury. Long-axis T2 fat-suppressed image shows edema and partial disruption at the attachment of the lateral flexor hallucis brevis tendon (*arrow*) to the sesamoid.

The orthopedic surgery literature describes a separate 5-stage grading system based on the degree of capsular disruption seen during arthroscopy.[3] The Anderson clinical classification includes both clinical and pertinent imaging findings (**Table 2**). Grade 1 injuries involve a minor sprain/tear to the ligamentous capsule with mild surrounding soft tissue edema.[3] The patient has limited range of motion, is able to bear weight, and is usually able to continue with activity.[21] Grade 2 injuries involve a partial tear of the capsuloligamentous complex with moderate surrounding soft tissue edema and ecchymosis.[21] The patient displays moderate pain, is barely able to bear weight on the affected joint, and has moderate limitation in range of motion. Grade 3 injury is a full-thickness tear of the capsuloligamentous complex, which involves a complete tear of the plantar plate.[21] Associated fractures of the sesamoids and impaction at the first MTP joint may be present. Significant swelling, ecchymosis, inability to bear weight, and complete restriction of motion are hallmarks of this injury severity.[21] A fourth grade was added by Coughlin and colleagues,[18] which involves debilitating injury to the osteocartilaginous component of the joint and eventual chondrolysis. This severity of injury is typically not amenable to surgical correction.

DIFFERENTIAL DIAGNOSIS

In the context of an ambiguous clinical history and presentation, other conditions affecting the first MTP joint also may be considered as part of the differential diagnosis. Such conditions include inflammatory processes like sesamoiditis, an isolated fracture of a sesamoid bone, arthritis, nerve impingement, and alternative injuries of the first MTP joint (**Table 3**).

Sesamoiditis, an inflammatory condition affecting the sesamoid bones, results in associated pain and with possible involvement of the surrounding tendons/ligaments.[22] Infection, repetitive trauma, and avascular necrosis of the sesamoids have all been implicated as possible etiologies for the development of sesamoiditis in young athletes.[22] Both nuclear medicine bone scan and MR imaging can be used to evaluate the sesamoids for inflammatory changes.

An isolated fracture of a sesamoid bone should be considered as part of the differential diagnosis. Other considerations include degenerative, inflammatory, and infectious arthropathies such as osteoarthritis, rheumatoid arthritis, crystal deposition disorders, and septic arthritis. Clinical correlation with history and laboratory findings may help the clinician arrive at the appropriate diagnosis.

Table 2
Diagnostic criteria for turf toe injury

Grade	Pathology	Clinical Signs and Symptoms	Radiographic Findings	MR Imaging Findings
1	Low-level sprain of the plantar plate and capsule	Ability to bear weight, normal range of motion, localized tenderness, no appreciable ecchymosis, minimal swelling	Normal	Surrounding soft tissue edema with intact bony and soft tissue structures
2	Partial tear of the plantar plate and capsule	Difficulty bearing weight, limited range of motion, diffuse tenderness, appreciable ecchymosis, moderate swelling	Normal	Soft tissue edema, high signal intensity within the plantar plate without evidence of full-thickness involvement
3	Frank tear with complete discontinuity of the plantar plate and capsule	Inability to bear weight, limited movement with severe tenderness, marked ecchymosis and swelling, (+) vertical Lachman test	May show avulsion fracture of the proximal phalanx, sesamoid fracture, proximally migrated sesamoid, dislocation of the first metatarsophalangeal joint	High signal throughout the capsuloligamentous complex, sesamoids, and chondral injury

Table 3
Summary of the differential diagnosis for turf toe

Pathology	Structures Involved
Sesamoiditis	Sesamoid bones
Isolated fracture of a sesamoid	Sesamoid bones
Degenerative, inflammatory, or infectious arthritis	Sesamoid bones, first metatarsal head, first proximal phalanx, hyaline cartilage
Nerve impingement	Medial branch of the plantar digital nerve, sesamoid bones
Sand toe	Extensor hallucis longus

Impingement of the medial branch of the plantar digital nerve by the medial/tibial sesamoid can contribute to pain at the first MTP joint.[9] "Sand toe," as described previously, also may be considered in the clinical differential diagnosis of first MTP joint pain following trauma. However, the mechanism involves forced hyperflexion of the joint, resulting in injury to the extensor mechanism, mainly the extensor hallucis longus.[4,6]

PEARLS, PITFALLS, VARIANTS

Pearls, pitfalls and variants are summarized in **Box 1**.

Fracture of the sesamoids may be difficult to differentiate from a variant bipartite/multipartite sesamoid bone. Making a distinction between a variant bipartite/multipartite sesamoid and sesamoid fracture often requires the application of MRI, in conjunction with radiographs and/or CT.[3]

The bipartite/multipartite sesamoid bone may undergo traumatic diastasis; one should be aware of the normal interval that typically separates the bipartite/multipartite sesamoid bone. In 2015, Favinger and colleagues[23] suggested the presence of traumatic diastasis of the bipartite/multipartite sesamoid when the dominant interval measures more than 2 mm on a routine frontal radiograph of the foot in the setting of recent hyperextension injury (**Fig. 15**).

Capsular avulsion at the first MTP joint should be suspected when an intra-articular/juxta-articular fragment is present adjacent to the proximal phalanx and/or sesamoids.

Traumatic hallux valgus occurs when a valgus force on the first MTP joint leads to rupture of the

medial collateral ligament complex, medial head of the FHB, and medial capsule.[4]

Injury to the plantar complex may result in proximal migration of a sesamoid. Proximal migration can be assessed by measuring the interval separating the distal aspect of the sesamoid from the proximal phalangeal base, or by comparing the uninjured interval of the contralateral foot with the affected side, as detailed previously.[4,10]

Finally, the plantar plate recess is a normal anatomic variant present at the phalangeal attachment, which may be mistaken for a partial-thickness tear.[3] This recess typically has a smooth and well-defined contour, occurs along the articular cartilage on the phalangeal aspect of the joint, and is less than half of the thickness of the plantar plate in depth (see **Fig. 4**).

WHAT THE REFERRING PHYSICIAN NEEDS TO KNOW

Once the diagnosis of plantar plate injury has been confirmed on imaging and accurately classified, the referring provider may opt for conservative management, including nonsteroidal anti-inflammatory drugs, RICE (rest, ice, compression, elevation), immobilization (taping), intra-articular steroid injections, and/or physical therapy. If

---

Box 1
Pearls, pitfalls, variants

- Making the distinction between a variant bipartite/multipartite sesamoid and sesamoid fracture may require the application of MR imaging in conjunction with radiographs and/or computed tomography.

- Traumatic diastasis of the bipartite/multipartite sesamoid can be inferred when the dominant interval measures more than 2 mm on a frontal radiograph of the foot in the setting of recent hyperextension injury.

- The presence of an intra-articular/juxta-articular fragment adjacent to the proximal phalanx and/or sesamoids suggests capsular avulsion.

- Traumatic hallux valgus deformity occurs from rupture of the medial collateral ligament, medial head of the flexor hallucis brevis, and medial capsule following a valgus force to the first metatarsophalangeal joint.

- Proximal migration of a sesamoid suggests injury to the plantar complex.

- The plantar plate recess is a normal anatomic variant that should not be confused for tear.

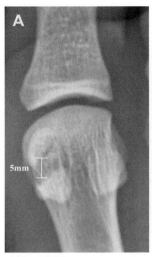
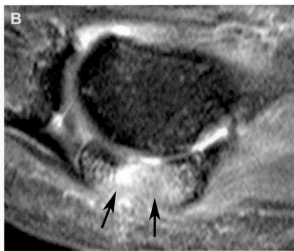

Fig. 15. Traumatic diastasis of a bipartite medial sesamoid in an 18-year-old woman with sports-related injury. (*A*) Dorsoplantar radiograph demonstrates diastasis of the bipartite medial sesamoid. (*B*) Sagittal PD fat-suppressed MR image demonstrates medial sesamoid diastasis with intervening soft tissue edema (*arrows*).

conservative management fails, operative treatment becomes the next logical step. The presence of traumatic hallux valgus, traumatic diastasis of the bipartite/multipartite sesamoid, proximal migration of one or both sesamoids, sesamoid fracture with or without an intra-articular body, vertical instability, osteochondral injury, and an unstable joint with a large capsular avulsion are all reportedly indications for potential surgical intervention (**Box 2**).[14,18,19,24] The decision to use an open repair approach versus arthroscopy is determined by the orthopedic surgeon. Osteochondral injuries have been successfully treated using both arthroscopic and open approaches.[14] Surgical complications include injury to the medial plantar hallucal nerve and avascular necrosis of the sesamoids.[14]

Box 2
What the referring physician needs to know

- The following features are reportedly possible surgical indications, and should be emphasized when identified on imaging:
  - Traumatic hallux valgus
  - Traumatic diastasis of a bipartite/multipartite sesamoid
  - Proximal migration of a sesamoid
  - Sesamoid fracture
  - Osteochondral injury
  - Large capsular avulsion

SUMMARY

Using the tools at our disposal, radiologists and clinicians are able to identify and treat the myriad of pathologies that comprise the turf toe spectrum. Accurate assessment of the first MTP joint on MR imaging requires a keen understanding of the complex anatomy. Failure to adequately diagnose and properly manage turf toe injury could lead to debilitating effects. Conservative and surgical interventions are used depending on the severity of injury identified.

REFERENCES

1. Bowers KD, Martin RB. Turf-toe: a shoe-surface related football injury. Med Sci Sports 1976;8:81–3.
2. Marchetti DC, Chang A, Ferrari M, et al. Turf toe: 40 years later and still a problem. Oper Tech Sports Med 2017;25:99–107.
3. Schein AJ, Skalski MR, Patel DB, et al. Turf toe and sesamoiditis: what the radiologist needs to know. Clin Imaging 2015;39:380–9.
4. Anderson R. Turf toe injuries of the hallux metatarsophalangeal joint. Tech Foot Ankle Surg 2002;1(2):102–11.
5. Coker TP, Arnold JA, Weber DL. Traumatic lesions of the metatarsophalangeal joint of the great toe in athletes. Am J Sports Med 1978;6:326–34.
6. Frey C, Andersen GD, Feder KS. Plantar flexion injury to the metatarsophalangeal joint ("sand toe"). Foot Ankle Int 1996;17:576–81.
7. Coughlin M. Athletic injury to the first metatarsal phalangeal joint. Médecine et Chirurgie du Pied 2005;21(2):65–72.

8. Rodeo SA, O'Brien S, Warren RF, et al. Turf-toe: an analysis of metatarsophalangeal joint sprains in professional football players. Am J Sports Med 1990;18: 280–5.

9. Sanders TG, Rathur SK. Imaging of painful conditions of the hallucal sesamoid complex and plantar capsular structures of the first metatarsophalangeal joint. Radiol Clin North Am 2008;46:1079–92, vii.

10. Waldrop NE, Zirker CA, Wijdicks CA, et al. Radiographic evaluation of plantar plate injury: an in vitro biomechanical study. Foot Ankle Int 2013;34:403–8.

11. Clanton TO, Butler JE, Eggert A. Injuries to the metatarsophalangeal joints in athletes. Foot Ankle 1986; 7:162–78.

12. Awh MH. Turf toe. MRI Web Clin; 2012. Available at: http://radsource.us/clinic-turf-toe/.

13. Srinivasan R. The hallucal-sesamoid complex: normal anatomy, imaging, and pathology. Semin Musculoskelet Radiol 2016;20:224–32.

14. Mason LW, Molloy AP. Turf toe and disorders of the sesamoid complex. Clin Sports Med 2015;34: 725–39.

15. Feuerstein CA, Weil L, Weil LS, et al. Static versus dynamic musculoskeletal ultrasound for detection of plantar plate pathology. Foot Ankle Spec 2014; 7:259–65.

16. Crain JM, Phancao JP. Imaging of turf toe. Radiol Clin North Am 2016;54:969–78.

17. Lepage-Saucier M, Linda DD, Chang EY, et al. MRI of the metatarsophalangeal joints: improved assessment with toe traction and MR arthrography. AJR Am J Roentgenol 2013;200:868–71.

18. Coughlin MJ, Kemp TJ, Hirose CB. Turf toe: soft tissue and osteocartilaginous injury to the first metatarsophalangeal joint. Phys Sportsmed 2010;38: 91–100.

19. McCormick JJ, Anderson RB. Turf toe: anatomy, diagnosis, and treatment. Sports Health 2010;2: 487–94.

20. Yao L, Do HM, Cracchiolo A, et al. Plantar plate of the foot: findings on conventional arthrography and MR imaging. AJR Am J Roentgenol 1994;163:641–4.

21. Clanton TO, Ford JJ. Turf toe injury. Clin Sports Med 1994;13:731–41.

22. Dedmond BT, Cory JW, McBryde A. The hallucal sesamoid complex. J Am Acad Orthop Surg 2006; 14:745–53.

23. Favinger JL, Porrino JA, Richardson ML, et al. Epidemiology and imaging appearance of the normal bi-/multipartite hallux sesamoid bone. Foot Ankle Int 2015;36:197–202.

24. George E, Harris AHS, Dragoo JL, et al. Incidence and risk factors for turf toe injuries in intercollegiate football: data from the National Collegiate Athletic Association Injury Surveillance System. Foot Ankle Int 2014;35:108–15.

Lisfranc Injury
Current Concepts

Hyojeong Mulcahy, MD*

KEYWORDS

• Lisfranc injury • Midfoot sprain • Midfoot fracture • Midfoot dislocation

KEY POINTS

• Prompt diagnosis and appropriate treatment of Lisfranc injury is the key to preventing osteoarthritis and chronic deformity.
• Radiographic evaluation of the Lisfranc joint requires a thorough search for subtle fractures and malalignment on all views.
• Computed tomography and MR imaging are primarily important for the diagnosis and management of low-energy Lisfranc injury.

INTRODUCTION

Lisfranc injury is named after Jacques Lisfranc de Saint-Martin, a French field surgeon during the Napoleonic wars, and refers to an injury to the tarsometatarsal (TMT) joints of the midfoot.[1] Lisfranc injuries include a broad spectrum of injuries ranging from sprain or subluxation to a grossly displaced fracture or fracture-dislocation of the TMT joints.[2] To avoid confusion, fractures of the tarsals or metatarsals without TMT joint subluxation should not be labeled as Lisfranc injuries.

Lisfranc injuries are uncommon and account for approximately 0.2% of all fractures.[3] They often coexist with tarsal or metatarsal fractures.[4] In the United States, the incidence has been reported to be 1 per 55,000 every year in the general population, although this can be an underestimation, as up to one-third of injuries can be missed during the initial assessment.[3]

Acute injuries can be separated into 2 major types. The more common high-energy injuries are secondary to crush injuries, falls, and motor vehicle accidents, whereas the low-energy injuries are often acquired in professional athletic trauma or during a misstep.[5] Lisfranc fracture-dislocation can also occur as part of the spectrum of neuropathic arthropathy.[6] Motor vehicle accidents are the most frequently cited mechanism, accounting for approximately 40% to 45% of injuries, and low-energy mechanisms account for approximately 30%.[7] Lisfranc injuries account for more than 15% of all athletic injuries.[8] Although the overall incidence is low, Lisfranc injuries have become the second most common athletic foot injury, following metatarsophalangeal joint injury.[6] The incidence of Lisfranc injuries is rising because of widespread high-performance athletic training.[9] They have been reported in various sports, including football, gymnastics, horse riding, and running.[10] Lisfranc injuries occur in 4% of football players and 29.2% of offensive linemen per year.[11] The "bunk bed" fracture is the pediatric equivalent of the TMT fracture-dislocation in adults.[12] Male individuals are 2 to 4 times more likely to sustain a Lisfranc joint injury, possibly due to a higher rate of participation in high-speed activities. The injury can occur at any age, but more commonly in the third decade of life.[3]

Disclosure: The author has nothing to disclose.
Department of Radiology, University of Washington, Seattle, WA, USA
* UWMC-Roosevelt Radiology, Box 354755, 4245 Roosevelt Way Northeast, Seattle, WA 98105.
E-mail address: hyomul@u.washington.edu

Radiol Clin N Am 56 (2018) 859–876
https://doi.org/10.1016/j.rcl.2018.06.003
0033-8389/18/© 2018 Elsevier Inc. All rights reserved.

ANATOMY
Osseous Structures

The midfoot is made up of 5 bones: navicular, cuboid, and 3 cuneiform bones. The Lisfranc joint includes the articulations between the 3 cuneiform bones and cuboid with the 5 metatarsals.[6] The 5 metatarsal bones contribute to the long plantar arch in the sagittal plane. The TMT articulations transition more proximally in the transverse plane from medial to lateral.[10] The second metatarsal base is recessed proximally relative to the remainder of the TMT articulations. Its design is a mortise configuration that provides resistance to medial or lateral shear forces across the joint complex. The trapezoidal shape of the metatarsal bases and their corresponding cuneiforms form a Roman arch, with the second metatarsal acting as the keystone, conferring coronal plane stability (**Fig. 1**).[13]

Biomechanically, the Lisfranc joint represents the transition from midfoot to forefoot and is, therefore, crucial for a normal gait pattern. Mobility within the joints of the TMT joint is, therefore, very important, particularly during weight bearing (WB) over uneven ground.[14] These joints also are classified into columns in the foot. The lateral column is the most mobile and made up of the articulation between the fourth and fifth metatarsals and the cuboid. Therefore, posttraumatic symptomatic arthritis is rare in this column. The medial column consists of the navicular, the medial cuneiform, and

the first metatarsal.[10] The middle column is the most rigid, made up of the second and third metatarsals and their respective TMT articulations (**Fig. 2**).[15] The relative stiffness on the

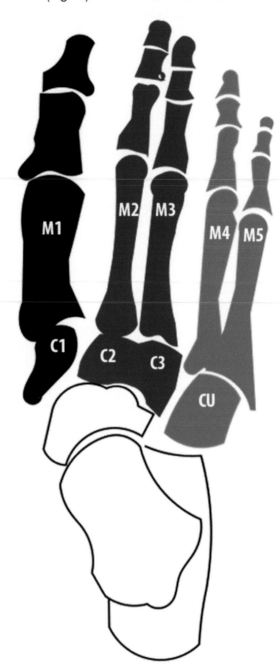

Fig. 2. Three columns. A diagram shows the normal 3-column anatomy of the midfoot. C1, medial cuneiform; C2, middle cuneiform; C3, lateral cuneiform; Cu, cuboid; M1–M5, metatarsals. The medial (*black*), middle (*blue*), and lateral (*red*) columns are shown. The stiff middle column acts as a rigid lever arm, with the medial and lateral columns providing appropriate adjustment as WB gait.

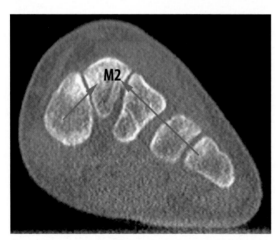

Fig. 1. Roman arch. Short-axis CT image through the level of proximal metatarsals demonstrates asymmetric Roman arch of the TMT joint. The middle cuneiform and second metatarsal base (M2) are shaped like a keystone in the coronal plane. M2 represents the "keystone" because of its dorsal-most position and trapezoidal articular surface, broad base dorsally, and apex at its plantar surface. This transverse arch is an inherently stable configuration mechanically, but predisposes to dorsal displacement (*red arrows; shear force vectors*).

medial side is possible because the center of mobility on the medial side of the foot is at the talonavicular joint. The stiff middle column acts as a rigid lever arm during WB, with the medial and lateral columns providing appropriate adjustment as WB forces pass through the mid-foot.[14] The Lisfranc ligament rigidly links the medial and middle columns while still allowing mobility between the first 2 metatarsals.[3]

Ligamentous Complex

The Lisfranc joint complex includes not only the TMT articular surfaces but also the intermetatarsal and anterior intertarsal surfaces. These ligaments reinforce and stabilize the articular capsules and skeletal elements. The ligamentous anatomy is complex and its complexity is reflected in the orthopedic and radiologic literature, which is inconsistent with respect to nomenclature and description.[16,17]

De Palma and colleagues[18] described Lisfranc ligament complex in terms of dorsal, plantar, and interosseous ligaments on the basis of location. Each set consists of longitudinal, oblique, and transverse fibers. The longitudinal fibers connect the TMT joint of the same rays. The oblique fibers connect the contiguous rays, and the transverse fibers connect the tarsals or the metatarsals.[18] Generally, the plantar ligaments are stronger than the dorsal ligaments, which may account for the dorsal direction of dislocations.[10]

The dorsal ligament system of the Lisfranc joint complex lies on the dorsal aspect of the foot. There are 7 TMT ligaments.[17] The dorsal ligament system includes also the intertarsal dorsal ligaments uniting the cuneiforms and the cuboid, and the intermetatarsal dorsal ligaments connecting the metatarsals (**Fig. 3**).

Interosseous TMT ligaments include the Lisfranc (medial), the central, and the lateral longitudinal ligaments. The Lisfranc ligament arises from the lateral surface of medial cuneiform. It extends distally, laterally, and slightly downward, inserting on the lower half of the medial aspect of second metatarsal. It is the largest ligament of the TMT joint and is 8 to 10 mm long and 5 to 6 mm thick. Although multiple ligamentous and capsular constraints exist to stabilize these complexes, isolated injury to the Lisfranc ligament has been shown to result in instability.[19] There are 2 more sets of interosseous ligaments. The intertarsal interosseous ligaments unite the cuneiforms and the cuboid and are the most powerful attachments of these bones. The 3 intermetatarsal interosseous ligaments unite from the second to the fifth

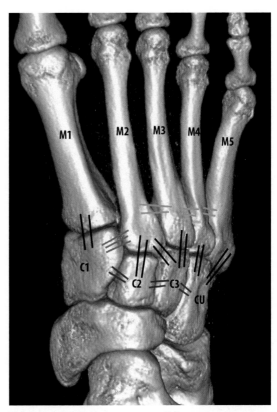

Fig. 3. Dorsal ligament system. Schematic representation of dorsal ligaments along the TMT joints. The dorsal ligament system of the Lisfranc joint complex lies on the dorsal aspect of the foot. There are 7 TMT ligaments. Black lines, TMT ligaments; blue lines, intertarsal ligaments; C, cuneiform; Cu, cuboid; green lines, intermetatarsal ligaments; M, metatarsal; red lines, Lisfranc ligament.

metatarsals, and they are uniquely absent between the first and second metatarsals.[18]

The plantar ligaments vary considerably in number and arrangement. The plantar TMT ligaments are located in the plantar region of the foot. The medial ligaments are stronger than the lateral. The plantar ligaments also include the intertarsal and intermetatarsal plantar ligaments, which are stronger than the corresponding dorsal ligaments. The second plantar ligament is called plantar Lisfranc ligament and is the strongest of the plantar ligaments. It arises inferolaterally from the medial cuneiform and separates into 2 bands inserting onto the second and third metatarsals. It is considered the keystone of the TMT arch (**Fig. 4**).[18]

MECHANISM OF INJURY AND CLASSIFICATIONS
Mechanism of Injury

Injuries to the TMT joints can be caused by direct or indirect forces. Direct injuries, most commonly

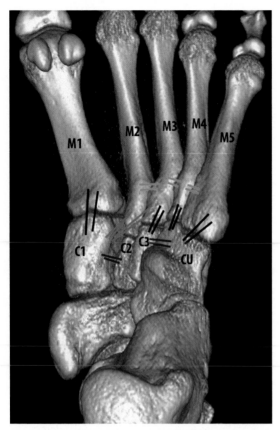

Fig. 4. Plantar ligament system. Schematic representation of plantar ligaments along the TMT joints. The plantar TMT ligaments are located in the plantar region of the foot. The second plantar ligament is called plantar Lisfranc ligament and is the strongest of the plantar ligaments. Black lines, TMT ligaments; blue lines, intertarsal ligaments; C, cuneiform; Cu, cuboid; green lines, intermetatarsal ligaments; M, metatarsal; red lines, plantar Lisfranc ligament.

crush injuries, are due to high-energy direct, blunt force applied to the dorsum of the foot. Direct injuries produce plantar or dorsal dislocation of metatarsals depending on the exact point of application of the force.[15] These injuries often are associated with multiple atypical tarsal fractures, and extensive surrounding soft tissue injuries, including vascular compromise and compartment syndrome. Direct injuries usually result in worse clinical outcome as compared with indirect injuries.[16]

Indirect injuries can occur due to either high-energy or low-energy force. High-energy indirect mechanism is usually related to motor vehicle accidents or falls from a height, whereas low-energy trauma typically occurs during sports.[20] These indirect mechanisms are much more common than direct mechanisms, and occur due to a longitudinal force applied to a plantar-flexed foot at the time of impact. Forefoot hyper-plantar flexion ruptures the weaker dorsal TMT ligaments, and the involved metatarsals assume a pathologic position in plantar flexion.[15] High-energy indirect injuries commonly occur in motor vehicle accidents when injury to the plantar-flexed foot occurs with a combination of deceleration and floorboard intrusion. Low-energy, indirect injuries are typically secondary to forced plantar flexion or forefoot abduction, and they account for most athletic injuries (a.k.a., midfoot sprain). This type of injury most commonly occurs in American football, when one player falls onto the heel of another whose foot is in equinus and planted.[21] Approximately 4% of professional football players sustain Lisfranc injuries each year.[22] This injury also can occur during running and jumping sports, falling from a horse with the foot fixed on the stirrup, or rolling the foot when stepping off a curb or step.[16,23]

Classifications

Several classification systems have been developed for Lisfranc injuries. The earliest was published by Quenu and Kuss[24] in 1909 and subsequently modified by Hardcastle and colleagues[25] in 1982 and Myerson and colleagues[15] in 1986. These classifications are all based on TMT joint congruency and displacement of the metatarsal bases. These classification systems are effective in standardizing terminology of Lisfranc injuries, and can be applied to high-energy and low-energy injuries; however, these classifications have not been found to be helpful in determining management and predicting outcomes.[7,15] These fracture-dislocation classification systems, however, are not useful for low-energy injuries without fractures. These low-energy Lisfranc injuries or midfoot sprains may involve the intercuneiform or the naviculocuneiform joints, and can be easily undiagnosed because of their subtle clinical and radiologic findings.[26] In 2002, Nunley and Vertullo[27] classified athletic midfoot injuries into 3 groups based on clinical findings, WB radiographs, and bone scintigraphy.

Quenu and Kuss[24] classified Lisfranc fracture-dislocations into 3 types, according to the direction of the metatarsal displacement: homolateral, isolated, and divergent. Homolateral type is the most common, and isolated type is the least common.[24] Because of its simplicity, this system formed the basis of many subsequent classification systems used in current clinical practice **(Fig. 5)**.[28]

A   **B**   **C**

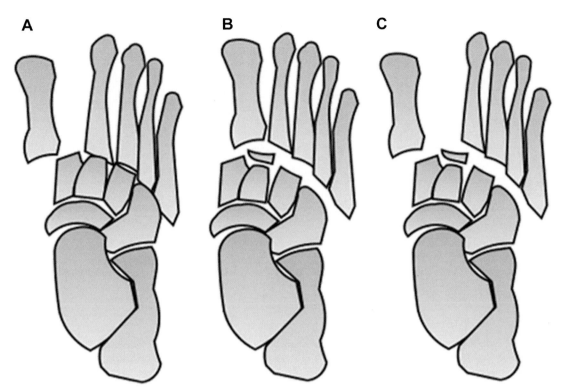

Fig. 5. Quenu classification. Lisfranc dislocations and fracture-dislocations as described by Quenu and Kuss.[24] (*A*) Isolated; unidirectional displacement of at least one but not all the metatarsals, typically the first or second rays. (*B*) Homolateral; uniform medial or more typically lateral subluxation or dislocation of all the metatarsals. (*C*) Divergent; separation of any combination of metatarsals in different directions or in more than one plane.

The Myerson classification system is the most common classification system currently used, and it divides Lisfranc fracture-dislocations into 3 large categories: types A, B, and C. In type A injury, all the TMT joints are disrupted with total incongruity (lateral or dorsoplantar). Type B injury involves 1 or more metatarsals being displaced with partial incongruity (B1, medial displacement of the first metatarsal, and B2, lateral displacement of the lesser metatarsals). Type C injury involves divergent displacement of metatarsals in opposite directions (partial or complete) (Fig. 6).[15]

Nunley and Vertullo[27] combined clinical, radiographic, and bone scintigraphy findings into a classification system to describe low-energy Lisfranc injuries with management implications. They categorized Lisfranc injuries into 3 stages: stage I, II, and III. Stage I is a low-grade sprain of the Lisfranc ligament complex and a dorsal capsular tear. The plain films are normal, but bone scans show uptake. Stage II is due to elongation or disruption of the Lisfranc ligament complex, with intact plantar capsular structures. Plain films show 1-mm to 5-mm diastasis between the first and second metatarsals on an anteroposterior

(AP) WB radiography. Stage III implies disruption of the dorsal Lisfranc and plantar ligament, with greater than 5-mm diastasis and loss of arch height on lateral WB radiography. Stage I injuries are treated conservatively. Stage III requires surgical treatment. Treatment of stage II is debatable, although the tendency is toward surgery (Fig. 7).[27,29]

DIAGNOSIS
Clinical Findings

Clinical findings in Lisfranc injury can be varied and high clinical suspicion is critical to diagnose subtle Lisfranc injury. In patients with high-energy injuries, such as crush injuries, the diagnosis is straightforward. Patients present with severe midfoot swelling, deformity, and a flat foot arch. Soft tissue injury, such as open fracture with skin defect, injury to the dorsalis pedis, and injury to the deep peroneal nerve, also may be present. Compartment syndrome can occur as a complication; it should be considered when severe pain and swelling are present. When clinically suspected, pressure measurements should be performed.

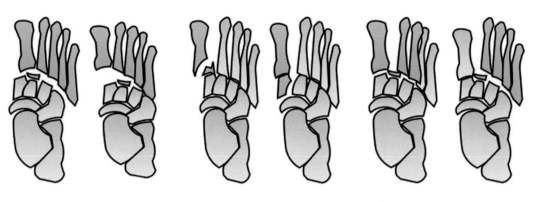

Type A: Total incongruity   Type B1: Partial incongruity , medial   Type B2: Partial incongruity , lateral

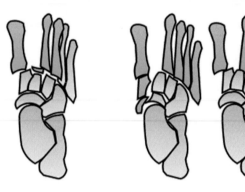

Type C1: Divergent, partial   Type C2: Divergent, total

Fig. 6. Meyerson Classification. Type A: Total incongruity of the TMT joint in any plane or direction. Type B1: Partial incongruity in which the displacement affects the first ray in relative isolation (partial-medial incongruity). Type B2: Partial incongruity in which the displacement affects 1 or more of the lateral 4 metatarsals in any plane (partial-lateral incongruity). Type C1: Divergent pattern, with the first metatarsal displaced medially and the lateral 4 in any other concomitant pattern of displacement with partial incongruity. Type C2: Divergent pattern with total incongruity.

Occasionally in the setting of multitrauma, Lisfranc fractures can reduce spontaneously. In those cases in which there is no gross deformity, clinical diagnosis is more difficult.[14,26]

Patients with low-energy Lisfranc injuries present with inability to bear weight and with variable degrees of swelling in the midfoot.[30] Pain with palpation or manipulation of the TMT joints is characteristic for Lisfranc injury.[3] The "piano key" test assesses TMT joint pain. In this test, the midfoot and hindfoot are manually secured and a plantar force is applied to the individual metatarsal head (as if one were striking a piano key). A positive test will produce localized pain at the involved metatarsal base (**Fig. 8**).[31] Plantar arch ecchymosis at the midfoot level is considered pathognomonic for Lisfranc injury, and should trigger a thorough clinical and radiographic evaluation; however, it may be absent in patients with

ligamentous strain or minor fracture (**Fig. 9**).[32] In patients with subtle Lisfranc injuries, a provocative test can be used to elicit midfoot pain, described by Curtis and colleagues.[33] Passive abduction and pronation of the forefoot is maneuvered with one hand while holding the hindfoot fixed with the other hand.

Radiographs

At our institution, the initial imaging evaluation of patients with a suspected Lisfranc injury consists of non-WB (NWB) AP, 30° internal oblique, and lateral radiographs of the injured foot. Although radiographs may readily demonstrate fracture or dislocation, Lisfranc injuries may be initially overlooked because of subtle findings in low-energy injuries, osseous overlap at TMT joint on traditional radiographs, and possible spontaneous reduction

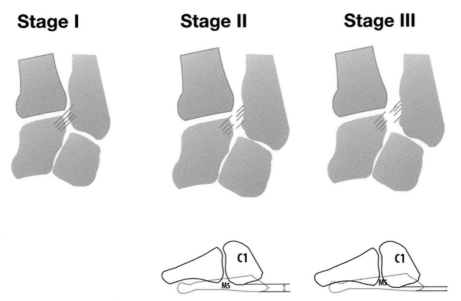

Fig. 7. Nunley classification. Stage I: Sprain of Lisfranc ligament with no diastasis or arch height loss on WB AP and lateral radiographs, but increased uptake on bone scan. Stage II: Intermetatarsal diastasis of 1 to 5 mm but no arch height loss. Stage III: Diastasis greater than 5 mm and loss of arch height (decreased distance between the plantar aspect of fifth metatarsal and plantar aspect of medial cuneiform). C1, medial cuneiform; M5, fifth metatarsal.

after trauma. In patients who had equivocal findings on NWB radiographs, or in patients who had normal findings on NWB radiographs with a high clinical suspicion, WB radiographs are recommended, including AP radiographs of both feet, and a lateral radiograph of the injured foot. WB radiographs are useful to better depict small fractures, and visualize malalignment of the Lisfranc joint.[26] Comparison radiographs of the uninjured foot increase detection of subtle malalignment when asymmetry of the Lisfranc joint becomes appreciable (**Fig. 10**). WB examinations could be difficult to obtain, however, due to pain and discomfort of

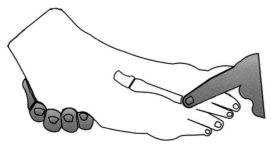

Fig. 8. "Piano key" test to assesses TMT joint pain. In this test, the midfoot and hindfoot are manually secured and plantar force is applied to the individual metatarsal head (as if one were striking a piano key). A positive test will produce localized pain at the involved metatarsal base.

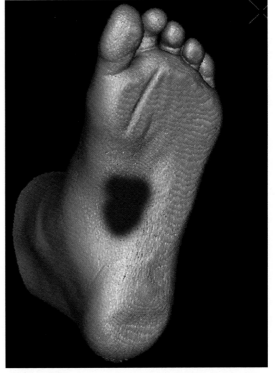

Fig. 9. Plantar bruise. Plantar arch ecchymosis at the midfoot level is considered pathognomonic for Lisfranc injury.

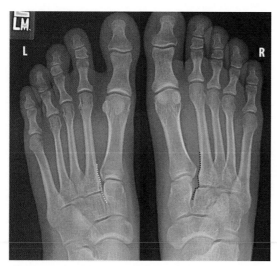

Fig. 10. Right-sided Lisfranc injury. Bilateral WB AP radiographs demonstrate normal alignment of C2-M2 on the comparison left foot (*dotted white line*), and malalignment of C2-M2 on the injured right foot (*dotted black line*).

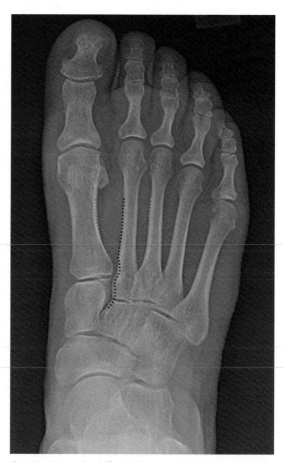

Fig. 11. Normal midfoot alignment on AP radiograph. On the AP view, the medial borders of M2-C2 (*dotted blue line*) as well as M3-C3 (*dotted green line*) should align. The lateral borders of M1-C1 (*dotted red line*) should align. The gap between C1 and M2 should be less than 2 mm.

patients. If patients cannot cooperate owing to pain, WB radiographs could be performed after administration of intra-articular local anesthetic, or after allowing the foot to rest for a week.[30]

On the AP view, the following relationships should be analyzed: (1) medial borders of the second metatarsal and middle cuneiform as well as third metatarsal and lateral cuneiform should align; (2) lateral borders of the first metatarsal and the medial cuneiform should align; and (3) gap between the medial cuneiform and second metatarsal should be less than 2 mm (**Fig. 11**).[28,34–36]

On the oblique view, the lateral borders of the middle cuneiform and second metatarsal as well as lateral cuneiform and the third metatarsal should align. The fourth and fifth metatarsals should align with the cuboid.[16] Occasionally, the second metatarsal base articulates with the lateral cuneiform, which should not be misinterpreted as a step-off. Another common variation is at the medial border of the M4 and cuboid, where a few millimeters of step-off is permitted (**Fig. 12**).[6]

On the WB lateral radiograph, the following relationships should be analyzed: (1) there should be no step-off at the dorsal margins of the tarsometatarsal joints[34]; (2) the talometatarsal angle (an angle formed by the long axes of the talus and M2) is less than 10°[15]; and (3) the plantar cortex of the medial cuneiform should project dorsal to the plantar cortex of the fifth metatarsal (**Fig. 13**).[37]

Diagnosis of Lisfranc fractures and Lisfranc injuries is challenging. Radiographic evaluation of the Lisfranc joint requires a thorough search for subtle fractures and malalignment on all views, as associated fractures occur in 39% of patients with Lisfranc injuries.[38] On NWB AP radiographs, small chip fragment between the second metatarsal and medial cuneiform may be the only indicator of an underlying Lisfranc injury ("fleck" sign).[15] Fractures are present in approximately 90% of these injuries,[3] are 3 times more common in patients with polytrauma than athletes,[15,33] and must be differentiated from the normal accessory ossicle (os intermetatarseum), which is typically smoothly corticated (**Fig. 14**).[16] Fractures associated with Lisfranc fracture-dislocation include those at the bases of the metatarsals, cuneiforms, cuboid, and, occasionally, navicular.[6] The nutcracker fracture, whereby the cuboid is fractured between the fourth and fifth metatarsals and the calcaneus, is critical to recognize, as

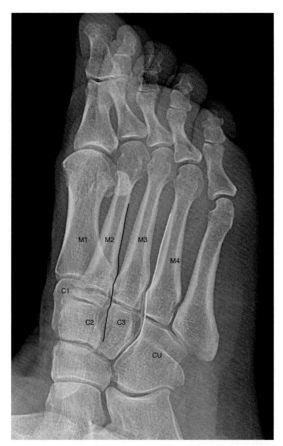

Fig. 12. Normal midfoot alignment on oblique radiograph. On the oblique view, the lateral borders of C2-M2 (*blue line*) as well as C3-M3 should align (*green line*). The M4 and M5 should align with the cuboid (*yellow line*).

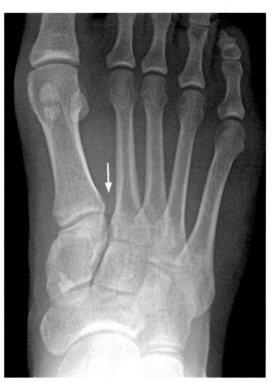

Fig. 14. Os intermetatarseum. AP radiograph shows well corticated ossicle between the first and second metatarsal bases with normal alignment of C2-M2 (*arrow*). The os intermetatarseum is well corticated and should be differentiated from fracture fragments seen in patients with Lisfranc injuries. Fracture fragments usually show irregular margins and indistinct cortices.

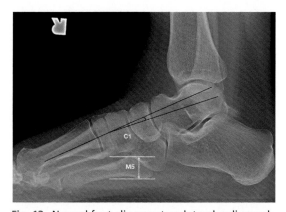

Fig. 13. Normal foot alignment on lateral radiograph. On the WB lateral radiograph, there should be no step-off at the dorsal margins of the TMT joints (*red dotted line*). The talometatarsal angle *(angle between the 2 black lines)* is less than 10°. Also, the plantar cortex of C1 should project dorsal to the plantar cortex of M5 *(double arrowed white line)*.

operative fixation is required and best performed for the lateral column first to restore length and aid in reduction of the middle and medial columns (**Fig. 15**).[39]

Radiographic findings indicative of Lisfranc injury on AP radiographs include (1) greater than 1 mm of widening between the first and second metatarsal bases or between the medial and middle cuneiforms; (2) greater than 2 mm widening between the medial cuneiform (C2) and second metatarsal base (M2) (along the Lisfranc ligament); and (3) any malalignment of the longitudinal line across C2-M2 and between the lateral cuneiform and third metatarsal (see **Fig. 15**).[6] On lateral WB radiographs, findings indicative of Lisfranc injury include (1) reduced distance between the plantar fifth metatarsal and medial cuneiform; (2) dorsal subluxation of the metatarsals at the TMT joints; and (3) talometatarsal angle greater than 15° (**Fig. 16**).[15,37] Generally, lateral step-off at the medial margin of the second TMT joint is accepted as the most common finding in Lisfranc injuries,[23]

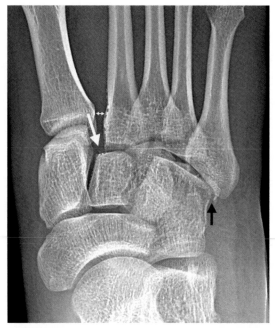

Fig. 15. "Fleck" sign. NWB AP radiograph shows malalignment of the longitudinal line across C2-M2 (*dotted red line*), widening of M1-2 (*double headed arrow*), and a small bone chip ("fleck" sign) between the M1-C2 (*white arrow*.) Also, there is a nutcracker type fracture of cuboid (*black arrow*).

Table 1	
Radiographic findings of Lisfranc injury	
Anteroposterior Radiograph	**Lateral Radiograph**
>1 mm of widening of M1-M2 or C1-C2	Dorsal subluxations of metatarsals at TMT joint
>2 mm widening of C1-M2	Reduced distance of plantar cortex between C1 and M5
Lateral step-off of medial cortex of M2 with respect of C2	
Bone fragment at C1-M2	>15° of talometatarsal angle

Abbreviations: C1, medial cuneiform; C2, middle cuneiform; C3, lateral cuneiform; M1-M5, first to fifth metatarsals; TMT, tarsometatarsal.

Computed Tomography

Computed tomography (CT) has several advantages over radiography, including visualization of unobscured osseous anatomy, and ability to demonstrate subtle fractures and malalignment in low-energy Lisfranc injuries.[9] A study with diastasis of 2 mm or more indicating instability (**Table 1**).[15,27]

When findings on WB radiographs are normal or equivocal but clinical suspicion remains high, stress radiographs (usually obtained under anesthesia) can be obtained to reveal dynamic instability. Abduction stress radiographs are performed by immobilizing the hindfoot and applying passive pronation and abduction to the forefoot (**Fig.17**). Again, a diastasis of more than 2 mm between the first and second metatarsal bases is considered abnormal.[15,30,33]

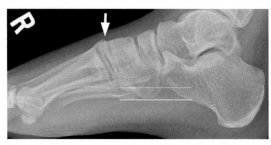

Fig. 16. Lisfranc injury. Lateral NWB radiograph shows reduced distance between the plantar fifth metatarsal (*white line*) and medial cuneiform (*dotted white line*), and dorsal subluxation of the metatarsals at the TMT joints (*white arrow*).

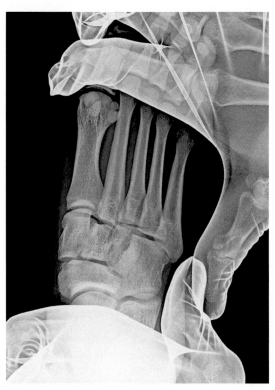

Fig. 17. Stress radiograph. Abduction stress radiograph is performed by immobilizing the hindfoot and applying passive pronation and abduction to the forefoot. Operator is wearing leaded gloves.

by Preidler and colleagues[40] showed that 50% more metatarsal and twice as many tarsal fractures were seen at CT than at radiography. Also, CT is an important tool for the assessment of fracture pattern, including their degree of comminution, intra-articular extension, displacement, and any interposed soft tissues, typically tendons, that could preclude reduction.[41,42] Multiplanar reformatted CT data are superior to MR imaging in detection of fractures or subtle displacement (**Fig.18**). Three-dimensional (3D) volume rendering (VR) images are especially beneficial for preoperative surgical planning in patients with complex fractures after high-energy trauma (**Fig.19**).[26] Therefore, CT is particularly recommended in patients who have high-energy midfoot injuries or when fractures other than simple fleck signs are identified on initial radiographs.[16]

The ideal imaging plane of the injured foot is with the CT beam angle oriented along the metatarsals as they meet with their corresponding tarsal bones. This can be accomplished by angling the CT gantry or performing multiplanar reconstructions from acquired data.[34] CT is also useful in evaluating arthritis and bony deformities in the undiagnosed injury.[43]

MR Imaging

MR imaging is primarily important for the diagnosis and management of low-energy Lisfranc injuries, and it is recommended when radiographic findings are normal or equivocal in the context of high clinical suspicion of Lisfranc injury. Similar to CT, the multiplanar capabilities of MR imaging allow optimal evaluation of malalignment at the midfoot, but unlike CT, MR is superior to other imaging modalities regarding direct visualization of soft tissue structures. Although MR imaging is sensitive for detecting subtle marrow edema, it may misdiagnose small avulsion fractures as bone bruise. Also, when tarsometatarsal malalignment is seen on MR imaging in the absence of ligamentous or osseous abnormality, its significance is uncertain.[44]

Imaging should be obtained with a small field of view, and a small surface coil centered in the midfoot. Sagittal, long axial (parallel to the metatarsals), and coronal planes (perpendicular to the metatarsals) are performed to visualize the ligament complex. Non–fat-saturated T1-weighted sequence is helpful to assess for fractures that might be difficult to identify, and the fluid-sensitive sequences (T2-weighted or proton-density fat saturation or short tau inversion recovery) are useful for detecting marrow and soft tissue signal abnormalities. Three-dimensional fast spin-echo volumetric SPACE (sampling perfection with application optimized contrasts using different flip-angle evolution) images can be helpful to assess the ligament complex by providing thin slices for multiplanar reformatted images.[45]

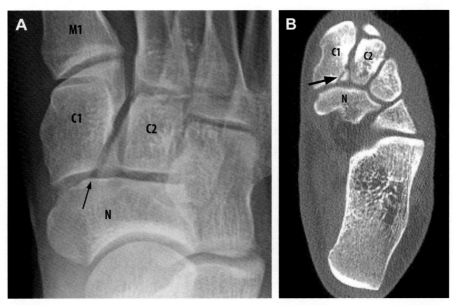

Fig. 18. Lisfranc injury. (*A*) NWB AP radiograph of foot demonstrates borderline widening of C1-M2 (*red lines*) and questionable lucency at the lateral cortex of C1 (*arrow*). (*B*) Axial CT image demonstrates fracture of the lateral, proximal aspect of C1 (*arrow*). N, navicula.

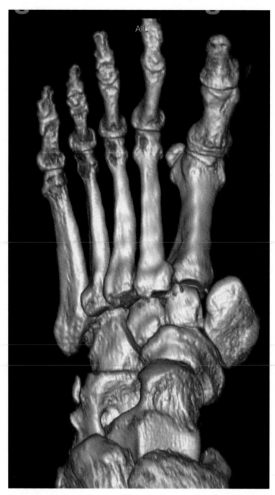

Fig. 19. Lisfranc injury. Three-dimensional VR image shows lateral total incongruity fracture-dislocation (Meyerson type A), with lateral dislocation of all metatarsals at the TMT joints.

Discrete dorsal, interosseous, and plantar bands should be identified as distinct structures on MR imaging. The normal Lisfranc ligament complex can be demonstrated in all 3 planes using MR imaging, and they appear as striated or homogeneous bands, with low to intermediate signal intensity on all sequences (**Fig. 20**).[17] The dorsal ligament is the first to tear in midfoot sprain, followed sequentially by the interosseous and plantar ligaments.[23] The dorsal intermetatarsal ligaments are best visualized in the coronal plane using thin slices, as they are thinner than the plantar ligaments.[34]

Lisfranc ligament injuries manifest as periligamentous fluid signal, waviness, irregularity, or disruption of the ligament. The presence of fluid surrounding the ligament, or isolated bone marrow edema can sometimes be the only clue to the presence of Lisfranc injury (**Fig. 21**).[26] Interruption of any one of the dorsal or plantar bands represents a partial tear, whereas disruption of both indicates a complete tear. Usually complete tears of the ligament are associated with diastasis of the articulation between the medial cuneiform and second metatarsal base to more than 2 mm.[26] In the chronic phase, diagnosis is more difficult because there may be thickening and signal heterogeneity of the injured ligament due to the fibrotic healing response.[46] MR is also useful for assessment of commonly associated injuries such as the intermetatarsal and intertarsal ligaments, as well as capsular tears. Other soft tissue injuries also may be encountered, including anterior tibialis tendon or deep peroneal nerve injuries.[6] In a study of American football players with suspected Lisfranc injury, Raikin and colleagues[47] noted that the plantar Lisfranc ligament was the most commonly injured. They compared MR imaging findings with intraoperative stress

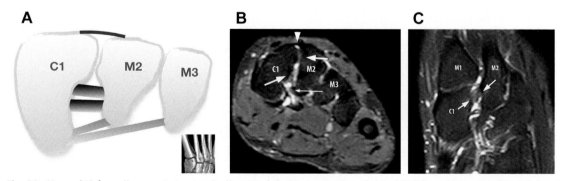

Fig. 20. Normal Lisfranc ligament. Anatomic diagram (*A*), short-axis T2-weighted FS (*B*), and long axis T2-weighted FS MR (*C*) images at the level of the second metatarsal (M2) demonstrate the 3 components of Lisfranc ligaments: interosseous or Lisfranc ligament *proper (graded black bands in A, and thick arrows in B)*, dorsal component (*black line in A, and arrowhead in B*), and plantar component (*graded gray bands in A, and thin arrow in B*). Axial T2-weighted FS MR image shows the Lisfranc ligament as a thick band from the C1 to M2 (*arrows in C*). FS, fat saturated.

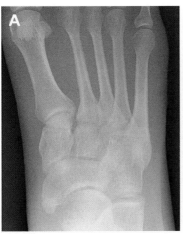 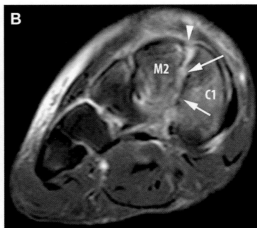

Fig. 21. Lisfranc injury. (*A*) WB AP radiograph shows normal alignment of TMT joint. (*B*) Short-axis T2-weighted FS MR image at the level of TMT joint demonstrates a partial tear of dorsal component (*arrowhead*) with increased signal, waviness, and indistinctness along the interosseous component (*arrows*). There is bone marrow edema at C1 and M2.

radiographs and surgical findings and concluded that normal appearance of plantar Lisfranc ligament on MR imaging is suggestive of a stable midfoot.

Diagnostic Imaging Decision Tree

The initial imaging evaluation of patients with a suspected Lisfranc injury consists of NWB radiographs of the injured foot. In patients with high-energy injuries, such as crush injuries with fracture or dislocation, the diagnosis is straightforward. Mostly patients will undergo CT for surgical planning. In patients who have equivocal findings on NWB radiographs, or in patients who have normal findings on NWB radiographs with a high clinical suspicion, WB radiographs are recommended. WB radiographs should be carefully scrutinized for subtle malalignment or asymmetries. Furthermore, initial normal radiographs do not exclude significant Lisfranc injury when there is high clinical concern for injury or symptoms persist. In those cases, further assessment should be performed with MR imaging. When MR imaging findings are equivocal, stress radiographs under anesthesia could play a role for the diagnose Lisfranc injury (**Fig. 22**).

MANAGEMENT

The key to successful management of Lisfranc injury is to determine whether to use surgical stabilization. Regardless of the severity of injury, the goal of treatment is to attain a painless, stable foot. Maintenance of anatomic alignment is the most important factor in achieving a satisfactory result. Other factors, such as energy of the injury, cartilage damage, and associated soft tissue injuries, can compromise the final outcome.[22]

Initial management of Lisfranc injuries varies depending on the nature of the injury. Patients with high-energy injuries should receive thorough evaluations for compartment syndrome with advanced imaging to assess for concomitant injuries and surgical planning. Open injuries should be managed with urgent irrigation, débridement, and stabilization. Dislocations of the TMT joints should undergo immediate closed reduction to protect the soft tissues from sustained tension.[13] Patients with low-energy injuries are managed based on the severity of the injury. Those with stable injuries (Nunley and Vertullo stage I) are treated conservatively, and those with unstable injuries (Nunley and Vertullo stages II and III) should be treated with open reduction and internal fixation (ORIF).[27]

Nonoperative Treatment

Nonoperative treatment is limited to stable Lisfranc joint complex injuries (Nunley and Vertullo, stage I), and includes those that are nondisplaced, and stable under radiographic stress examination.[27] Also, the patient with minimal ambulatory ability, an insensate foot, or preexisting inflammatory arthritis may be best treated nonsurgically.[22]

Treatment involves protected WB in a controlled ankle motion walking boot. Serial physical examinations and repeat WB radiographs should be performed 2 weeks from initial presentation to rule out occult instability. If the injury is stable, WB can be progressed and immobilization discontinued with

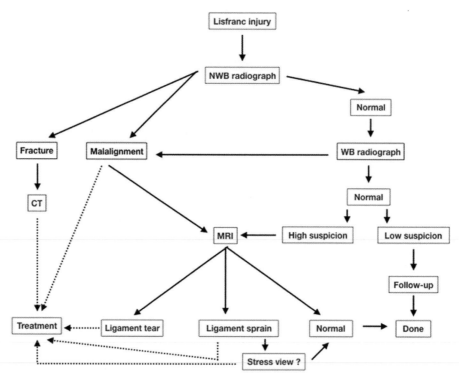

Fig. 22. Diagnostic imaging decision tree for foot injuries.

gradual return to regular activity. If symptoms persist, occult foot injuries should be assessed for, and further imaging modalities may be indicated. It takes approximately 4 months to recover from a nonoperative Lisfranc injury.[3,21]

Operative Treatment

Surgery is indicated for displaced fractures and dislocations as well as unstable ligamentous injuries. Unstable injuries, even subtle ones, are managed surgically. Subtle Lisfranc injuries are occurring with increasing frequency, likely because of greater participation in high-demand sports. Obvious injuries in patients with multiple trauma are not often missed, but more subtle injuries are a common source of continued disability.[22]

The timing of surgery should be determined based on several factors. In open injuries, impending compartment syndrome, and a threatened soft tissue envelope, are considered surgical emergencies. Dislocations always should be reduced urgently by either closed or open means because they may occlude distal perfusion. In closed injuries, the status of the soft tissue guides the timing of surgical intervention. The timing of surgery is predicated on resolution of swelling, when the skin begins to wrinkle.[13]

Operative treatment can take many forms, including ORIF and open reduction with hybrid internal and external fixation, closed reduction with percutaneous internal or external fixation, or open arthrodesis. Under fluoroscopic visualization, closed reduction should be attempted for all patients with dislocations regardless of the type of fixation that is to be used (**Fig. 23**). When closed reduction fails, the failure is usually due to a bone fragment or soft tissue interposed at the base of the second metatarsal.[39] Several studies have reported that restoration of anatomic reduction is best achieved via open reduction.[48,49]

Several different methods of internal fixation of Lisfranc injuries have been described. The 3 basic implements include Kirschner wires (K-wires), screws, or small plates. Recently, the use of suture button devices has been examined (**Fig. 24**).[50,51] Because of the higher rate of complications of K-wire fixation, including pin migration, and pin site infection, current recommendations are for more rigid fixation with transarticular screws.[20,52,53] The medial column is fixed first, then the middle column is reduced while the lateral column may be pinned with K-wires.[21,22] One exception to the order of reduction is in the presence of a fractured and shortened cuboid. The length of the cuboid and the lateral column of the foot must be restored first to avoid a permanent

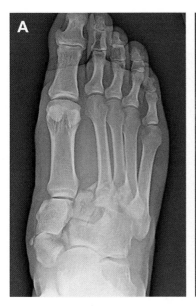
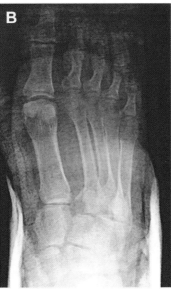

Fig. 23. Closed reduction of Lisfranc fracture-dislocation. (*A*) Initial radiograph demonstrates Meyerson Type C2 total divergent type Lisfranc fracture-dislocation. Also, there is fracture subluxation of navicular. (*B*) AP radiograph after closed reduction demonstrates near anatomic alignment.

abduction deformity of the forefoot.[39] Disadvantages of transarticular screw fixation include the need to remove the screws, articular damage to involved joints, and the potential for screw breakage.[3] Another operative treatment option is dorsal plating, and dorsal plating has ability to reduce the joints and resist joint displacement similar to intra-articular screws. Also, it minimizes additional soft tissue damage and intra-articular wear that occurs with transarticular screw placement. However, plates cannot be inserted percutaneously and require longer operating time to insert.[50,54] Primary arthrodesis has recently been advocated for some Lisfranc injuries, and it may be an alternative treatment for severely comminuted intra-articular fractures.[48,55] However, when a primary arthrodesis is performed, more dissection is required, more bone is removed, larger defects may require bone grafting, and it is more difficult to achieve fixation. Primary arthrodesis is rarely performed in an athlete.[39] Internal fixation is maintained for a

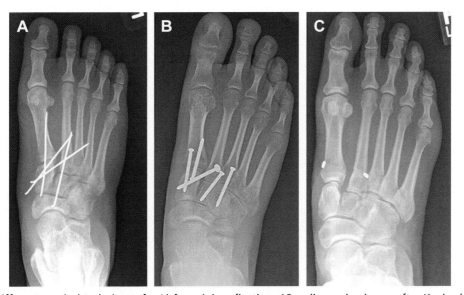

Fig. 24. Different surgical techniques for Lisfranc injury fixation. AP radiographs shown after K-wire (*A*), screw (*B*), and tightrope (*C*) fixation of medial and middle columns in patients with Lisfranc injury.

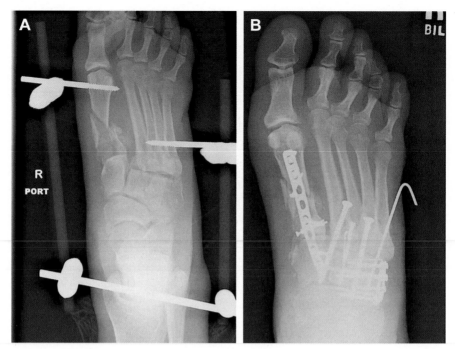

Fig. 25. Surgical fixation of a patient with Lisfranc fracture-dislocation. (*A*) Initial injury was temporarily stabilized by an external fixator placement. (*B*) Postoperative radiograph 1 month after original injury demonstrates ORIF using a bridging plate, screws, and K-wire.

minimum of 4 months to allow ligamentous healing. The hardware can be left in permanently if the patient is asymptomatic. If there is any concern about the midfoot stability, then the patient should start wearing the boot again and the rehabilitation should be decreased until the symptoms fully resolve.[15] External fixation can be used for severe soft tissue injury precluding internal fixation, preliminary alignment of a grossly unstable injury, and as an adjunct to internal fixation when the bone is comminuted or osteopenic (**Fig. 25**).[13]

SUMMARY

Although Lisfranc injuries are relatively uncommon, they encompass a wide spectrum of injury, ranging from sprain to fracture-dislocation. Misdiagnosed or undertreated Lisfranc injuries commonly result in instability, which leads to early osteoarthritis and chronic deformity. It is important, therefore, for radiologists to have thorough understanding of anatomy, and mechanisms and patterns of these injuries to diagnose and to help clinicians to assess treatment options and prognosis. Imaging modalities, such as conventional, WB, and stress radiographs, as well as CT and MR imaging can allow detection of these injuries and assess the degree of injury. Stable injuries may be treated conservatively, whereas all other injuries require surgical interventions.

REFERENCES

1. Fischer LP. Jacques Lisfranc de Saint-Martin (1787-1847). Hist Sci Med 2005;39(1):17–34 [in French].
2. Welck MJ, Zinchenko R, Rudge B. Lisfranc injuries. Injury 2015;46(4):536–41.
3. Desmond EA, Chou LB. Current concepts review: Lisfranc injuries. Foot Ankle Int 2006;27(8):653–60.
4. Wright MP, Michelson JD. Lisfranc injuries. BMJ 2013;347:f4561.
5. Richter M, Wippermann B, Krettek C, et al. Fractures and fracture dislocations of the midfoot: occurrence, causes and long-term results. Foot Ankle Int 2001; 22(5):392–8.
6. Cheung Y. Soft tissue injury to the ankle: ligament injuries. In: Pope TL, Bloem HL, Beltran J, et al, editors. Musculoskeletal imaging. 2nd edition. Philadelphia: WB Saunders; 2015. p. 455–73.
7. Thompson MC, Mormino MA. Injury to the tarsometatarsal joint complex. J Am Acad Orthop Surg 2003;11(4):260–7.
8. Garrick JG, Requa RK. The epidemiology of foot and ankle injuries in sports. Clin Sports Med 1988;7(1): 29–36.
9. Kalia V, Fishman EK, Carrino JA, et al. Epidemiology, imaging, and treatment of Lisfranc fracture-dislocations revisited. Skeletal Radiol 2012;41(2): 129–36.
10. DeOrio M, Erickson M, Usuelli FG, et al. Lisfranc injuries in sport. Foot Ankle Clin 2009;14(2):169–86.

11. Meyer SA, Callaghan JJ, Albright JP, et al. Midfoot sprains in collegiate football players. Am J Sports Med 1994;22(3):392–401.

12. Johnson GF. Pediatric Lisfranc injury: "bunk bed" fracture. AJR Am J Roentgenol 1981;137(5):1041–4.

13. Richter M, Kwon JY, Digiovanni CW. Foot injuries. In: Browner B, Jupiter J, Krettek C, et al, editors. Skeletal trauma: basic science, management, and reconstruction, vol. 2, 5th edition. Philadelphia: WB Saunders; 2015. p. 2251–387.

14. Lau S, Bozin M, Thillainadesan T. Lisfranc fracture dislocation: a review of a commonly missed injury of the midfoot. Emerg Med J 2017;34(1):52–6.

15. Myerson MS, Fisher RT, Burgess AR, et al. Fracture dislocations of the tarsometatarsal joints: end results correlated with pathology and treatment. Foot Ankle 1986;6(5):225–42.

16. Hatem SF. Imaging of Lisfranc injury and midfoot sprain. Radiol Clin North Am 2008;46(6):1045–60.

17. Castro M, Melao L, Canella C, et al. Lisfranc joint ligamentous complex: MRI with anatomic correlation in cadavers. AJR Am J Roentgenol 2010;195(6):W447–55.

18. De Palma L, Santucci A, Sabetta SP, et al. Anatomy of the Lisfranc joint complex. Foot Ankle Int 1997;18(6):356–64.

19. Panchbhavi VK, Andersen CR, Vallurupalli S, et al. A minimally disruptive model and three-dimensional evaluation of Lisfranc joint diastasis. J Bone Joint Surg Am 2008;90(12):2707–13.

20. Stavlas P, Roberts CS, Xypnitos FN, et al. The role of reduction and internal fixation of Lisfranc fracture-dislocations: a systematic review of the literature. Int Orthop 2010;34(8):1083–91.

21. Rosenbaum A, Dellenbaugh S, Dipreta J, et al. Subtle injuries to the Lisfranc joint. Orthopedics 2011;34(11):882–7.

22. Watson TS, Shurnas PS, Denker J. Treatment of Lisfranc joint injury: current concepts. J Am Acad Orthop Surg 2010;18(12):718–28.

23. Crim J. MR imaging evaluation of subtle Lisfranc injuries: the midfoot sprain. Magn Reson Imaging Clin N Am 2008;16(1):19–27, v.

24. Quenu E, Kuss G. Etude sur les luxations du metatarse. Rev Chir Paris 1909;39:281.

25. Hardcastle PH, Reschauer R, Kutscha-Lissberg E, et al. Injuries to the tarsometatarsal joint: incidence, classification and treatment. J Bone Joint Surg Br 1982;64(3):349–56.

26. Llopis E, Carrascoso J, Iriarte I, et al. Lisfranc injury imaging and surgical management. Semin Musculoskelet Radiol 2016;20(2):139–53.

27. Nunley JA, Vertullo CJ. Classification, investigation, and management of midfoot sprains: Lisfranc injuries in the athlete. Am J Sports Med 2002;30(6):871–8.

28. Siddiqui NA, Galizia MS, Almusa E, et al. Evaluation of the tarsometatarsal joint using conventional radiography, CT, and MR imaging. Radiographics 2014;34(2):514–31.

29. Sandlin MI, Taghavi CE, Charlton TP, et al. Lisfranc injuries in the elite athlete. Instr Course Lect 2017;66:275–80.

30. Seybold JD, Coetzee JC. Lisfranc injuries: when to observe, fix, or fuse. Clin Sports Med 2015;34(4):705–23.

31. Keiserman LS, Cassandra J, Amis JA. The piano key test: a clinical sign for the identification of subtle tarsometatarsal pathology. Foot Ankle Int 2003;24(5):437–8.

32. Ross G, Cronin R, Hauzenblas J, et al. Plantar ecchymosis sign: a clinical aid to diagnosis of occult Lisfranc tarsometatarsal injuries. J Orthop Trauma 1996;10(2):119–22.

33. Curtis MJ, Myerson M, Szura B. Tarsometatarsal joint injuries in the athlete. Am J Sports Med 1993;21(4):497–502.

34. Gupta RT, Wadhwa RP, Learch TJ, et al. Lisfranc injury: imaging findings for this important but often-missed diagnosis. Curr Probl Diagn Radiol 2008;37(3):115–26.

35. Chiodo CP, Myerson MS. Developments and advances in the diagnosis and treatment of injuries to the tarsometatarsal joint. Orthop Clin North Am 2001;32(1):11–20.

36. Foster SC, Foster RR. Lisfranc's tarsometatarsal fracture-dislocation. Radiology 1976;120(1):79–83.

37. Faciszewski T, Burks RT, Manaster BJ. Subtle injuries of the Lisfranc joint. J Bone Joint Surg Am 1990;72(10):1519–22.

38. Vuori JP, Aro HT. Lisfranc joint injuries: trauma mechanisms and associated injuries. J Trauma 1993;35(1):40–5.

39. Myerson MS, Cerrato RA. Current management of tarsometatarsal injuries in the athlete. J Bone Joint Surg Am 2008;90(11):2522–33.

40. Preidler KW, Peicha G, Lajtai G, et al. Conventional radiography, CT, and MR imaging in patients with hyperflexion injuries of the foot: diagnostic accuracy in the detection of bony and ligamentous changes. AJR Am J Roentgenol 1999;173(6):1673–7.

41. Thordarsen DB. Fractures of the midfoot and forefoot. In: Myerson MS, editor. Foot and ankle disorders, vol. 2. Toronto: WB Saunders; 1999. p. 1265–96.

42. Philbin T, Rosenberg G, Sferra JJ. Complications of missed or untreated Lisfranc injuries. Foot Ankle Clin 2003;8(1):61–71.

43. Kaplan JD, Karlin JM, Scurran BL, et al. Lisfranc's fracture-dislocation. A review of the literature and case reports. J Am Podiatr Med Assoc 1991;81(10):531–9.

44. Delfaut EM, Rosenberg ZS, Demondion X. Malalignment at the Lisfranc joint: MR features in asymptomatic patients and cadaveric specimens. Skeletal Radiol 2002;31(9):499–504.

45. Ulbrich EJ, Zubler V, Sutter R, et al. Ligaments of the Lisfranc joint in MRI: 3D-SPACE (sampling perfection with application optimized contrasts using different flip-angle evolution) sequence compared to three orthogonal proton-density fat-saturated (PD fs) sequences. Skeletal Radiol 2013;42(3): 399–409.

46. Kitsukawa K, Hirano T, Niki H, et al. MR imaging evaluation of the Lisfranc ligament in cadaveric feet and patients with acute to chronic Lisfranc injury. Foot Ankle Int 2015;36(12):1483–92.

47. Raikin SM, Elias I, Dheer S, et al. Prediction of midfoot instability in the subtle Lisfranc injury. Comparison of magnetic resonance imaging with intraoperative findings. J Bone Joint Surg Am 2009;91(4): 892–9.

48. Rammelt S, Schneiders W, Schikore H, et al. Primary open reduction and fixation compared with delayed corrective arthrodesis in the treatment of tarsometatarsal (Lisfranc) fracture dislocation. J Bone Joint Surg Br 2008;90(11): 1499–506.

49. Perez Blanco R, Rodriguez Merchan C, Canosa Sevillano R, et al. Tarsometatarsal fractures and dislocations. J Orthop Trauma 1988;2(3):188–94.

50. Pelt CE, Bachus KN, Vance RE, et al. A biomechanical analysis of a tensioned suture device in the fixation of the ligamentous Lisfranc injury. Foot Ankle Int 2011;32(4):422–31.

51. Brin YS, Nyska M, Kish B. Lisfranc injury repair with the TightRope device: a short-term case series. Foot Ankle Int 2010;31(7):624–7.

52. Kuo RS, Tejwani NC, Digiovanni CW, et al. Outcome after open reduction and internal fixation of Lisfranc joint injuries. J Bone Joint Surg Am 2000;82-A(11): 1609–18.

53. Ly TV, Coetzee JC. Treatment of primarily ligamentous Lisfranc joint injuries: primary arthrodesis compared with open reduction and internal fixation. A prospective, randomized study. J Bone Joint Surg Am 2006;88(3):514–20.

54. Alberta FG, Aronow MS, Barrero M, et al. Ligamentous Lisfranc joint injuries: a biomechanical comparison of dorsal plate and transarticular screw fixation. Foot Ankle Int 2005;26(6):462–73.

55. Sheibani-Rad S, Coetzee JC, Giveans MR, et al. Arthrodesis versus ORIF for Lisfranc fractures. Orthopedics 2012;35(6):e868–73.

Metatarsalgia

Aaron Hodes, MD[a], Hilary Umans, MD[b],*

KEYWORDS

- Metatarsalgia • Plantar plate tear • Interdigital neuroma • Morton neuroma • Stress fracture
- Stress reaction • Freiberg infraction

KEY POINTS

- Metatarsal stress injuries are common, although radiography is relatively insensitive for fracture detection.
- Osseous "stress reaction" describes bone stress injury as a spectrum from periosteal edema, increasing marrow edema, and ultimately, fracture.
- Freiberg infraction is a subset of stress injury affecting the subchondral bone of the lesser metatarsal head that is often complicated by superimposed osteonecrosis.
- Interdigital neuroma and plantar plate tear (typically associated with "pseudoneuroma" in the adjacent interspace) can be difficult to differentiate clinically and by imaging.

INTRODUCTION

Metatarsalgia is a term that refers to pain regardless of cause located in the region of the metatarsal (MT), metatarsophalangeal joint (MTPJ), intermetatarsal space (IS), and submetatarsal soft tissues. This article focuses on osseous stress injury, plantar plate (PP) tear with reactive pericapsular soft tissue thickening ("pseudoneuroma" = PN), and interdigital neuroma (IN), because these present diagnostic challenges.

Foot radiographs are useful to evaluate bone mineral density, foot alignment, arthropathy, fracture, bone lesions, and swelling. Three views are standard, with alignment accurately evaluated only on weight-bearing. Ultrasound (US) provides high-resolution imaging in a small field of view, best combined with dynamic or provocative maneuvers.

MR imaging permits a larger overview of the forefoot, providing superior soft tissue contrast for assessing wide range of pathologic conditions that manifest as metatarsalgia. Imaging parameters vary with field strength and surface coil selection. The field of view ranges from 6 to 10 cm, centered at the MTPJs or MT shafts depending on the indication. Slice thickness and gap generally vary between 2 to 3.5 mm and 0 to 0.3 mm, respectively. At the authors' institution, proton-density-weighted fat-suppressed (PDFS) and T1-weighted images are obtained in long-axis, short-axis, and sagittal planes. Adequate resolution in small joint imaging requires 1.5- or 3.0-T units. Toes are ideally padded in neutral position. Long-axis images are aligned along the axis of the lesser MTs (**Fig. 1**A), and short-axis images are prescribed perpendicular to either the MT heads or the MTPJ (**Fig. 1**B). Sagittal images are oriented along the second MT axis, using the axial and coronal localizers, to optimize imaging of PP tear (**Fig. 1**C).

STRESS INJURIES OF THE LESSER METATARSALS

MT stress injury results from cyclic loading forces that exceed the strength of the bone. Stress injury occurs in normal bone subjected to supraphysiologic force (fatigue injury) or weakened bone subjected to normal physiologic force (insufficiency injury). MT fatigue stress injuries are common among elite athletes and military recruits with rapid

Disclosure Statement: The authors have nothing to disclose.
[a] Department of Radiology, Jacobi Medical Center, 1400 Pelham Parkway South, Bronx, NY 10461, USA;
[b] Department of Radiology, Albert Einstein College of Medicine, 1300 Morris Park Avenue, Bronx, NY 10461, USA
* Corresponding author. 71 East 77th Street, New York, NY 10075.
E-mail address: hilary.umans@gmail.com

Radiol Clin N Am 56 (2018) 877–892
https://doi.org/10.1016/j.rcl.2018.06.004
0033-8389/18/© 2018 Elsevier Inc. All rights reserved.

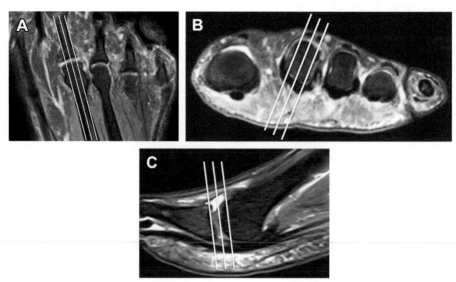

Fig. 1. MR imaging plane localization. Long- (*A*) and short-axis (*B*) scout images illustrate scan plane orientation (*lines*) along the second MT axis for sagittal imaging. (*C*) Sagittal localizer illustrates scan plane orientation (*lines*) perpendicular to the MT head and MTPJ.

increase in training intensity or distance or changes in shoe gear or terrain.[1–3] Insufficiency stress injuries occur in individuals with low bone mass, especially estrogen-deficient women, including postmenopausal women or high-performance athletes with female athlete triad, which is defined by menstrual dysfunction and low-energy availability often related to an eating disorder.[1] Lesser MT stress injuries most commonly occur in the second followed by the third rays.[2] Symptoms of MT stress reaction and fracture include vague forefoot pain with weight-bearing and dorsal swelling.

BIOMECHANICS

MTPJ, MT axial load, and MT bending moment forces are greatest on the first followed by the second MTs and then third through fifth MTs.[4,5] Unlike the first MT, lesser MTs experience disproportionately greater force relative to their size and do not routinely have sesamoids to dissipate load.[4] Hallux valgus, high-heeled shoe gear, or muscle fatigue alter the normal foot biomechanics and shift stress, normally borne by the first ray to the lesser MTs and MTPJ region.[5–8] Many believe that relative elongation of the second MT shifts stress from the first to the second ray and predisposes to injury.[9] Some surgeons perform shortening second MT osteotomy to achieve a more normal MT parabola.

RADIOGRAPHIC FINDINGS

Radiographic findings of MT stress fracture are subtle and frequently occult. Mulligan[10] reported the "gray cortex" as an early sign of tibial stress fracture, with vague intracortical lucency but no discrete linear defect. Graying of the cortex occurs in the resorption phase of bone remodeling, before development of mineralized periosteal and endosteal callus.[11,12] The gray cortex sign is a subtle finding in MT stress fracture, often detectable only in retrospect (see **Fig. 4**D).

STRESS INJURY DIAGNOSTIC SCHEMA WITH MR IMAGING

Fredericson and colleagues[13] devised a grading system that stratifies tibial stress reaction as a continuum from periosteal edema to marrow edema and ultimately fracture. Although devised to characterize tibial stress injury, it is commonly used to grade all osseous stress injury (**Figs. 2–5, Table 1**). Using this schema to grade osseous stress injury throughout the skeleton in collegiate athletes, Nattiv and coauthors[1] reported a minor increase in recovery time comparing grade I to II, moderately longer recovery in grade III, and longest recovery time with grade IV stress reaction. Although computed tomography is useful to detect radiographically occult MT stress fracture, MR imaging is preferred because it permits detection of grade I–III osseous stress reaction and soft tissue injury (see **Figs. 2–4**).

US can be used to screen for cortical defect to confirm fracture. In the proper clinical setting with corresponding focal tenderness, periosteal thickening and hyperemia are virtually diagnostic of stress MT stress injury (see **Fig. 5**).

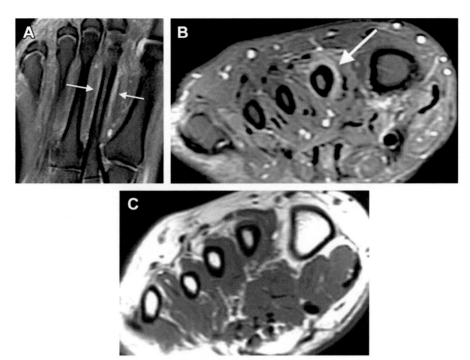

Fig. 2. Grade 2 stress reaction of the second MT shaft in a female runner with metatarsalgia. PDFS images in the long (*A*) and short (*B*) axes demonstrate periosteal edema (*arrows*) as well as subtle stress-related marrow edema. (*C*) Note that marrow edema is not clearly visible in the corresponding short axis T1-weighted image.

FREIBERG INFRACTION: EPIDEMIOLOGY AND MR IMAGING FINDINGS

Initially recognized in adolescents, Freiberg infraction most commonly occurs in women in their third to seventh decades.[14–16] Freiberg infraction is a confusing eponym that remains in common usage. Although cause is debated, "infraction" is an elision of "infarction" and "fracture," which is apt because imaging and histologic findings suggest

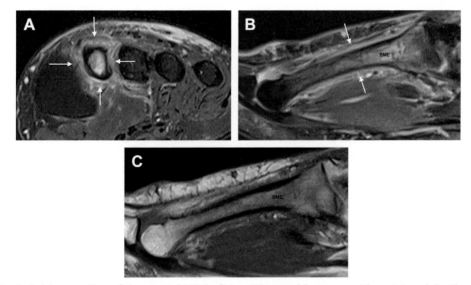

Fig. 3. Grade 3 stress reaction of the second MT shaft in a 70-year-old woman with metatarsalgia. Short-axis (*A*) and sagittal (*B*) PDFS images demonstrate severe periosteal edema (*arrows*) and bone marrow edema (BME). (*C*) BME is also evident on sagittal T1-weighted image. Grade 3 stress reaction is differentiated from grade 4 stress reaction by the absence of a linear cortical defect or fracture line.

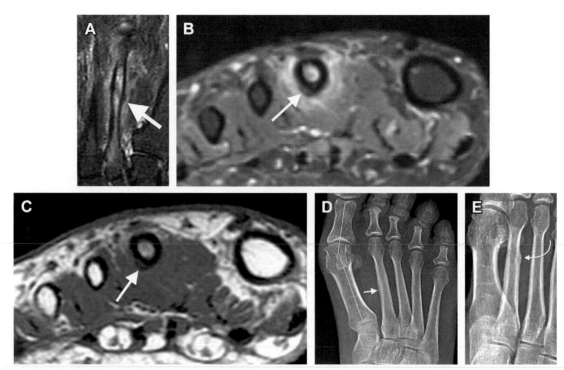

Fig. 4. A 47-year-old woman with second MT pain on ambulation. Long-axis STIR (*A*), short-axis PDFS (*B*), and short-axis T1-weighted (*C*) MR images demonstrate marrow edema (hyperintense on *A* and *B*, and hypointense on *C*) and hyperintense periosteum (*A*, *B*). Hypointense fracture line is evident on (*A*) (*arrow*). Small, thin arrows on (*B*, *C*) indicate faint, dark signal peripheral callus. Anteroposterior (*D*) and oblique (*E*) radiographs obtained 8 weeks after MR imaging demonstrate a "gray cortex sign" (*arrow* in *D*) and peripheral bridging mineralized callus and residual linear intracortical lucency (*arrow* in *E*). Note the hallux valgus deformity (*straight lines* in *D*) and 2nd to 5th proximal interphalangeal resection arthroplasties.

a combination of both. Lesser MT heads are exclusively affected, with a predilection for the second and third.[6,14,15] Torriani and colleagues[14] provide compelling evidence that subchondral fracture is the inciting injury that may progress to subarticular osteonecrosis with articular collapse and end-stage degenerative arthrosis. Late-stage Freiberg infraction results in limited range of motion at the lesser MTPJ.[17] The Smillie radiographic classification system (**Table 2**) stratifies progressive MT head deformity and secondary degenerative arthrosis.[18] Although devised before the advent of MR imaging, this classification system is still used to grade lesions and guide treatment.[6,15,18] The earliest radiographic finding is smooth MT head flattening, although asymptomatic, presumably normal variant flattening of the second MT head has been reported in up to 10% of individuals.[19] Superimposed subchondral bone sclerosis and cystlike change indicate Freiberg infraction.[14] Late-stage disease is evident on radiographs. MR imaging is sensitive for detection of subchondral marrow signal alteration, radiographically occult fracture, and subtle subarticular collapse in earlier stages, but elucidates the full extent of pathologic condition in all stages (**Figs. 6–8**).[14]

PLANTAR PLATE TEAR
Normal Anatomy

The PP is a rectangular to trapezoidal fibrocartilaginous structure that inserts onto the plantar margin of the proximal phalanges of the lesser MTPJs. Comprising primarily type I collagen,[20] it measures 2 to 5 mm in thickness, 16 to 23 mm in length, and 8 to 13 mm in width,[21] but must withstand tremendous compressive and tensile stresses. The terminal plantar fascia, deep transverse intermetatarsal ligament (DTML), tendons of dorsal and plantar interossei, accessory and main collateral ligaments, indirect insertions of the dorsal capsule, and extensor hood by way of the accessory collateral ligament all blend with the PP, which is the primary stabilizer of the lesser MTPJs (**Fig. 9**). A midline plantar groove accommodates and stabilizes the flexor digitorum tendons in their course deep to the MT heads at the MTPJs.[20]

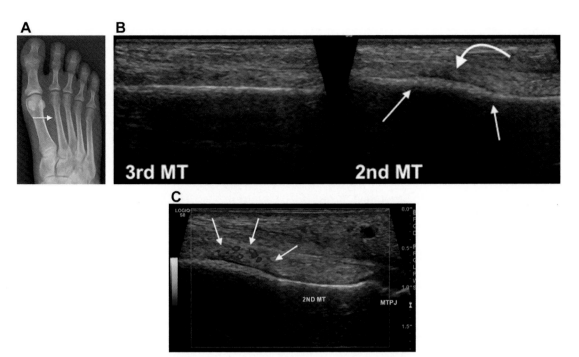

Fig. 5. A 36-year-old woman with 3 weeks of second MT pain and tenderness. (*A*) Anteroposterior radiograph was reported as negative for fracture, but demonstrates subtle peripheral mineralized callus (*arrow*) at the distal medial second MT shaft. (*B*) Long-axis sonographic images obtained 3 days after radiography demonstrate contour distortion (*thin arrows*) corresponding to peripheral callus of the second MT shaft, and superimposed periosteal edema (*curved arrow*), which are absent in the comparison image of the asymptomatic third MT. (*C*) Power Doppler illustrates periosteal hyperemia (*arrows*) at the site of this healing stress fracture.

Biomechanics

PP tear destabilizes the lesser MTPJ and results in acquired toe deformity and dysfunction. Because the second MT bears the greatest relative stress

Table 1
MR imaging features of grade 1–4 stress reaction

	Fluid-Sensitive Sequences		T1-Weighted	
Grade	Periosteal Edema	Marrow Edema	Marrow Edema	Fracture Line
1	Yes	No	No	No
2	Yes	Yes	No	No
3	Yes	Yes	Yes	No
4	Yes	Yes	Yes	Yes

Note. Increasing severity of stress injury is reflected in relative conspicuity of marrow edema on fluid-sensitive and T1-weighted sequences. Fluid sensitive sequences include proton-density or T2-weighted fat-suppressed as well as STIR sequences. Grade 4 stress reaction is synonymous with stress fracture.
Data from Fredericson M, Bergman AG, Hoffman KL, et al. Tibial stress reaction in runners. Correlation of clinical symptoms and scintigraphy with a new magnetic resonance imaging grading system. Am J Sports Med 1995;23:478.

per unit area after the first MT,[4,5] stress is potentiated by hallux valgus and relative elongation of the second MT,[9] and the second MTPJ PP is most prone to tear. Because the lesser MTs are relatively supinated and the larger lateral condyle of the MT heads withstands the greatest degree of stress, tears tend to originate laterally and propagate medially.[22,23] These tears are typically chronic, microdegenerative tears, most commonly in middle-aged and older women, owing to chronic stress in MTPJ hyperextension due to high-heeled shoe gear.[7] Acute traumatic tears occur much less commonly without as strict female predominance.

Because the PP receives insertions from the accessory collateral ligaments and dorsal capsule and shares an insertion with the proper phalangeal ligament, tears of the PP affect all the static stabilizers of the lesser MTPJs. The interossei and lumbricals are the primary dynamic flexors of the MTPJs.[7] With PP failure, static resistance to extension is diminished. The axis of the interossei shifts dorsally, and they become ineffective flexors, resulting in increasing extension, subluxation, and, ultimately, dislocation of the affected toe.[21] As the lateral PP and capsule fail, the lumbricals contribute an unopposed adduction force resulting in superimposed tibial deviation and subluxation of the toe. As the second toe is most

Table 2
Radiographic and MR imaging features of Freiberg infraction according to Smillie system

Smillie Stage	Smillie Stage Features	Bone Marrow Edema on MR Imaging	XR Findings	Deformity on MR Imaging and XR
1	Subtle MT head epiphysis fissure	Yes	None	None
2	Subchondral resorption, mild MT head flattening; intact dorsal and plantar cartilage	Yes	Questionable	Mild sinking
3	Further subchondral resorption, MT head flattening; collapsed dorsal articular cartilage; intact plantar cartilage ± bony projections	Yes	Yes	Sunken head with ± intact bony projections
4	Severely MT head collapse; collapsed dorsal and plantar articular cartilage; broken bony projections	Yes	Yes	Sunken head and broken bony projections
5	MT head articular collapse and secondary degenerative arthrosis	Yes	Yes	Arthrosis with flattened and deformed MT head

Note. All stages will show MT subchondral marrow edema on fluid-sensitive and T1-weighted images, allowing detection of low-grade injury. Severity of MT head collapse and articular damage ultimately determines the stage.

Data from Torriani M, Thomas BJ, Bredella MA, et al. MRI of metatarsal head subchondral fractures in patients with forefoot pain. AJR Am J Roentgenol 2008;190:570–5; and Smillie IS. Treatment of Freiberg's infraction. Proc R Soc Med 1967;60:29–31.

commonly affected, there is typically tibial deviation and extension of the second toe with splaying of the second and third toes.

CLINICAL EVALUATION AND MANAGEMENT

Affected individuals present with submetatarsal pain commonly localized to the site of tear (most commonly at the lateral base of the second toe), which may extend into the adjacent IS and toes (**Fig. 10**A). Pain is often maximal just before

rupture, diminishing as toe deformity worsens.[24] PN accompanies almost all PP tears and may impinge upon the digital nerve, resulting in pain indistinguishable from IN.[25,26] Acquired weakness of toe flexion and superimposed toe extension contribute to loss of "toe purchase" (dynamic ability of the toe to push against the ground), worsening with increasing grade of PP tear.[24] Sagittal plane instability of the MTP joint is assessed by the "vertical stress test."[24] A positive test subluxes the toe and reproduces pain. Grade I lesions are

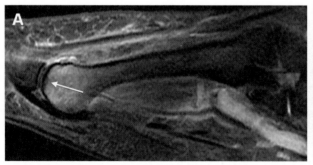
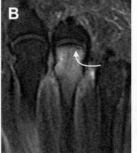
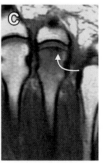

Fig. 6. A 50-year-old woman with third MT pain after fifth MT exostectomy. Marrow edema is hyperintense on sagittal PDFS (*A*) and long-axis PDFS (*B*) images and hypointense on long-axis T1-weighted (*C*) images with low signal inseparable from the subchondral cortex (*arrow* in *A*) and preserved articular contour, consistent with Smillie grade 1 Freiberg infraction. Low signal focus (*B, C*) is clearly a subchondral fracture (*arrow*).

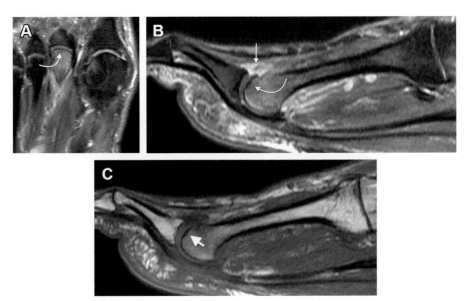

Fig. 7. A 63-year-old woman with second MTPJ pain and swelling and MR imaging features of Smillie grade 2 Freiberg infraction. On long-axis PDFS image (*A*), there is suggestion of a small subchondral fracture (*arrow*). Subtle articular cortical flattening is indicated by curved arrow on sagittal PDFS (*B*) and arrow on T1-weighted images (*C*). In (*B*), arrow indicates MTPJ synovitis.

stable to vertical stress, with worsening instability accompanying higher-grade lesions.[24] MTPJ instability on vertical stress testing is the most specific clinical examination finding of PP tears.[24]

First-line treatment of low-grade lesions that focuses on off-loading and stabilization of lesser MTPJs typically mitigates painful symptoms, but PP tears, toe dysfunction, and deformity tend to worsen over time.[7] Although surgical procedures have historically combined soft tissue transfers and arthroplasty to correct to deformity, only procedures that repair the PP restore function.[27] Because more recent surgical innovations have enabled PP repair via a dorsal capsular approach, PP repair has become a first-line surgical option with reported excellent outcomes.[28] Plantar plate repair is most commonly performed with a shortening MT osteotomy that permits exposure to the PP, although newer systems have been

devised that enable unilateral or bilateral PP repair without osteotomy.[29]

INTERDIGITAL NEUROMA

IN is a nonneoplastic lesion characterized by perineural fibrosis, vascular proliferation, endoneural edema, and axonal degeneration.[30] Although "Morton neuroma" is used synonymously to describe a neuroma in any IS, that eponym specifically refers to neuroma in the third IS.[31] Surgical series report the incidence to be greatest in the third (64%–91%), followed by the second (18%–31%), and rare in the fourth (0%–6%) and first (0%–2.5%) IS.[32–35]

Cause is favored to be due to a combination of mechanical irritation, ischemia, neural entrapment, and tethering. Relative tightness of the third IS and the tendency for the third common digital nerve to

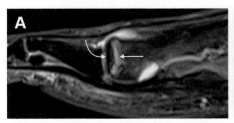
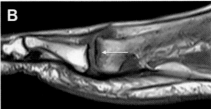
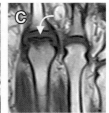

Fig. 8. A 54-year-old woman with second MTPJ pain. Sagittal PDFS (*A*), sagittal T1-weighted (*B*) and long-axis T1-weighted (*C*) MR images demonstrate hyperintense signal subchondral cleft (*straight arrows* in *A* and *B*) with moderate collapse of the overlying articular cortex of the second MT head (*curved arrows* in *A* and *C*).

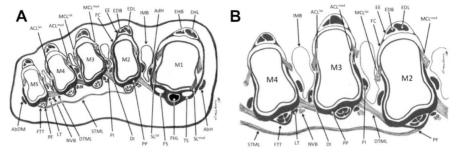

Fig. 9. Short-axis anatomy through the MTs. Short-axis anatomic diagrams at the level of the MT head in all (*A*) and second to fourth (*B*) MTPJs. AbDM, abductor digiti minimi tendon; AbH, abductor hallucis tendon; ACL^lat, lateral accessory collateral ligament, lateral component; ACL^med, medial accessory collateral ligament, medial component; AdH, adductor hallucis tendon; DI, dorsal interosseous tendon; EDB, extensor digitorum brevis tendon; EDL, extensor digitorum longus tendon; EE, extensor expansion (ie, extensor hood); EHB, extensor hallucis brevis tendon; EHL, extensor hallucis longus tendon; FC, fibrous capsule; FHL, flexor hallucis longus tendon; FS, fibular sesamoid (lateral); FTT, flexors tendons tunnel for flexor digitorum longus and brevis; IMB, intermetatarsal bursa; MCL^lat, main collateral ligament, lateral component; MCL^med, main collateral ligament, medial component; NVB, neurovascular bundle; PF, plantar fascia (vertical fibers); PI, plantar interosseous tendon; SL^lat, sesamoid ligament, lateral component; SL^med, sesamoid ligament, medial component; STML, superficial transverse intermetatarsal ligament; TS, tibial sesamoid bone (medial). (*Courtesy of* Caio Nery, MD, São Paulo, Brazil; with permission.)

form from communicating branches of the medial and lateral plantar nerve (**Fig. 10**B), as well as shearing stress from the relatively mobile fourth MT, might explain the predilection for the third IS.[36] Although men may be affected, symptomatic IN most commonly affects women in the fourth to eighth decades.[30,36–39]

Although INs may be multiple, not all are symptomatic[40,41]; only symptomatic IN warrants therapeutic intervention. Symptoms, including sharp, burning pain and numbness, may localize to the IS, the MTPJ, or the toes. Many describe the sensation of "walking on marbles."

CLINICAL EVALUATION AND MANAGEMENT

Provocative maneuvers designed to re-create typical symptoms of IN include forefoot squeeze or compressing each individual IS. These maneuvers are sensitive, but nonspecific. The less sensitive Mulder maneuver is considered the most specific provocative clinical test for IN.[42] It involves simultaneous forefoot and IS compression, which forces the IN out of the plantar aspect of the IS often with a palpable click, only considered positive if the maneuver reproduces pain. Although many use anesthetic injections to confirm or

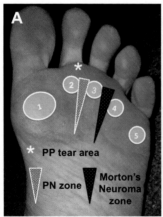
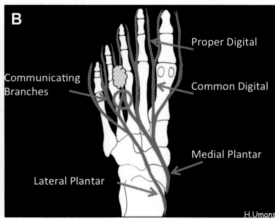

Fig. 10. Schematic depictions of forefoot pain and neural anatomy. (*A*) Schematic image depicts most common areas of tenderness for PP tear (*asterisk*), PN (*checkered triangle in second IS*), and Morton neuroma (*black triangle in third IS*). MT heads are indicated by numbered circles. Pain over the third IS usually is suspect for typical third IS IN (*black triangle*), called Morton neuroma. (*B*) Schematic of plantar and digital nerve anatomy in the foot with common branching pattern, with the commonest location of IN (Morton neuroma) illustrated in the third IS (*yellow mass*) distal to the confluence of communicating branches (*red circle*) from the 2nd and 4th IS common digital nerves.

exclude IN, this will not differentiate IN from PN (which accompanies most PP tear). Caution is advised in injecting steroids into the IS without fully assessing the integrity of the adjacent PP, because it may precipitate or exacerbate a degenerative PP tear.[43]

Conservative therapy (shoe-gear modification and submetatarsal padding) is effective in most individuals. IS injection with anesthetic and steroid is commonly performed. Ethanol or radiofrequency ablation and surgical neurectomy are options when conservative therapy fails. INs greater than 5 mm in transverse dimension have been reported to fare better after surgery than smaller ones.[37] Postablation or neurectomy numbness is expected, although most consider this acceptable should pain abate.[37,44,45] Postsurgical IS pain may persist in a subset, resulting from stump neuroma, scarring, and bursitis. Stump neuroma is reported in up to 24% and may mimic IN on MR imaging and US.[38] Of course, ablation or neurectomy may fail due to misdiagnosis and mistreatment of a suspected IN that was actually PN with adjacent PP tear.[46]

METATARSOPHALANGEAL JOINT, PLANTAR PLATE, AND INTERMETATARSAL SPACE EVALUATION BY ULTRASOUND AND MR IMAGING

Radiographs are the first-line screening examination, and they may reveal hallux valgus or relative elongation of the second MT that may shift stress to the lesser MTPJ region and predispose to PP tear.[7,9] Tibial deviation and extension of the lesser toes (most commonly the second with splaying of the second and third) suggest PP tear. Toe deformity does not indicate IN.

Along with superior resolution in a small field of view, advantages of US over MR imaging include the ability to talk with and examine the patient. Forefoot squeeze, IS compression and Mulder maneuvers, and MTPJ vertical stress test may be combined with US to help distinguish between IN and PP tear with adjacent PN.[42]

US of the MTPJ and IS region is a nuanced examination, heavily influenced by operator experience. Anisotropy due to nonparallel probe positioning at the insertion of the PP results in spurious hypoechogenicity that may be misinterpreted as degeneration or tear (Fig. 11A, B). Ideally the toe should be brought to neutral position. If there is fixed toe extension, care should be taken to alter the plane of the probe footplate along the plantar MTPJ to remain parallel to the PP insertion. Tight interspaces and plantar callosities can pose technical challenges to even experienced sonographers.

Forefoot US is performed in the long and short axis through the second to fourth PP and each IS (Fig. 11C). The normal PP appears as a compact, fibrillar, slightly echogenic thin rectangular to trapezoidal structure (see Fig. 11A), inserting onto the base of the lesser toes.[47] A normal, discrete, midline anechoic recess ($\leq$2.5 mm) must not to be mistaken for tear.[22] Because the axis of the MT and toe may vary, especially with acquired deformity, the PP is scanned in short increments from side to side, to differentiate a tear from the capsular recess. Tears are best evaluated in the long axis and appear as anechoic or hypoechoic defects at the insertion (most commonly laterally) (Fig. 12A) with variable extension to or across midline.[47] US permits sensitive detection of PP tear, although distinguishing tear from degeneration is difficult and contributes to low reported specificity.[47]

Chronic PP tear may appear to heal with scarring but remain symptomatic.[48] In these cases, correlated signs of PP tear are most useful.[25,47]

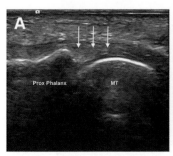
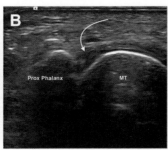
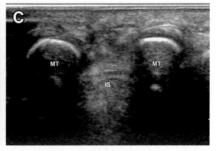

Fig. 11. Normal PP on sonography. Long-axis US images through the intact second PP obtained with probe positioned parallel to the PP insertion with the toe in neutral (A) and nonparallel to the PP insertion with the toe positioned in extension (B). Arrows (A) indicate echogenic, fibrillar appearance of the normal PP, anchored onto plantar base of proximal (Prox) phalanx at the MTPJ. Arrow (B) indicates spurious intrasubstance hypoechogenicity at the insertion due to anisotropy. (C) Short-axis US image obtained plantar to the MT heads with counterpressure at the dorsum of the IS shows normal echogenic fat in IS, with no hypoechoic mass.

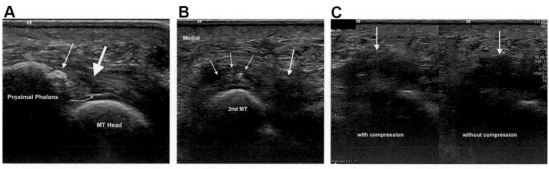

Fig. 12. Chronic PP tears with scarring on sonography. (*A*) Long-axis image of the lateral second PP demonstrates full-thickness insertional tear (*straight bold arrow*), with correlated findings of insertional enthesophytes (*straight thin arrow*) and a thin echogenic line along the hyaline cartilage of the MT head ("cartilage interface sign") (*curved thin arrow*), supporting the diagnosis of PP tear. Short-axis (*B*) image plantar to the second MT head and IS and long-axis (*C*) image through the second IS demonstrate a noncompressible hypoechoic IS mass (*arrows*), supporting diagnosis of PP tear with adjacent PN. Straight, short, thin arrows on (*B*) indicate thickening and hypoechogenicity of the torn second PP.

Enthesophytes at the phalangeal insertion of the PP (more conspicuous on US than MR imaging) favor tear (see **Fig. 12**A). The most consistent correlated sign is eccentric, pericapsular mass (PN) that forms along the surface of the PP near the site of tear, with extension along the capsule in the IS (**Fig. 12**B, C). During US scanning, recognition of acquired toe deformity (typically tibial deviation of the second toe with splaying of the second and third with or without toe hyperextension) should suggest the diagnosis of PP tear (**Fig. 13**). In some cases of full-thickness PP tear, there may be a detectable sonographic "cartilage interface sign" with an echogenic interface between the hyaline cartilage MT head and the overlying hypoechoic or anechoic PP defect (see **Fig. 12**A). The cartilage interface sign has been a useful US sign of supraspinatus tendon tear that may have utility in US imaging of the PP.[49]

Hypoechoic IS masses should be imaged without and with firm digital counter-pressure opposite the probe location in the IS to differentiate solid mass from compressible bursae (**Fig. 14**). Firm counter-pressure splays the MT heads and pushes echogenic fat into the IS (see **Fig. 11**C), helping distinguish a centrally located IN (**Fig. 15**A) from an eccentric PN (see **Fig. 12**B, C). IN appears as a well-defined, ovoid/fusiform hypoechoic mass centered in the plantar aspect of the IS.[30,40] Pressure on the dorsal IS while scanning along the sole may result in displacement and expansion of the IN, which assumes the shape of a gingko leaf; this sign is reportedly insensitive but specific for IN.[50] Diagnostic specificity for IN is improved if the common digital nerve can be identified entering and exiting the mass in long-axis images (see **Fig. 15**A), although a large PN may similarly appear to encase the digital nerve (**Fig. 15**B).[39]

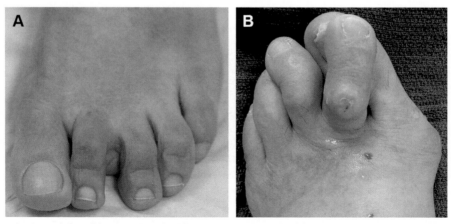

Fig. 13. Acquired toe deformities associated with PP tears. Low-grade (*A*) and end-stage (*B*) second MTPJ PP tear. Tibial deviation of the second toe is seen in (*A*) and second toe extension with tibial deviation crossing over the hallux is seen in (*B*).

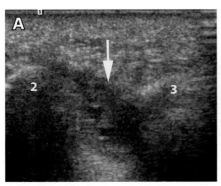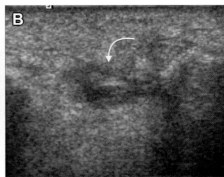

Fig. 14. Intermetatarsal bursitis. Short-axis US images of the second IS without (*A*) and with (*B*) compression demonstrate a hypoechoic mass (*straight arrow*) in (*A*), which compresses (*curved arrow*) in (*B*), indicative of intermetatarsal bursitis.

Short-axis US is essential for determining whether an IS mass is centrally or eccentrically located; long-axis imaging alone can be misleading. Even in the short axis, it can be difficult to appreciate the eccentric origin of a large PN using US. In that case, identification of an adjacent PP tear should favor PN, and MTPJ instability should confirm PP tear with PN. PP tear and adjacent IS IN were exceedingly rare in the recent surgical series by Yamada and colleagues.[26] PP tear (most commonly of the second MTPJ with second IS PN) often coexists with third IS neuroma.[43]

MR imaging is less operator dependent than US and permits simultaneous visualization of the IS along with the surrounding osseous, articular, caspuloligamentous, and myotendinous structures.

The normal PP inserts firmly onto the plantar base of the proximal phalanx without an intervening bright signal defect (**Fig. 16**A).[51] A normal capsular recess, which appears as a discrete high-signal zone undercutting the midline insertion of the PP and measures less than 2.5 mm, must

not be mistaken for tear (**Fig. 16**B). On MR imaging, PP tear appears as a bright signal defect at the PP insertion onto the base of the proximal phalanx (**Figs. 17**A and **18**A).[22,52] Tears typically originate laterally and propagate medially. Although tears may extend longitudinally with MT protrusion into the defect (**Fig. 19**), this is relatively uncommon.[53]

MTPJ effusion/synovitis commonly accompanies acute or subacute PP tear but is nonspecific and common with metatarsalgia from any cause.[43] Fluid signal simultaneously in the MTPJ and flexor tendon sheath may imply pathologic communication through an intervening PP tear, but is not specific for tear without MTPJ arthrography.[23,52] Although some favor MTPJ arthrography (a quick and easy procedure using US guidance), it is invasive and considered by most to be unnecessary for detection of tear.[51,54]

Correlated findings strongly associated with PP tear include reactive pericapsular soft tissue thickening (PN) (**Figs. 17**B and **18**C), insertional enthesophytes (± reactive marrow edema) (**Fig. 17**C),

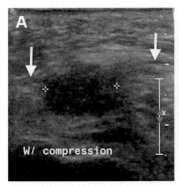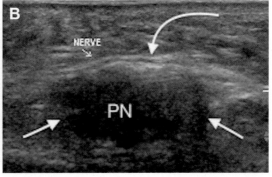

Fig. 15. IS masses. (*A*, *B*) Long-axis US images of noncompressible, hypoechoic IS masses. In (*A*), the digital nerve enters and exits the mass (*straight arrows*), supporting the likelihood of IN. In (*B*), the nerve (*curved arrow*) courses plantar to the mass (*straight arrows*, PN), excluding IN.

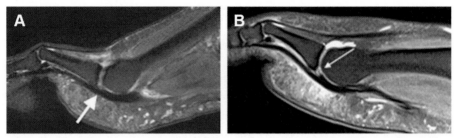

Fig. 16. Intact PP on MR imaging. (*A, B*) Sagittal PDFS images demonstrate an intact PP. Arrow (*A*) indicates intact paramedian insertion for the dark signal PP. Arrow (*B*) indicates the normal (<2.5 mm) midline capsular recess.

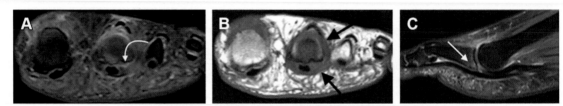

Fig. 17. PP tear. Short-axis PDFS (*A*) and short-axis T1-weighted (*B*) images through the base of the second toe proximal phalanx and sagittal PDFS (*C*) image through the second MTPJ demonstrate a linear bright signal tear at the lateral insertion of the second PP (*arrow in A*), with eccentric pericapsular intermediate signal PN (*arrows in B*) and enthesitis (marrow edema deep to the tear indicated by arrow in *C*).

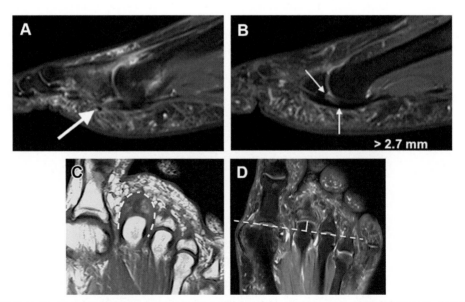

Fig. 18. PP tear. Sagittal (*A, B*) PDFS, long-axis T1-weighted (*C*) and long-axis PDFS (*D*) images demonstrate a linear bright signal tear (*arrow in A*) at the lateral second PP insertion with elongation of the PPPP greater than 2.7 mm indicating tear at midline (*arrows in B*). Curved, dashed line (*C*) delineates the PN. In (*D*), hallux valgus and second MT elongation (>4.5 mm protrusion of the second MT head [*solid line*] beyond a baseline between the first and third MT heads [*dashed line*]) predispose to PP tear.[25]

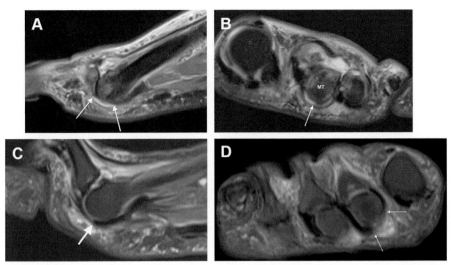

Fig. 19. PP tear. Sagittal (*A*) and short-axis (*B*) PDFS images demonstrate a large full-thickness tear (*arrows*) with longitudinal extension of the lateral second MTPJ PP, with buttonhole protrusion of the MT head into the defect. In another patient who is a runner, sagittal (*C*) and short-axis (*D*) PDFS images demonstrate a large full-thickness tear with longitudinal extension of the medial second MTPJ PP (*arrows*) with buttonhole protrusion of the MT head into the defect. Note hyperextension and marked dorsal subluxation of the toe at the MTPJ.

flexor tendon subluxation, and MT axis supination.[25] These correlated MR imaging findings have proved accurate for diagnosis of PP tear even without a clearly visible bright T2 signal defect. Yamada and colleagues[26] recently reported that a "plantar plate-proximal phalanx" (PPPP) distance greater than 2.7 mm is specific for PP tear, which appears to be particularly helpful for detection of more chronic tears without clearly visible bright T2 signal defects (**Fig. 18**B).

PN is evident as an intermediate T1 signal mass (see **Figs. 17**B and **18C**), of variable signal on fluid-sensitive sequences depending on chronicity.[43] PN is typically intermediate-dark signal on fluid-sensitive sequences, but reactive inflammation and granulation tissue, which diminish over time,

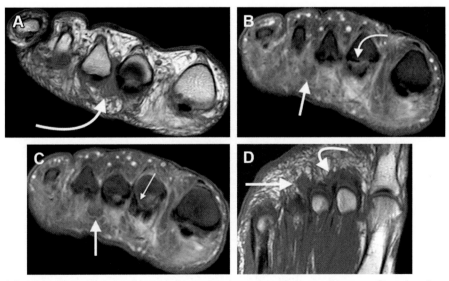

Fig. 20. IN. (*A*) Short-axis T1-weighted image demonstrates a centrally located intermediate signal mass centered in the plantar second IS (*arrow*) indicative of IN. Short-axis PDFS (*B, C*) and long-axis T1-weighted (*D*) images in another individual with dark signal third IN (*straight bold arrows* in *B, C*) poorly seen due to surrounding fat suppression, but more conspicuous on T1-weighting (*straight bold arrow* in *D*). There is degenerative thickening of the lateral second PP (*straight thin arrow* in *C*) and a superimposed lateral insertional tear (*curved thin arrow* in *B*), with adjacent eccentrically located second IS PN (*curved bold arrow* in *D*).

are bright. Although intravenous contrast may enhance conspicuity of PP tear and PN may enhance, this is inconsistent.[55] Contrast-enhanced imaging is typically reserved for complicated cases in which nonenhanced MR imaging is not definitive.

IN is evident as a round to ovoid mass centered within the plantar IS. It is isointense to muscle on T1-weighting.[40] T2 signal is variable, but is often intermediate to dark signal, limiting visualization in fat-suppressed, fluid-sensitive sequences (Fig. 20).[40] Inasmuch as IN may or may not enhance, intravenous contrast does not reliably improve detection of IN.[56] Note that IS bursitis commonly accompanies IN and PN, although pericapsular reactive soft tissue edema typically only accompanies PP tear with PN (Table 3).

Table 3
Comparison between common clinical and imaging features for plantar plate tear, pseudoneuroma, and interdigital neuroma

Disease Entity	PP Tear	IN
Most common location	Second > third MTPJ	Third IS > second IS at level of MTPJ
Important physical examination findings	Tibial deviation of toe Crossover deformity Vertical subluxability Reduced toe purchase and ground touch	If symptomatic: Mulder sign and click Note: pain in IS may be elicited due to PN next to PP tear
Key US features	Hypoechoic defect at base of proximal phalanx *Affects lateral > medial bundles*	Hypoechoic, noncompressible ovoid mass *CENTERED in IS*
Major US associated findings	1. *PN = ECCENTRIC, noncompressible IS mass adjacent to PP tear* 2. Insertional enthesophytes 3. Flexor tendon dislocation from PP groove 4. "Cartilage interface sign" = echogenic interface between MT head cartilage and overlying hypoechoic PP defect Note: IS bursitis is COMPRESSIBLE, hypoechoic ovoid structure centered ABOVE DTML	1. Rarely occurs in IS adjacent to PP tear 2. Common digital nerve can be seen entering mass, because IN occurs at common digital nerve bifurcation Note: IS bursitis is COMPRESSIBLE, hypoechoic ovoid structure centered ABOVE DTML
Key MR imaging features	*Fluid-weighted sequences*: bright signal defect at 1. PP lateral > medial bundle insertion into proximal phalanx 2. Midline distal capsular recess >2.5 mm	1. T1: Isointense to muscle 2. Fluid-weighted sequences: dark 3. Round/ovoid-shaped mass *centered in IS*
Major MR imaging–associated findings	1. *PN = ECCENTRIC IS mass adjacent to PP tear*, intermediate signal on T1 and variable signal on fluid-sensitive sequences 2. Insertional enthesophytes at proximal phalangeal base 3. Flexor tendon subluxation 4. MT axis supination 5. PP-proximal phalanx distance >2.75 mm	1. CENTRALLY LOCATED in IS 2. Rarely occurs in IS adjacent to PP tear

SUMMARY

Variations of forefoot morphology, body habitus, shoe-gear preference, and physical demands of daily living and sport contribute to metatarsalgia, which is a common clinical complaint that accompanies a wide range of injury and pathologic condition. Radiographs are useful for first-line screening of injury and assessment of anatomic variations that might predispose to pathologic condition. US permits sensitive, high-resolution imaging of the forefoot, but it is most useful in the hands of experienced practitioners, especially in combination with physical examination and provocative dynamic maneuvers and interpreted along with comparison radiographs. MR imaging provides a larger overview of the osseous and soft tissue structures of the forefoot with unparalleled tissue contrast for detection of marrow and soft tissue signal abnormalities, which may be occult to detection by radiography and US.

REFERENCES

1. Nattiv A, Kennedy G, Barrack MT, et al. Correlation of MRI grading of bone stress injuries with clinical risk factors and return to play: a 5-year prospective study in collegiate track and field athletes. Am J Sports Med 2013;41:1930–41.
2. Niva MH, Sormaala MJ, Kiuru MJ, et al. Bone stress injuries of the ankle and foot: an 86-month magnetic resonance imaging-based study of physically active young adults. Am J Sports Med 2007;35:643–9.
3. Arendt E, Agel J, Heikes C, et al. Stress injuries to bone in college athletes: a retrospective review of experience at a single institution. Am J Sports Med 2003;31:959–68.
4. Stokes IA, Hutton WC, Stott JR. Forces acting on the metatarsals during normal walking. J Anat 1979;129: 579–90.
5. Donahue SW, Sharkey NA. Strains in the metatarsals during the stance phase of gait: implications for stress fractures. J Bone Joint Surg Am 1999;81: 1236–44.
6. Gauthier G, Elbaz R. Freiberg's infraction: a subchondral bone fatigue fracture. A new surgical treatment. Clin Orthop Relat Res 1979;142:93–5.
7. Coughlin MJ. Subluxation and dislocation of the second metatarsophalangeal joint. Orthop Clin North Am 1989;20:535–51.
8. Weist R, Eils E, Rosenbaum D. The influence of muscle fatigue on electromyogram and plantar pressure patterns as an explanation for the incidence of metatarsal stress fractures. Am J Sports Med 2004;32: 1893–8.
9. Fleischer AE, Klein EE, Ahmad M, et al. Association of abnormal metatarsal parabola with second

10. metatarsophalangeal joint plantar plate pathology. Foot Ankle Int 2017;38:289–97.
10. Mulligan ME. The "gray cortex ": an early sign of stress fracture. Skeletal Radiol 1995;24:201–3.
11. Daffner RH. Anterior tibial striations. AJR Am J Roentgenol 1984;143:651–3.
12. Lassus J, Tulikoura I, Konttinen YT, et al. Bone stress injuries of the lower extremity: a review. Acta Orthop Scand 2002;73:359–68.
13. Fredericson M, Bergman AG, Hoffman KL, et al. Tibial stress reaction in runners. Correlation of clinical symptoms and scintigraphy with a new magnetic resonance imaging grading system. Am J Sports Med 1995;23:472–81.
14. Torriani M, Thomas BJ, Bredella MA, et al. MRI of metatarsal head subchondral fractures in patients with forefoot pain. AJR Am J Roentgenol 2008;190: 570–5.
15. Edmondson MC, Sherry KR, Afolayan J, et al. Case series of 17 modified Weil's osteotomies for Freiberg's and Kohler's II AVN, with AOFAS scoring pre- and post-operatively. Foot Ankle Surg 2011; 17:19–24.
16. Freiberg AH. The so-called infraction of the second metatarsal bone. J Bone Joint Surg 1926;8:257–61.
17. Lewin P. Juvenile deforming metatarsophalangeal osteochondritis: Freiberg's infraction of the metatarsal head. J Am Med Assoc 1923;81:189–92.
18. Smillie IS. Treatment of Freiberg's infraction. Proc R Soc Med 1967;60:29–31.
19. Jensen EL, de Carvalho A. A normal variant simulating Freiberg's disease. Acta Radiol 1987;28:85–6.
20. Johnston RB 3rd, Smith J, Daniels T. The plantar plate of the lesser toes: an anatomical study in human cadavers. Foot Ankle Int 1994;15:276–82.
21. Nery C, Umans H, Baumfeld D. Etiology, clinical assessment, and surgical repair of plantar plate tears. Semin Musculoskelet Radiol 2016;20:205–13.
22. Umans HR, Elsinger E. The plantar plate of the lesser metatarsophalangeal joints: potential for injury and role of MR imaging. Magn Reson Imaging Clin N Am 2001;9:659–69.
23. Kier R, Abrahamian H, Caminear D, et al. MR arthrography of the second and third metatarsophalangeal joints for the detection of tears of the plantar plate and joint capsule. AJR Am J Roentgenol 2010;194:1079–81.
24. Nery C, Coughlin MJ, Baumfeld D, et al. Classification of metatarsophalangeal joint plantar plate injuries: history and physical examination variables. J Surg Orthop Adv 2014;23:214–23.
25. Umans RL, Umans BD, Umans H, et al. Predictive MRI correlates of lesser metatarsophalangeal joint plantar plate tear. Skeletal Radiol 2016;45:969–75.
26. Yamada AF, Crema MD, Nery C, et al. Second and third metatarsophalangeal plantar plate tears: diagnostic performance of direct and indirect MRI

features using surgical findings as the reference standard. AJR Am J Roentgenol 2017;209:W100–8.

27. Coughlin MJ, Schenck RC Jr, Shurnas PS, et al. Concurrent interdigital neuroma and MTP joint instability: long-term results of treatment. Foot Ankle Int 2002;23:1018–25.

28. Nery C, Coughlin MJ, Baumfeld D, et al. Prospective evaluation of protocol for surgical treatment of lesser MTP joint plantar plate tears. Foot Ankle Int 2014;35: 876–85.

29. Baravarian B. Current concepts in hammertoe correction. Podiatry Today 2015;28:36–44.

30. Read JW, Noakes JB, Kerr D, et al. Morton's metatarsalgia: sonographic findings and correlated histopathology. Foot Ankle Int 1999;20:153–61.

31. Lee S, Scardina RJ. Morton neuroma. In: Frontera WR, Silver JK, Rizzo TD, editors. Essentials of physical medicine and rehabilitation: musculoskeletal disorders, pain, and rehabilitation. 3rd edition. Philadelphia: Elsevier Saunders; 2015. p. 459–62.

32. Addante JB, Peicott PS, Wong KY, et al. Interdigital neuromas. Results of surgical excision of 152 neuromas. J Am Podiatr Med Assoc 1986;76:493–5.

33. Bartolomei FJ, Wertheimer SJ. Intermetatarsal neuromas: distribution and etiologic factors. J Foot Surg 1983;22:279–82.

34. Bennett GL, Graham CE, Mauldin DM. Morton's interdigital neuroma: a comprehensive treatment protocol. Foot Ankle Int 1995;16:760–3.

35. Friscia DA, Strom DE, Parr JW, et al. Surgical treatment for primary interdigital neuroma. Orthopedics 1991;14:669–72.

36. Kim JY, Choi JH, Park J, et al. An anatomical study of Morton's interdigital neuroma: the relationship between the occurring site and the deep transverse metatarsal ligament (DTML). Foot Ankle Int 2007; 28:1007–10.

37. Biasca N, Zanetti M, Zollinger H. Outcomes after partial neurectomy of Morton's neuroma related to preoperative case histories, clinical findings, and findings on magnetic resonance imaging scans. Foot Ankle Int 1999;20:568–75.

38. Espinosa N, Schmitt JW, Saupe N, et al. Morton neuroma: MR imaging after resection–postoperative MR and histologic findings in asymptomatic and symptomatic intermetatarsal spaces. Radiology 2010; 255:850–6.

39. Quinn TJ, Jacobson JA, Craig JG, et al. Sonography of Morton's neuromas. AJR Am J Roentgenol 2000; 174:1723–8.

40. Zanetti M, Strehle JK, Zollinger H, et al. Morton neuroma and fluid in the intermetatarsal bursae on MR images of 70 asymptomatic volunteers. Radiology 1997;203:516–20.

41. Bencardino J, Rosenberg ZS, Beltran J, et al. Morton's neuroma: is it always symptomatic? AJR Am J Roentgenol 2000;175:649–53.

42. Torriani M, Kattapuram SV. Technical innovation. Dynamic sonography of the forefoot: the sonographic Mulder sign. AJR Am J Roentgenol 2003;180: 1121–3.

43. Umans H, Srinivasan R, Elsinger E, et al. MRI of lesser metatarsophalangeal joint plantar plate tears and associated adjacent interspace lesions. Skeletal Radiol 2014;43:1361–8.

44. Pace A, Scammell B, Dhar S. The outcome of Morton's neurectomy in the treatment of metatarsalgia. Int Orthop 2010;34:511–5.

45. Hughes RJ, Ali K, Jones H, et al. Treatment of Morton's neuroma with alcohol injection under sonographic guidance: follow-up of 101 cases. AJR Am J Roentgenol 2007;188:1535–9.

46. Haddad SL, Sabbagh RC, Resch S, et al. Results of flexor-to-extensor and extensor brevis tendon transfer for correction of the crossover second toe deformity. Foot Ankle Int 1999;20:781–8.

47. Gregg J, Silberstein M, Schneider T, et al. Sonographic and MRI evaluation of the plantar plate: a prospective study. Eur Radiol 2006;16:2661–9.

48. Umans H, Wolf J, Elsinger E. Follow up MRI of untreated or nonoperatively treated plantar plate tear. American Roentgen Ray Society Annual Meeting. New Orleans, LA, May 1, 2017.

49. Jacobson JA, Lancaster S, Prasad A, et al. Full-thickness and partial-thickness supraspinatus tendon tears: value of US signs in diagnosis. Radiology 2004;230:234–42.

50. Park HJ, Kim SS, Rho MH, et al. Sonographic appearances of Morton's neuroma: differences from other interdigital soft tissue masses. Ultrasound Med Biol 2011;37:1204–9.

51. Mohana-Borges AV, Theumann NH, Pfirrmann CW, et al. Lesser metatarsophalangeal joints: standard MR imaging, MR arthrography, and MR bursography–initial results in 48 cadaveric joints. Radiology 2003;227:175–82.

52. Yao L, Do HM, Cracchiolo A, et al. Plantar plate of the foot: findings on conventional arthrography and MR imaging. AJR Am J Roentgenol 1994;163:641–4.

53. Nery C, Coughlin MJ, Baumfeld D, et al. MRI evaluation of the MTP plantar plates compared with arthroscopic findings: a prospective study. Foot Ankle Int 2013;34:315–22.

54. Lepage-Saucier M, Linda DD, Chang EY, et al. MRI of the metatarsophalangeal joints: improved assessment with toe traction and MR arthrography. AJR Am J Roentgenol 2013;200:868–71.

55. Dinoa V, von Ranke F, Costa F, et al. Evaluation of lesser metatarsophalangeal joint plantar plate tears with contrast-enhanced and fat-suppressed MRI. Skeletal Radiol 2016;45:635–44.

56. Lee MJ, Kim S, Huh YM, et al. Morton neuroma: evaluated with ultrasonography and MR imaging. Korean J Radiol 2007;8:148–55.

Imaging Manifestations of Ankle Impingement Syndromes

Gary M. LiMarzi, MD[a],*, Omar Khan, MD[b],
Yashesh Shah, MD[b], Corrie M. Yablon, MD[a]

KEYWORDS

- Ankle impingement • Ankle pain in athletes • Impingement review • MR imaging ankle impingement
- Anterior impingement • Posterior impingement • Anterolateral impingement
- Anteromedial impingement

KEY POINTS

- Ankle impingement can be categorized based on the portion of the ankle affected as anterior, anterolateral, posterior, anteromedial, and posteromedial.
- Impingement syndromes include a variety of pathologic conditions that result in pain and limited range of motion due to abnormal contact of bone or soft tissue.
- Different types of impingement have unique findings on imaging examinations that may suggest the diagnosis when correlated with the clinical examination.
- Multiple imaging modalities provide useful information in the evaluation of impingement, including radiography, computed tomography, MR imaging, and ultrasound.

INTRODUCTION

Ankle impingement syndromes encompass various pathologic entities that contribute to ankle pain with limited range of motion. Although classically described in athletes, these changes can occur in individuals of all ages, often with a history of prior ankle trauma. Ankle impingement is broadly categorized as anterolateral, anterior, posterior, anteromedial, and posteromedial, depending on the area of the ankle affected. Both osseous and soft tissue abnormalities can contribute to impingement symptoms, and a combination of these is often present. Although ankle impingement is largely a clinical diagnosis, imaging is often used to evaluate suspected ankle impingement in order to confirm the presence of typical changes and as a tool for preoperative planning. Imaging can also help differentiate impingement from alternative diagnoses that may have overlapping clinical presentations.

Conventional radiographs are a universal starting point for evaluation of ankle impingement. Characteristic osseous changes are often apparent radiographically, although may be obscured by overlapping structures. Computed tomography (CT) with multiplanar reformatted images provides excellent osseous resolution and improved characterization of osseous changes than do conventional radiographs. CT also provides a degree of soft tissue detail not possible on radiographs but is still markedly inferior to MR imaging, which possesses excellent soft tissue

Disclosure: The authors have nothing to disclose.
[a] Department of Radiology, MSK Division, University of Michigan Health System, 1500 Medical Center Drive–TC2910Q, Ann Arbor, MI 48109, USA; [b] Department of Radiology, University of Michigan Health System, 1500 Medical Center Drive–TC2910Q, Ann Arbor, MI 48109, USA
* Corresponding author.
E-mail address: gary.limarzi.md@flhosp.org

Radiol Clin N Am 56 (2018) 893–916
https://doi.org/10.1016/j.rcl.2018.06.005
0033-8389/18/

contrast resolution. Soft tissue changes are also well depicted with sonography; however, characterization of osseous pathologic condition is very limited.

Routine MR imaging protocols should include a combination of fluid-sensitive sequences (eg, T2 fat saturation (FS), proton density (PD) FS, or short tau inversion recovery [STIR]) and at least one anatomic sequence, usually T1, performed in 3 anatomic planes. Sagittal T1 and fat-suppressed, fluid-sensitive sequences are optimal for detection of osseous changes, whereas axial and sagittal fat-suppressed fluid-sensitive sequences allow for targeted evaluation of any soft tissue abnormalities.[1-3] The added value of direct or indirect MR arthrography compared with conventional MR imaging is subject to debate. Direct arthrography is usually avoided due to the invasive nature of the examination and need for an additional fluoroscopic procedure before the MR imaging. Indirect MR arthrography entails the intravenous injection of gadolinium-based contrast followed by several minutes of activity before MR imaging, during which contrast diffuses into the articular soft tissues. This technique was hypothesized to increase conspicuity of synovitis or granulation tissue due to differences in vascularity of these tissues. However, a series by Haller and colleagues[4] demonstrated poorer performance of indirect MR arthrography compared with conventional MR imaging for detecting synovitis and scar tissue, using arthroscopy as the gold standard.

ANTEROLATERAL IMPINGEMENT
Normal Anatomy and Imaging Technique

The anterolateral recess of the ankle, also known as the anterolateral gutter, is a triangular space defined by both osseous and soft tissue boundaries. The tibia and fibula comprise the posteromedial and lateral borders, respectively, while the remaining margins consistent of supporting ligaments. Anteriorly, the recess is bound by the anterior talofibular ligament (ATFL), which blends with the joint capsule. The inferior margin is defined by the calcaneofibular ligament and the superior margin by the anterior inferior tibiofibular ligament (AITFL) (**Fig. 1**).[5-9] During dorsiflexion, the anterolateral talus occupies the anterolateral recess and may be obstructed by abnormal soft tissue or osseous changes.

The clinical syndrome of anterolateral impingement is the most commonly described soft tissue impingement process in the lower extremity and is attributed to prior episodes of inversion

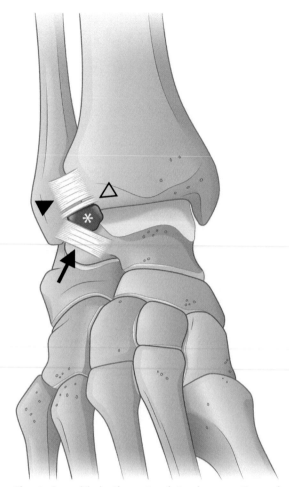

Fig. 1. Synovitis in the anterolateral recess. Coronal color illustration of anterolateral impingement shows synovitis in the anterolateral recess (*asterisk*) bound superiorly by the AITFL (*arrowhead*) and ATFL (*arrow*). A separate fascicle of the AITFL represents Basset ligament (*open arrowhead*).

injury resulting in trauma to the lateral and syndesmotic ligament complexes.[6-10] Approximately 2% to 3% of ankle inversion injuries may progress to clinical manifestations of anterolateral impingement.[7,11,12]

Conventional radiographs of the ankle may provide limited diagnostic information if there is an osseous component to the patient's impingement symptoms.[5] In cases of osseous impingement, lateral radiographs may demonstrate anterior spur formation arising from the tibial plafond; dedicated impingement views obtained with the ankle at an extreme range of dorsiflexion may show bony abutment but are not routinely used. Precise localization of these spurs to the anterolateral recess on the basis of radiography alone can be difficult, and further characterization with CT is often helpful.[5] Conventional radiographs, CT, or MR imaging may also prove useful in cases of impingement related to the presence of posttraumatic ossicles in the anterolateral recess (**Fig. 2**).

Over the past 2 decades, there have been conflicting reports with regards to the usefulness of MR imaging in diagnosing anterolateral impingement, using arthroscopy as the gold standard.[5] Rubin and colleagues[13] reported limited accuracy of conventional MR imaging in the absence of a joint effusion due to decreased conspicuity of abnormal soft tissue in the anterolateral recess. Liu and colleagues[14] reported poor sensitivity and specificity of routine MR imaging, measuring 39% and 50%, respectively, are markedly inferior to clinical examination. When comparing patients with and without symptoms of anterolateral impingement, Schaffler and colleagues[10] demonstrated a high sensitivity and specificity of MR imaging for detecting lateral ligament abnormalities

(89% and 100%, respectively). Although there was no significant difference when compared with the asymptomatic group, abnormal findings were more frequent in symptomatic patients. In a prospective investigation of MR arthrography, Robinson and colleagues[6] reported 100% sensitivity, specificity, and accuracy for detecting soft tissue changes in the anterolateral recess in patients with a clinical diagnosis of impingement; this was confirmed arthroscopically. However, similar MR imaging and arthroscopic findings were present in patients without clinical features of impingement.

Ultrasound of patients with clinically suspected anterolateral impingement has also been reported in the literature and is of particular interest due to its relatively low cost and shorter examination duration compared with MR imaging. Ultrasound also allows application of dynamic maneuvers to increase conspicuity of abnormal soft tissue.[8] McCarthy and colleagues[8] used ultrasound to evaluate 10 male soccer players with a clinical diagnosis of anterolateral impingement and demonstrated abnormal soft tissue within the anterolateral gutter in all cases, with sensitivity and specificity of 100%. They proposed a minimum synovial mass size of 10 mm to diagnose a positive examination. However, when investigating a general, nonathlete population with clinical symptoms of anterolateral impingement, Cochet and colleagues[15] suggested a limited utility of ultrasound with sensitivity and specificity of 76.5% and 57.1%, respectively. The diagnostic criteria they proposed included a nonhyperechoic mass in the anterolateral gutter with a minimum size of 4 mm, with increased flow on color Doppler imaging.[15] Posttraumatic changes of the lateral ligaments can also be detected and suspected pathologic condition can easily be compared with the contralateral asymptomatic ankle.

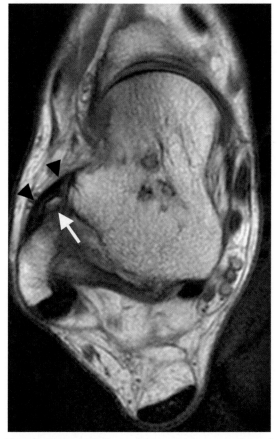

Fig. 2. Posttraumatic ossicle causing anterolateral impingement in 37-year-old woman with prior inversion injury. Axial T1 image at the level of the anterolateral recess shows a corticated intra-articular body in the joint recess (*arrow*) causing outward bulging of the ATFL (*arrowheads*).

Differential diagnosis of anterolateral ankle pain
Soft tissue causes
• Synovial proliferation/synovitis
• Fibrous "meniscoid lesion"
• Partial/full-thickness injury of the ATFL
• Ganglion cysts
Osseous causes
• Intra-articular bodies
• Anterolateral ankle spurs
• Osteochondral lesions

Pathogenesis

Ankle inversion injury is the most common inciting event contributing to the development of anterolateral impingement. Although the initial injury may be subclinical and may not be recalled by the patient, injury to the lateral ligament complex can contribute to instability and predispose to repetitive trauma.[9,11,16,17] Over time, recurrent sprains and tears of the lateral ligaments result in hemorrhage within the anterolateral gutter, which then contribute to reactive synovitis, organizing fibrosis, and eventually, masslike scar formation.[9,16] In its most advanced stage, the scar can mold itself to the confines of the anterolateral gutter and is referred to as a "meniscoid lesion," due to its arthroscopic resemblance to meniscal fibrocartilage of the knee (**Fig. 3**).[9,18] Over time, repetitive dorsiflexion can result in injury to the anterolateral talar dome articular cartilage.[17]

A structural cause of anterolateral impingement has been attributed to a thickened inferior fascicle of the AITFL, also known as Basset ligament.[9,19] This fascicle is considered a normal anatomic variant and has been identified in up to 97% of ankles oriented in parallel to the AITFL but separated from the main ligament by a fibrofatty septum.[9,19] Both the AITFL and Basset ligament have an obliquely inferior course from the distal tibia to the distal fibula; contact between Basset ligament and the talus, usually during dorsiflexion, can contribute to symptoms of impingement.

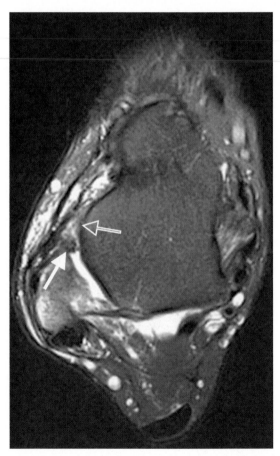

Fig. 3. Meniscoid lesion causing anterolateral impingement in a 40-year-old man with a history of multiple prior inversion injuries. Axial T2 FS image through the anterolateral recess shows a nodular hypointense mass of scar tissue (*arrow*), located deep to an abnormal appearing ATFL (*open arrow*).

Repetitive abutment can lead to thickening of the ligament, which in turn contributes to greater limitation of dorsiflexion.[9] Soft tissue laxity due to prior ankle inversion injury can allow increased anterior translation of the talar dome, allowing increased contact with Basset ligament. Resulting inflammatory and hypertrophic changes to the ligament can further limit the range of dorsiflexion and worsen impingement symptoms.[9,17]

Clinically, patients commonly complain of anterolateral ankle pain worsened by inversion or eversion while the foot is in dorsiflexion. For the examiner, differentiation of impingement from cartilaginous or osteochondral injury can be difficult. A positive "impingement sign," in which pain is elicited by direct pressure over the anterolateral ankle while the foot is moved into dorsiflexion, has a reported sensitivity and specificity of 94.8% and 88%, respectively.[11,20] Exacerbation of pain during a single-leg squat and during dorsiflexion and eversion are considered to have the highest correlation with abnormal findings at arthroscopy.

Imaging Findings

The presence of an anterior tibial plafond spur or ossicles in the region of the lateral gutter on radiography or CT in a patient with lateral ankle pain should prompt suggestion that these may contribute to symptoms of anterolateral impingement. CT can demonstrate the exact location of the spur, which can impinge on the anterolateral capsule and talar dome cartilage, as well as complicating features such as spur fracture.[5] Subsequent evaluation with MR imaging is important to identify the presence of marrow edema or focal osteochondral abnormality in the talus, findings seen in approximately 17% of cases (**Fig. 4**).[21]

Synovitis on MR imaging is typically seen as a nodular or masslike area of intermediate signal on fat-saturated, fluid-sensitive sequences and intermediate to low signal on T1 or non-fat-saturated PD sequences (**Fig. 5**).[5] It is most easily visualized on axial fluid-sensitive images, although both sagittal and coronal sequences can provide useful information. The presence of synovitis should prompt close examination of the adjacent ligaments, especially the ATFL and AITFL, for post-traumatic changes, including signal heterogeneity, thickening, attenuation, or complete disruption (**Fig. 6**). Synovitis may evolve over time to the well-organized, uniformly low signal meniscoid lesion that conforms to the boundaries of the anterolateral gutter.[5,17]

Ultrasound findings in anterolateral impingement closely follow those found on MR imaging. There is usually underlying abnormality of the

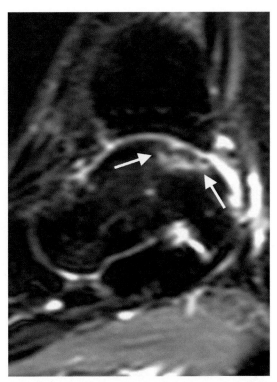

Fig. 4. Osteochondral abnormality of the talar dome. Sagittal STIR MR imaging shows a defect of the talar dome articular cartilage and irregularity of the articular surface with adjacent bone marrow edema (*arrows*).

ATFL, which overlies a region of hypoechoic synovial thickening in the anterolateral gutter (**Fig. 7**). Depending on the chronicity of the abnormality, increased flow on Doppler imaging may or may not be present. In equivocal cases, the operator can pinch the distal fibula and tibia together, which can cause the abnormal synovial tissue to extrude further into the joint recess and improve sonographic visualization.[9]

Clinical correlation remains of paramount importance because of the fact that abnormal findings on MR imaging do not invariably correlate with signs of impingement on clinical examination.[1] Providing a detailed description of suspicious MR imaging findings and their potential contribution to anterolateral impingement is a preferred reporting style rather than claiming a firm diagnosis of impingement based solely on imaging.[10,17] Alternative diagnoses that may mimic symptoms of impingement include sinus tarsi syndrome, peroneal tendon abnormalities, and tarsal coalition.[11]

ANTERIOR IMPINGEMENT SYNDROME
Normal Anatomy and Imaging Technique

The anterior recess of the ankle joint is bordered by the distal tibia, talar dome, and anterior joint

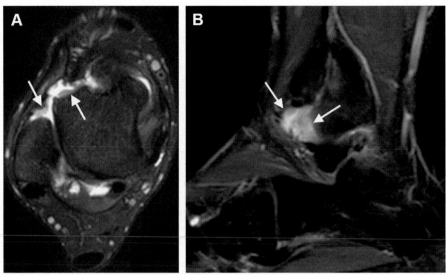

Fig. 5. Anterolateral impingement in 16-year-old male skateboarder with recurrent inversion injuries. Axial T2 FS (A) and sagittal STIR (B) images show nodular areas of hyperintense synovitis (arrows) lining the anterolateral recess, outlined by a joint effusion.

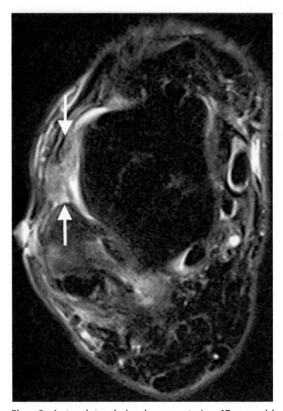

Fig. 6. Anterolateral impingement in 45-year-old woman with a history of chronic lateral ankle pain. Axial T2 FS image through the anterolateral recess shows complete disruption of the ATFL. The recess is nearly filled by hyperintense synovial tissue (arrows), outlined by a small effusion.

capsule. Normally, this space contains mostly fat, synovial tissue, and sometimes a small amount of physiologic joint fluid.[22] The anterior joint capsule extends from the distal tibia to the dorsal neck of the talus (Fig. 8). Anterior impingement syndrome, less common than anterolateral impingement, is a source of anterior ankle pain in athletes, with both osseous and soft tissue components.

Standard lateral ankle radiographs can provide a clue to the diagnosis if osteophytes are seen arising from the anterior tibial plafond and dorsal talus (Fig. 9).[12] Specialized radiographic views obtained in maximal dorsiflexion, known as the

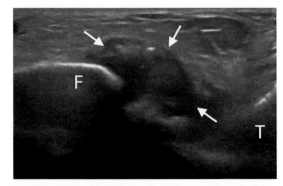

Fig. 7. Anterolateral impingement in 34-year-old man with focal pain over the anterolateral recess. Longitudinal grayscale ultrasound over the anterolateral ankle shows a hypoechoic mass of synovial tissue (arrows) in the anterolateral recess in the expected region of the ATFL. No hyperemia was present on color Doppler imaging. F, fibula; T, talus.

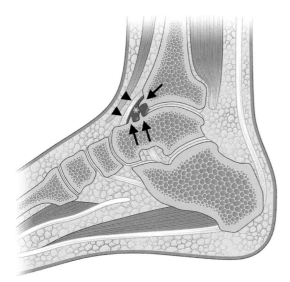

Fig. 8. Anterior impingement. Sagittal color illustration of anterior impingement shows synovitis (*asterisk*) within the anterior tibiotalar recess, bound anteriorly by the joint capsule (*arrowheads*). The potential locations of osteophyte development are demonstrated within the joint capsule (*arrows*).

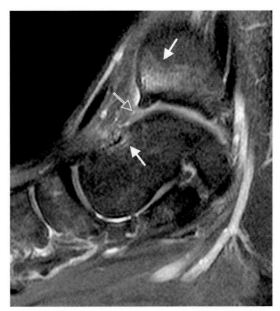

Fig. 10. Anterior impingement in 16-year-old male basketball player with pain worsened by dorsiflexion. Sagittal T2 FS image shows spurs arising from the anterior tibial plafond and dorsal talus, with subjacent bone marrow edema (*white arrows*). Synovitis in the anterior recess is visible as mildly hyperintense soft tissue (*black arrow*). Note that the tibiotalar joint space is otherwise preserved.

"plié view," can better quantify the degree of limited motion, whereas oblique images can more accurately depict the size of the tibiotalar osteophytes.[1,2,12,22] CT allows better characterization of osseous productive changes, and MR imaging can reveal the degree of associated synovitis as well as the presence of bone marrow edema (**Fig. 10**).[12,23] MR imaging is most useful to evaluate associated soft tissue changes and bone marrow edema that may accompany the productive changes seen on radiographs and CT.

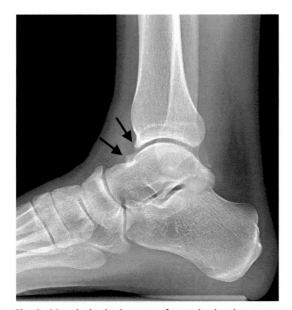

Fig. 9. Morphologic changes of anterior impingement in 27-year-old female dancer. Lateral standing radiograph of the ankle shows spurs arising from the anterior tibia and dorsal talus (*arrows*) with preservation of the tibiotalar joint space.

Criteria to diagnose anterior impingement
Clinical criteria
• Anterior ankle pain worsened by dorsiflexion with limited range of motion
• History or prior inversion injury
• Palpable bone spurs over the anterior ankle
• Pain exacerbated by forced dorsiflexion and relieved with plantarflexion
Imaging criteria
• Synovitis in the anterior recess
• Anterior ankle spurs
• Injury to the talar dome cartilage
• Intra-articular bodies/posttraumatic ossicles

Pathogenesis

Initially, the development of anterior impingement was attributed to repetitive plantarflexion of the tibiotalar joint, leading to anterior capsular avulsion injuries and subsequent osteophyte formation at the capsular attachments.[11,12,19] More recent evidence indicates that these osteophytes actually form within the anterior joint recess distant from the capsular attachment, likely due to repeated, forceful ankle dorsiflexion or direct impact on the anterior ankle causing microfractures of the anterior tibial plafond and dorsal talus. Healing of these microfractures, often with superimposed recurrent injury, results in fibrosis and eventually leads to osteophyte formation. These osteophytes in turn limit the range of ankle dorsiflexion.[1,11,12,19,22,24]

Anterior impingement is commonly associated with soccer players and ballet dancers due to the common mechanisms of direct impact and forceful dorsiflexion, respectively. Asymptomatic anterior ankle osteophytes have been reported in 45% of soccer players and 59% of dancers.[22] Therefore, the presence of synovitis in the anterior recess is thought to be the finding most indicative of symptomatic impingement.[22] In one series, anterior osteophytes were found in up to 60% of professional soccer players; the condition is also classically referred to as "soccer ankle" or "footballer's ankle."[5,9,12,22,25,26]

Patients commonly present clinically with symptoms of anterior ankle pain associated with limited dorsiflexion, stiffness, and swelling after activity. There may be a history of repeated ankle inversion injuries. Palpable osteophytes may or may not be detectable on examination, but their presence can help confirm the diagnosis of anterior impingement.[5,12,16,22,24] Pain is commonly exacerbated by forced dorsiflexion (anterior impingement test) on clinical examination and relieved with plantarflexion.[3,12,24,26]

Imaging Findings

Radiographic findings in anterior impingement syndrome usually include anterior tibiotalar osteophytes in the absence of significant joint space loss and a decreased angle between the tibia and talus.[1,3,26,27] Interestingly, the osteophytes seen on radiographs do not actually overlap or abut one another when evaluated on CT with multiplanar reformatted images. In a series of 10 ankles by Berberian, CT demonstrated that the tibial and talar spurs are located medial and lateral to midline, respectively. This finding also mirrors that of a cadaveric study by Tol and van Dijk.[22,26]

Synovitis in the anterior recess is classically hyperintense on sagittal fat-saturated T2 or STIR sequences and may be hypointense to intermediate-signal on T1 or PD images performed without FS (**Fig. 11**). Changes of synovitis in the anterior recess are usually best depicted by fluid-sensitive images in the sagittal plane. Conventional MR imaging was shown to have a sensitivity of 92% and specificity of 64% for detecting synovitis by Huh and colleagues.[26] MR imaging can also provide a thorough evaluation of associated cartilage injury as well as ligament or tendon pathologic condition that may mimic symptoms of anterior impingement (**Figs. 12** and **13**). Ultrasound of the anterior joint recess can reveal synovitis

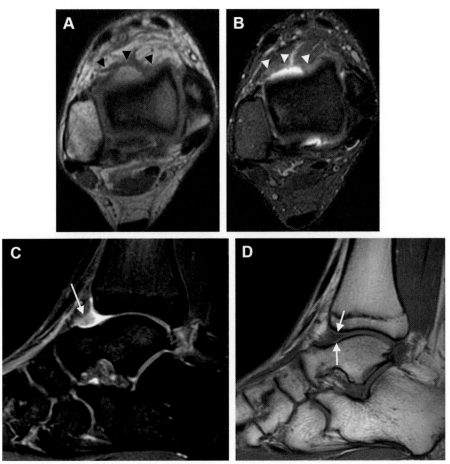

Fig. 11. Anterior synovitis in 15-year-old soccer player with symptoms of impingement. Axial T1 (*A*) and T2 FS (*B*) images show synovial thickening in the anterior joint recess (*arrowheads*). Sagittal STIR (*C*) and T1 (*D*) images of the ankle demonstrate a masslike area of synovitis in the anterior tibiotalar recess (*arrows*) adjacent to the area of synovitis seen on the axial images.

filling the joint capsule and is best visualized in the sagittal plane. Synovial tissue is typically mostly hypoechoic, and increased flow on Doppler imaging is present to a variable degree (**Fig. 14**).[28]

Anterior ankle impingement is generally a diagnosis of exclusion, with symptoms that can closely resemble other more common entities with disparate therapies. The primary differential diagnoses of anterior impingement syndrome include fractures, osteoarthrosis with or without intra-articular bodies, and osteochondral lesions. In a series of 105 arthroscopies performed on patients with painful ankle dorsiflexion, Rasmussen and colleagues[26] found 30 cartilage lesions and 16 intra-articular bodies. Differentiating among these entities requires integration of the clinical history and imaging features.[2,5,12,26]

POSTERIOR IMPINGEMENT SYNDROME
Normal Anatomy and Imaging Technique

Posterior impingement of the ankle encompasses a range of osseous and soft tissue pathologic conditions that cause painful limitation of plantar flexion (**Fig. 15**). Relevant osseous structures include the posterior tibial plafond, posterior process of the talus, and the superior tuberosity of the calcaneus. The posterior process of the talus normally has a medial and lateral tubercle separated by a groove, which contains the FHL tendon traveling through a fibro-osseous tunnel.[29,30] The posterior ankle ligaments, including the posterior talofibular ligament (PTFL), intermalleolar ligament (IML), the tibial slip, and the posterior inferior tibiofibular ligament (PITFL), play important roles in stabilizing the posterior tibiofibular

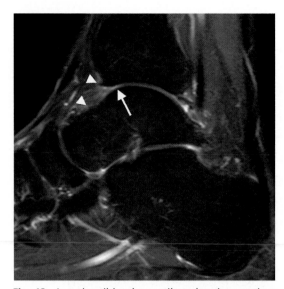

Fig. 12. Anterior tibiotalar cartilage loss in a patient with anterior impingement. Sagittal STIR image shows anterior tibial plafond and dorsal talar spurs (*arrowheads*) with focal cartilage loss along the anterior aspect of the talar dome (*arrow*).

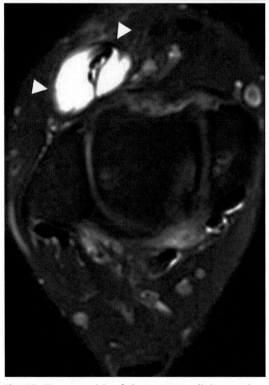

Fig. 13. Tenosynovitis of the extensor digitorum longus tendon sheath mimicking symptoms of anterior impingement. Axial T2 FS image shows a large amount of fluid within the tendon sheath (*arrowheads*) highlighting the individual extensor tendons in this patient with painful dorsiflexion and tenderness over the anterior ankle.

syndesmosis and can also contribute to some cases of impingement.[31] The PTFL originates from the posterior surface of the lateral malleolus and normally inserts on the lateral tubercle of the posterior talar process. A small band of tissue extends from the PTFL to the medial malleolus, known as the tibial slip. The IML is located proximal to the PTFL and runs in oblique fashion between the posterior surfaces of the medial and lateral malleoli; the IML is present in between 60% to 80% of normal ankles (**Fig. 16**).

The most common anatomic variants in this location are an elongated posterior talar process (Stieda process) and an unfused secondary ossification center of the lateral posterior talar tubercle, known as an os trigonum (**Fig. 17**).[29,30,32] An os trigonum is a common asymptomatic anatomic variant that can be seen in 14% to 25% of the normal adult population and is commonly bilateral; its presence does not imply a diagnosis of posterior impingement syndrome in the absence of clinical symptoms.[33,34] When an os trigonum is present, it serves as the attachment site of the PTFL. The FHL tendon and, on occasion, accessory muscles can also play an important role in posterior ankle impingement.[5,16,29,32,35]

Radiographs are the standard first step in imaging of patients with a clinical diagnosis of posterior ankle impingement, due to the frequent association with either an unfused os trigonum or a Stieda process, best seen on the lateral projection.[33,35] Additional morphologic abnormalities may be present, including a prominent superior calcaneal tuberosity and exaggerated downsloping of the posterior tibial plafond (**Fig. 18**). Although less common than an os trigonum or Stieda process, prominence of the superior calcaneal tuberosity had the highest association with posterior impingement symptoms in a study of affected ballet dancers.[35,36] Although the detection of these anatomic variants in isolation should not prompt a radiographic diagnosis of posterior ankle impingement, their presence in association with characteristic clinical examination findings can be highly suggestive of the diagnosis.

MR imaging is excellent for depiction of associated soft tissue changes, including synovitis, ligamentous injury, and the presence of bone marrow edema.[33,35] Abnormalities of the PTFL, PITFL, or IML can also contribute to impingement symptoms because of thickening of these structures as a result of prior injury, which in turn can be pinched by opposing bone

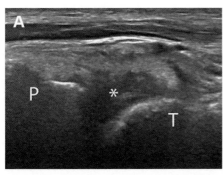 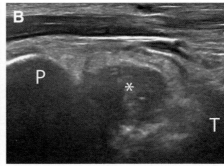

Fig. 14. Anterior impingement in 24-year-old male soccer player with anterior ankle tenderness and limited dorsiflexion. Longitudinal grayscale ultrasound of the anterior tibiotalar joint imaging with the ankle in neutral (*A*) and dorsiflexion (*B*) shows a heterogeneous mass of synovial tissue (*asterisks*) located between the anterior tibial plafond (P) and the dorsal talus (T). Dynamic imaging shows bulging of the synovial tissue, limiting the range of maximal dorsiflexion.

interfaces during plantar flexion (**Fig. 19**). Ganglion cysts arising from the posterior ankle ligaments are not uncommon, and depending on their size, can exert mass effect on adjacent soft tissues.[17]

Ultrasound can be useful in cases of posterior impingement for both diagnostic and therapeutic purposes. Ultrasound can depict the presence of an os trigonum and other osseous changes associated with posterior impingement, in addition to soft tissue abnormalities such as synovitis or fluid in the posterior joint recess. Targeted anesthetic injection at the site of abnormality under ultrasound can confirm the origin of the patient's symptoms as well as provide therapeutic relief.[37]

Differential diagnosis of posterior ankle pain
Soft tissue causes
• Synovial proliferation/synovitis
• Flexor tendon tenosynovitis/tendinosis
• Achilles tendinosis/paratenonitis
• Accessory muscles
• Ganglion cysts
• Posterior ligament injuries/degeneration
Osseous causes
• Os trigonum/Stieda process
• Intra-articular bodies
• Shepherd fracture
• Haglund deformity

Pearls, pitfalls, and variants
• Os trigonum is common in asymptomatic individuals
• Accessory muscles may create impingement symptoms due to local mass effect
• Bone marrow edema adjacent to a synchondrosis correlates with symptoms

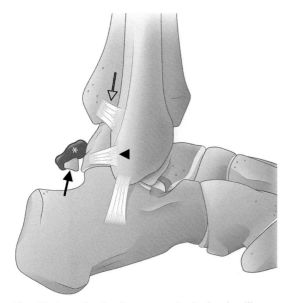

Fig. 15. Posterior impingement. Sagittal color illustration shows changes of posterior ankle impingement with an unfused os trigonum (*arrow*) and adjacent synovitis (*asterisk*). The PITFL (*open arrow*) and PTFL (*arrowhead*) can also contribute to symptoms of impingement.

Criteria to diagnose posterior impingement

Clinical criteria

- Posterior ankle pain and swelling
- Pain worsened by forced plantar flexion (positive plantar flexion test)
- Focal posterolateral ankle tenderness

Imaging criteria

- Presence of os trigonum or Stieda process
- Flexor hallucis longus (FHL) tenosynovitis
- Space-occupying lesions (ganglia, accessory muscles, and similar)
- Abnormalities of the posterior ligaments

What the referring physician needs to know

- Is an os trigonum present? Is there evidence of instability at the synchondrosis?
- What is the state of the flexor tendons? Could an abnormality of the Achilles tendon be causing symptoms?
- Are the posterior ligaments abnormal? Is there an injury of the posterior syndesmosis?
- Are there accessory muscles?

Pathogenesis

Posterior impingement syndrome is a common source of ankle pain in athletes and is also referred to as os trigonum syndrome, talar compression syndrome, and posterior block of the ankle. It encompasses several processes that result from acute traumatic or repetitive plantar flexion of the foot. Repetitive and extreme degrees of plantar-flexion can cause impaction between posterior osseous interfaces with compression of the intervening soft tissues resulting in limited range of motion and pain during plantar flexion. Symptoms of posterior impingement are classically associated with athletes who routinely perform repetitive plantar flexion, including ballet dancers, soccer players, and downhill runners.[11,19,33] Prompt diagnosis and early treatment are invaluable in improving the patients overall functional ability. Approximately 40% of affected patients will require surgical intervention due to persistent hindfoot symptoms.[33]

Accessory muscles in the posterior ankle, most commonly the accessory soleus, can also cause symptoms of posterior impingement, most commonly due to mass effect on adjacent soft tissues, including the tibial neurovascular bundle. The accessory soleus is more commonly described in athletes than the general population, possibly because of exercise-induced hypertrophy of the muscle increasing local mass effect (**Fig. 20**).[38]

An athlete presenting with a history of acute or chronic posterior ankle pain along with soft tissue swelling and limited plantar flexion should raise clinical suspicion for posterior impingement syndrome. Symptoms may develop after only a single acute episode of forced plantar flexion, although more commonly they develop over time because of repetitive motion. Distinguishing between acute

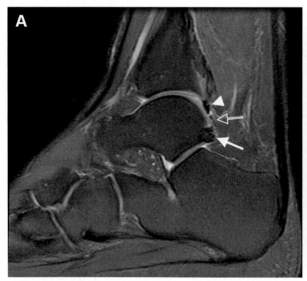
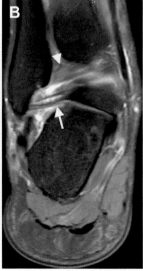

Fig. 16. Normal posterior ligaments of the ankle depicted on sagittal PD FS (*A*) and coronal T2 FS (*B*) images. The PTFL (*solid arrow*), IML (*arrowhead*), and tibial slip (*open arrow*) can contribute to symptoms of posterior impingement in cases of degenerative thickening or prior injury.

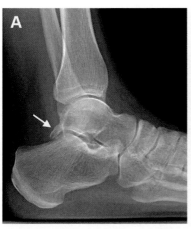
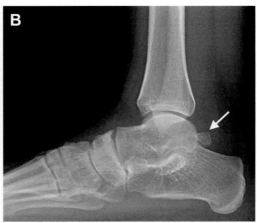

Fig. 17. Stieda process and os trigonum. Lateral standing radiographs demonstrate Stieda process (*A*) and os trigonum (*B*) (*arrows*). Elongated posterior process of the talus (*A*) and unfused ossification center (*B*) of the lateral posterior talar tubercle are frequently asymptomatic but can contribute to symptoms of posterior impingement.

and chronic presentations is important because chronic impingement has an overall better prognosis.[29,33] Reproducible pain with forced plantar flexion is a characteristic finding on physical examination and is referred to as a positive plantar flexion test; a negative test significantly decreases the likelihood of posterior impingement. Focal tenderness may also be elicited over the posterolateral aspect of the ankle.[30,33,35] Targeted anesthetic injection into the posterior ankle capsule with relief of pain is a helpful diagnostic sign of posterior impingement.[29,30]

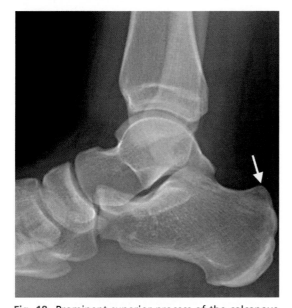

Fig. 18. Prominent superior process of the calcaneus. Lateral standing ankle radiograph shows a prominent superior process of the calcaneus (*arrow*) in a collegiate lacrosse player with posterior ankle pain.

Imaging Findings

Osseous causes of posterior impingement can often be identified with conventional radiography, CT, or MR imaging. Decreased joint mobility can be inferred by the presence of a decreased tibiocalcaneal angle, which is normally between 60° and 90°.[3] An osteochondroma extending into the posterior ankle soft tissues can also lead to posterior impingement, especially if it abuts the FHL tendon or tibial neurovascular bundle (Fig. 21). If no obvious bony abnormality is identified or if there is suspicion for concomitant soft tissue abnormality, MR imaging should be pursued.

CT and MR imaging can identify other sources of ankle pain that may mimic symptoms of posterior impingement, such as osteochondral injuries, tenosynovitis, or inflammatory arthritis. Fracture of the posterior talar process, commonly referred to as a Shepherd fracture, can cause acute onset posterior impingement symptoms and is particularly associated with soccer players.[17] In patients with an os trigonum, CT can characterize changes of the bone adjacent to the synchondrosis, including the presence of sclerosis or cystic degeneration, which may be associated with symptomatic instability (Fig. 22).

The presence of bone marrow edema on MR imaging is a consistent finding in cases of symptomatic posterior ankle impingement. Edema is visible as hypointense signal changes on T1 and non-fat-saturated PD sequences and as hyperintense signal on fat-saturated, fluid-sensitive sequences, usually STIR, T2 FS, or PD FS. Marrow edema is most frequently seen within an os trigonum and the adjacent posterior process of the talus, usually centered around the

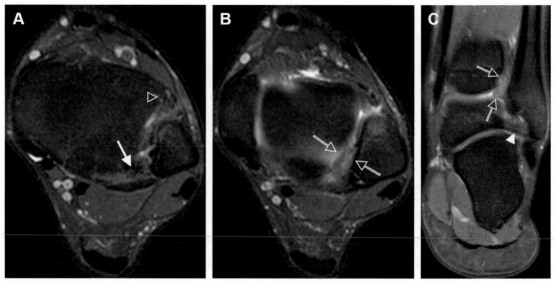

Fig. 19. Injury of the tibiofibular syndesmosis in a 19-year-old American college football player, resulting in impingement symptoms. (*A*) Axial T2 FS image shows injury of the AITFL (*open arrowhead*) and PITFL (*arrow*), which are irregular and heterogeneous. Additional axial T2 FS (*B*) and coronal PD FS (*C*) images show masslike synovial tissue in the posterior syndesmosis protruding into the posterior soft tissues (*open arrows*). Note the normal PTFL (*solid arrowhead*).

synchondrosis (**Fig. 23**).[29,30] Lee and colleagues[35] observed bone marrow edema in 84% of patients with posterior impingement symptoms. Fluid within the synchondrosis may also be present and suggests instability of the os trigonum. Bureau and colleagues[35] described a series of 7 patients with posterior impingement symptoms, in which the most common MR imaging finding was edema within the posterior talus/os trigonum. Additional sites of marrow edema can include the posterior tibial plafond and posterosuperior calcaneus, implying their involvement with repetitive impaction injury.[29]

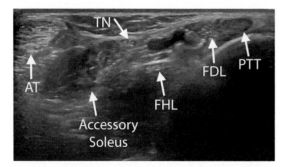

Fig. 20. Accessory soleus muscle causing posterior impingement symptoms in a 13-year-old ballet dancer. Transverse grayscale ultrasound of the posterior ankle shows an accessory soleus muscle located between the Achilles tendon (AT) and FHL tendon. FDL, flexor digitorum longus tendon; PTT, posterior tibialis tendon; TN, tibial nerve.

Abnormalities of the Achilles tendon, including tendinosis or paratenonitis, can mimic symptoms of posterior impingement and have characteristic features on MR imaging and ultrasound that allow differentiation from impingement (**Fig. 24**).

Inflammatory or posttraumatic soft tissue changes are also well demonstrated on MR imaging, including synovitis in the posterior joint recess, often adjacent to the posterior and superior margin of an os trigonum. These findings are usually best seen on sagittal and occasionally axial images. Lee and colleagues[35] observed synovitis in 100% of cases of symptomatic patients evaluated with MR imaging. Synovitis usually appears as low to intermediate signal intensity on T1 and non-FS PD sequences, with corresponding increased signal on fluid-sensitive images. Ultrasound can accurately depict these changes while also allowing dynamic examination.

Abnormalities of the posterior ankle ligaments are also often visible on MR imaging, depicted as thickening and increased intrasubstance signal, usually with loss of the normal fibrillar architecture. The PTFL may appear thickened from either prior injury or myxoid degeneration.[5] Ganglia arising from the posterior ligaments can be caused by prior injury or degenerative changes. Ganglia are identifiable as fluid signal intensity structures with internal septations and possibly debris that can often be traced to a point of origin from one of the posterior ligaments (**Fig. 25**). Because of the

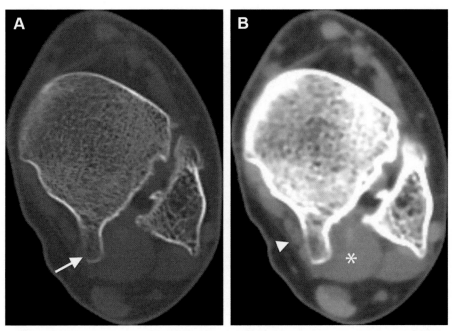

Fig. 21. Osteochondroma causing posterior impingement symptoms in a 15-year-old girl. Axial CT images in bone (*A*) and soft tissue (*B*) windows show an osteochondroma (*arrow*) arising from the posterior tibia. The osteochondroma exerts mass effect on the FHL muscle (*asterisk*) and tibial neurovascular bundle (*arrowhead*).

close relationship of the FHL tendon to the posterior talus, FHL tendinosis and tenosynovitis are common associated findings, described in up to two-thirds of cases. Tenosynovitis is visible as high-intensity fluid distending the FHL tendon sheath, with either a normal or abnormal appearance of the tendon itself (**Fig. 26**). On ultrasound, hypoechoic or anechoic fluid is interposed between the hyperechoic tendon and its sheath, which is normally closely apposed to the tendon surface.[5,29,30,35]

ANTEROMEDIAL AND POSTEROMEDIAL IMPINGEMENT
Normal Anatomy and Imaging Techniques

The anteromedial ankle recess is bordered by the talus laterally, medial malleolus medially, the anterior tibiotalar component of the deltoid ligament inferiorly, anteromedial joint capsule superficially, and posterior tibiotalar component of the deltoid ligament posteriorly.[5,11] The posteromedial recess is bound anteriorly by the medial malleolus and the

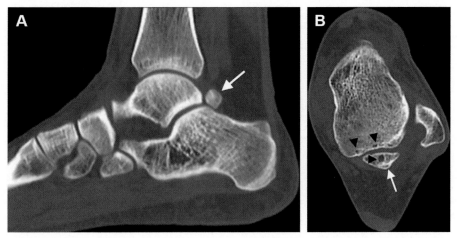

Fig. 22. Os trigonum with instability at the synchondrosis. Sagittal (*A*) and axial (*B*) CT images of the ankle show an os trigonum (*arrows*) with cystic changes (*arrowheads*) bordering the synchondrosis, suggesting symptomatic instability.

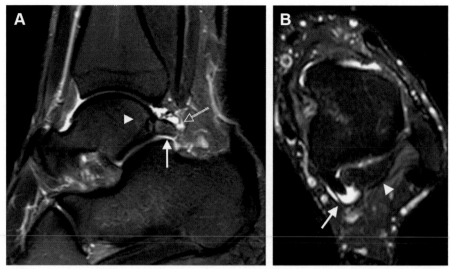

Fig. 23. Posterior ankle impingement in a 20-year-old male track athlete. (*A*) Sagittal STIR image of the ankle shows an os trigonum (*arrow*) with marrow edema on both sides of the synchondrosis (*arrowhead*) and fluid in the posterior joint recess (*open arrow*). (*B*) Axial T2 FS image of the ankle shows an os trigonum (*arrowhead*) with tenosynovitis of the adjacent FHL tendon (*arrow*).

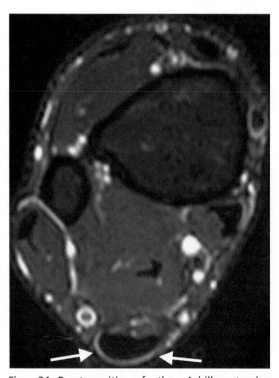

Fig. 24. Paratenonitis of the Achilles tendon mimicking symptoms of posterior impingement in a 22-year-old track athlete. Axial T2 FS image shows hyperintense signal surrounding the Achilles tendon (*arrows*), consistent with paratenonitis.

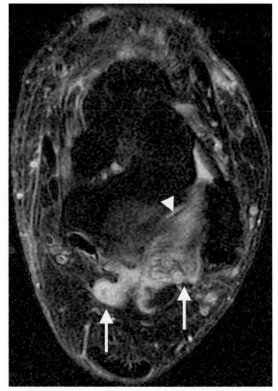

Fig. 25. Posterior ankle ganglion causing impingement symptoms in a 50-year-old woman. Axial T2 FS image of the ankle shows a large, lobulated ganglion (*arrows*) arising from the posterior aspect of the PTFL (*arrowhead*).

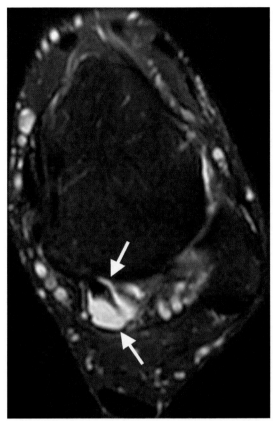

Fig. 26. Isolated FHL tenosynovitis without additional findings of posterior impingement. Axial T2 FS image shows fluid distending the FHL tendon sheath (*arrows*).

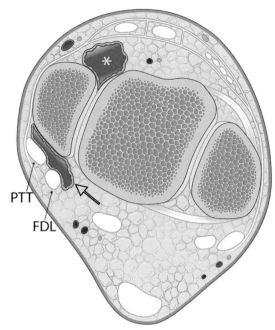

Fig. 27. Anteromedial and posteromedial synovitis. Axial color illustration through the level of the medial ankle recesses shows synovitis in the anteromedial (*asterisk*) and posteromedial (*arrow*) recesses. The posteromedial synovitis abuts the PTT and FDL tendons.

posterior tibiotalar deltoid ligament, posteriorly by the posteromedial joint capsule, with the medial margin of the talus and the posteromedial talar process forming the medial and deep margins of the recess.[5,11,17] The posteromedial recess is a small space deep to the interval separating the flexor digitorum longus and FHL tendons (**Fig. 27**).[5]

The anterior and posterior tibiotalar ligaments (ATTL and PTTL, respectively) comprise the deep components of the deltoid ligament, while the superficial components include the tibiocalcaneal, tibionavicular, tibiospring, and superficial posterior tibiotalar ligaments. The deep ligaments, of which the PTTL is the larger and more mechanically robust, help prevent lateral shifting of the talus and function together with the superficial ligaments to maintain rotational stability.[39–41] The PTTL extends inferiorly and posteriorly from the medial malleolus to the medial talar body, whereas the ATTL has a shorter course from the medial malleolus to the talus. Both the superficial and the deep components of the deltoid ligament complex have been implicated in the development of impingement symptoms, although involvement of the ATTL and PTTL is most often described.[39]

Conventional ankle radiographs may be of limited utility to detect changes of anteromedial or posteromedial impingement. Dedicated oblique radiographs with elevation of the tube angle to 45° and the patient's foot in 30° of external rotation have been described in the literature as more sensitive for detecting small anteromedial spur formation (**Fig. 28**).[5,42] CT may improve detection of subtle bone changes such as osteophyte formation or loose bodies and can better depict osteochondral injuries of the talus, which may be associated with or mimic symptoms of impingement.[5] However, most impingement lesions develop secondary to soft tissue injury, making radiography and CT often inadequate because of their relatively poor soft tissue contrast resolution.[9,11,43]

MR imaging has an excellent ability to detect abnormalities of the deltoid ligament complex, with a sensitivity of 83% and specificity of 94% for detecting superficial ligament injury and a sensitivity of 96% and specificity of 98% for detecting injuries to the deep components.[39]

Using contrast-enhanced 3-dimensional gradient echo imaging, Lee and colleagues[35] reported 96.3% sensitivity for identifying synovitis or soft tissue impingement in the anteromedial gutter. In a limited prospective analysis, Robinson and colleagues[1,44] evaluated MR arthrography in 2 patients with clinical symptoms of anteromedial

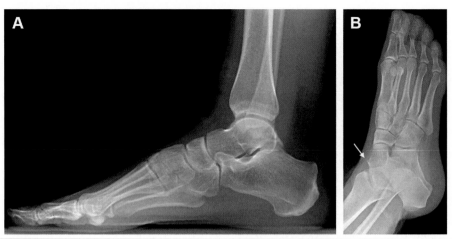

Fig. 28. A 29-year-old woman with pain and tenderness over the anteromedial ankle. (*A*) Lateral standing radiograph of the foot does not show any notable osseous irregularity of the ankle joint. (*B*) Oblique radiograph of the foot reveals a dorsal spur (*arrow*) arising from the medial neck of the talus.

impingement and detected abnormalities of the anteromedial soft tissue in both cases, including synovitis, ATTL thickening, capsular hypertrophy, and chondral injuries. These findings were subsequently confirmed arthroscopically. However, because of the invasive nature of the examination, MR arthrography is not widely used. MR imaging is also excellent for depicting bone marrow edema associated with either anteromedial bone spurs or "kissing contusions" from medial ankle impaction injury (**Fig. 29**).

MR imaging has proven to be effective in evaluating abnormalities of the PTTL and posteromedial joint capsule, as well as scar tissue and synovitis, which in extensive cases may abut or surround the posteromedial flexor tendons.[40,41,45] Messiou and colleagues[45] identified displacement of the flexor tendons as a finding seen in all patients with symptomatic posteromedial impingement in addition to synovitis. Similar findings were reported in a survey of 25 patients by Koulouris and colleagues.[41] Involvement of the flexor tendons, although not present in all cases, seems to have a high association with symptomatic cases of posteromedial impingement when compared with the presence of synovitis alone.[45] MR imaging is of particular utility in cases of equivocal clinical diagnosis due to its ability to localize both osseous and soft tissue pathologic condition, as well as being able to exclude other coincident injuries.

Criteria to diagnose anteromedial/posteromedial impingement

Clinical criteria

- Anteromedial/posteromedial tenderness to palpation
- Limited range of motion with dorsiflexion and inversion

Imaging criteria

- Injury to the deep deltoid ligaments
- Contusions involving the medial malleolus and medial talus (kissing contusions)
- Thickening of the anteromedial joint capsule or flexor retinaculum
- Soft tissue surrounding the flexor tendons
- Intra-articular bodies

Differential diagnosis of medial ankle pain

Soft tissue causes

- Synovial proliferation/synovitis
- Injury to the deep/superficial deltoid ligament fibers
- Thickening of the anteromedial/posteromedial joint capsule
- Injury to the flexor retinaculum
- Ganglion cysts

Osseous causes

- Intra-articular bodies
- Anteromedial ankle spurs
- Contusions of the medial malleolus/medial talus
- Osteochondral lesions

Pearls, pitfalls, and variants

- Thickening of the anteromedial capsule is often associated with symptoms
- Posteromedial soft tissue surrounding or displacing flexor tendons are often symptomatic

---

What the referring physician needs to know

- Are changes present that could predispose to either anteromedial or posteromedial impingement?
- Are the tendons involved? Could symptoms be caused by abnormalities of the tendons or injury to the flexor retinaculum?
- Is there an osteochondral injury of the medial talus?

Pathogenesis

The cause of both anteromedial and posteromedial impingement is usually described as acute or repetitive ankle inversion injury, often with a rotational component, leading to the development of abnormal soft tissue in the joint recesses. Eversion injuries have also been implicated, but are thought to be less common than inversion mechanisms.[1,5,40] Inversion causes compression of the

tibiotalar ligaments between the medial malleolus and medial border of the talus resulting in kissing contusions and injury of the tibiotalar ligaments. There may also be compression of the medial joint capsule during ankle inversion.[5,17,39,42,46]

Thickening and fibrosis of the ATTL, PTTL, and joint capsule may result, especially in cases of recurrent injury, usually with associated synovial proliferation and synovitis. In more advanced or chronic cases, the recurrent episodes of fibrosis can lead to formation of fibrous meniscoid lesions.[1,5,32,41,43] A series of 11 patients with anteromedial impingement undergoing arthroscopy found that thickening of the anteromedial joint capsule was the most consistent finding.[46] In posteromedial impingement, the flexor tendons can become involved by hypertrophic soft tissue or capsular thickening (**Fig. 30**).[9,11]

Repetitive impaction trauma can lead to bony hypertrophy and spur formation along the talar neck, anterior margin of the medial malleolus, or anteromedial tibial plafond (**Fig. 31**).[1,5,17] These osseous spurs can impair range of motion and thus also contribute to development of anteromedial impingement.[11] Posttraumatic ossifications in the anteromedial or posteromedial recesses can also lead to impingement symptoms, due to either prior avulsion injury or dystrophic mineralization within the injured ligaments (**Fig. 32**).[5] In some cases of posteromedial impingement, an avulsion fracture may occur from the posteromedial talus at the PTTL insertion, which can incite a proliferative healing response and lead to impingement symptoms.[5]

Anteromedial ankle impingement classically presents as pain and limited range of motion with dorsiflexion and inversion. Pain and swelling in the anteromedial ankle are common, and the presence of focal tenderness to palpation along the anteromedial joint line can suggest a diagnosis of anteromedial impingement.[42] Patients with posteromedial impingement typically present with pain along the posteromedial aspect of the ankle, localized to the space between the posteromedial talus and medial malleolus, that is worsened by inversion.[5,40] A classic clinical sign of posteromedial impingement is evocation of pain during inversion with the ankle held in plantar flexion. This finding also helps to differentiate symptoms related to posteromedial impingement from those related to dysfunction of the posterior tibialis tendon.[43] However, because of the frequent coincidence of injury to the medial and lateral ankle ligaments, pain may be more diffuse, making precise localization difficult.[42]

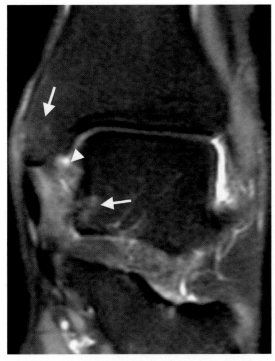

Fig. 29. Injury to the deep deltoid ligament in a 33-year-old female runner with ankle pain following inversion injury. Coronal PD FS image through the medial ankle demonstrates an abnormal tibiotalar ligament (*arrowhead*) with interstitial tearing and increased intrasubstance signal. Marrow edema in the medial malleolus and medial talus (*arrows*) is consistent with "kissing contusions" from impaction injury.

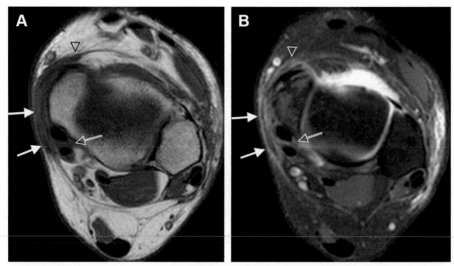

Fig. 30. Injury of the posteromedial and anteromedial joint capsule in a 24-year-old woman. Axial T1 (*A*) and T2 FS (*B*) images show thickening of the anteromedial capsule (*open arrowheads*) and flexor retinaculum (*solid arrows*). Synovitis is present in the posteromedial recess (*open arrows*) extending between the PTT and FDL tendons.

Imaging Findings

In cases of anteromedial impingement with an osseous component, anteromedial spur formation may be seen arising from the medial talar neck, anteromedial tibial plafond, or anterior aspect of the medial malleolus. These spurs may be occult on conventional ankle radiographs because of overlapping contours, but can often be seen on dedicated oblique radiographs.[5] Spurs may also be readily apparent on CT and MR imaging. Bone productive changes are less common in cases of posteromedial impingement; however, small cortical avulsion fractures from the PTTL attachment may be present, which are best demonstrated on CT.[5,17]

MR imaging can demonstrate other signs of symptomatic impingement, including marrow edema at the site of spur formation, ligament

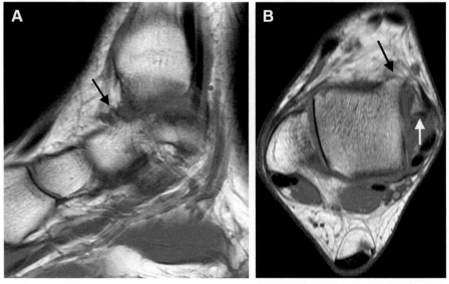

Fig. 31. Anteromedial ankle spurs in a 29-year-old woman with focal ankle tenderness. Sagittal (*A*) and axial (*B*) T1 images show osteophytes arising from the dorsal medial talus (*black arrows*) and from the medial malleolus (*white arrow*).

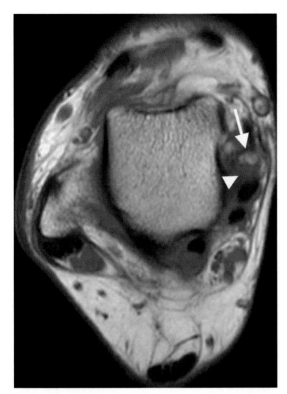

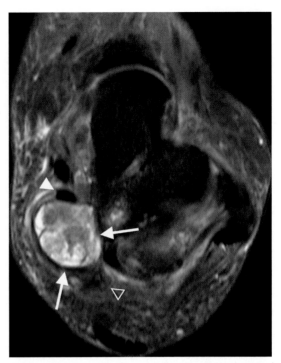

Fig. 34. Large posteromedial ganglion causing impingement symptoms in a 50-year-old woman. Axial T2 FS image shows a soft tissue ganglion with internal debris (*arrows*) extending between the FDL tendon (*arrowhead*) and the tibial neurovascular bundle (*open arrowhead*).

Fig. 32. Posttraumatic ossicles and scar tissue causing posteromedial impingement in a 28-year-old man. Axial T1 image shows corticated bone fragments (*arrow*) in the posteromedial ankle recess with adjacent intermediate signal-intensity scar tissue (*arrowhead*) abutting the anterior surface of the PTT.

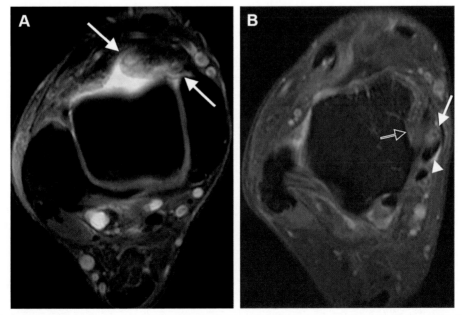

Fig. 33. Anteromedial and posteromedial synovitis causing impingement. (*A*) Axial T2 FS image in 21-year-old male American football player shows a large, ovoid mass of hyperintense synovial tissue (*arrows*) in the anteromedial recess of the ankle, with an adjacent joint effusion. (*B*) Axial T2 FS image in 24-year-old man shows nodular synovial tissue in the posteromedial recess (*arrow*) abutting the anterior surface of the PTT (*arrowhead*). There is also prior injury of the PTTL (*open arrow*), with increased intrasubstance signal.

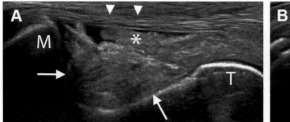
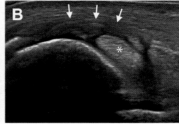

Fig. 35. Ultrasound of anteromedial and posteromedial impingement. (*A*) Longitudinal grayscale ultrasound of the anteromedial recess in a 24-year-old male basketball player shows a lobulated area of echogenic synovial tissue (*asterisks*) located superficial to the tibiotalar ligament (*arrows*) and deep to the PTT (*arrowheads*). Transverse ultrasound (*B*) of the posteromedial recess shows thickening of the flexor retinaculum (*arrows*) overlying the PTT (*asterisks*). M, medial malleolus; T, talus.

injury, synovitis in the anteromedial or posteromedial recess, or thickening of the joint capsule (**Fig. 33**).[47] In cases of prior ligament injury, there is typically loss of the normal fibrillar architecture of the ATTL or PTTL, often with increased intrasubstance signal on MR imaging, lending the ligament an amorphous appearance.[19,39,41] Abnormalities of the tibiotalar ligaments are usually best visualized in the coronal and sometimes sagittal planes, especially using fluid-sensitive sequences with FS. Large ganglion cysts arising from the injured ligament or extending from the subtalar joint can extend into the anteromedial or posteromedial recess and create impingement symptoms (**Fig. 34**). Fluid-sensitive sequences also increase conspicuity of synovitis, which stands out as focal increased signal relative to adjacent tissue. Fibrosis and scar formation, conversely, stand out as areas of low signal on non-fat-saturated sequences, including T1- and PD-weighted images. In cases of posteromedial impingement, synovitis or fibrosis may extend into the space between the posterior tibialis and flexor digitorum longus tendons, although the tendons themselves typically appear normal. MR imaging can also help characterize nonimpingement pathologic condition that may mimic clinical symptoms of impingement, including osteochondral injuries of the talus, acute or chronic deltoid ligament injuries without synovitis, or abnormalities of the adjacent tendons.[5,17]

Ultrasound may show expected changes of scar formation, synovitis, or ligament pathologic condition in the anteromedial or posteromedial recess, with the sonographic appearance typically mirroring what is seen on MR imaging.[5] Ultrasound can reliably depict an abnormal appearance of the injured tibiotalar ligament, thickening of the joint capsule, synovitis, and entrapment of the flexor tendons (**Fig. 35**).[41,45]

SUMMARY

Ankle impingement syndromes are a diverse spectrum of abnormalities that are most often described in athletes but can also affect the general population, often following an inversion injury. Although they remain a largely clinical diagnosis, imaging has an established role in characterizing changes associated with the various types of impingement as well as identifying clinical mimics. Knowledge of the imaging manifestations of impingement is important for the interpreting radiologist, as is the frequency of certain changes in asymptomatic individuals. Suspicious findings should motivate the radiologist to suggest an association with impingement rather than rendering a firm diagnosis of impingement based on imaging alone.

ACKNOWLEDGMENTS

The authors thank Danielle Dobbs for creating the color illustrations.

REFERENCES

1. Robinson P, White L, Salonen D, et al. Anteromedial impingement of the ankle. AJR Am J Roentgenol 2002;178:601–4.
2. Mansour R, Jibri Z, Kamath S, et al. Persistent ankle pain following a sprain: a review of imaging. Emerg Radiol 2011;18:211–25.
3. Spiga S, Vinci V, Tack S, et al. Diagnostic imaging of ankle impingement syndromes in athletes. Muscuoskelet Surg 2013;97:145–53.
4. Haller J, Bernt R, Seeger T, et al. MR-imaging of anterior tibiotalar impingement syndrome: agreement, sensitivity and specificity of MR-imaging and indirect MR-arthrography. Eur J Radiol 2006;58:450–60.
5. Dimmick S, Linklater J. Ankle impingement syndromes. Radiol Clin North Am 2013;51:479–510.
6. Robinson P, White L, Salonen D, et al. Anterolateral ankle impingement: MR arthrographic assessment

of the anterolateral recess. Radiology 2001;221: 186–90.

7. Meehan T, Martinez-Salazar E, Torriani M. Aftermath of ankle inversion injuries. Magn Reson Imaging Clin N Am 2017;25:45–61.

8. McCarthy C, Wilson D, Coltman T. Anterolateral ankle impingement: Findings and diagnostic accuracy with ultrasound imaging. Skeletal Radiol 2007; 37:209–16.

9. Hopper M, Robinson P. Ankle impingement syndromes. Radiol Clin N Am 2008;46:957–71.

10. Schaffler G, Tirman P, Stoller D. Impingement syndrome of the ankle following supination external rotation trauma: MR imaging findings with arthroscopic correlation. Eur Radiol 2003;13:1357–62.

11. Berman Z, Tafur M, Ahmed S, et al. Ankle impingement syndromes: an imaging review. Br J Radiol 2017;90(1070):20160735.

12. Umans H, Cerezal L. Anterior ankle impingement syndromes. Sem Musculoskelet Radiol 2008;12: 146–53.

13. Rubin DA, Tishkoff NW, Britton CA, et al. Anterolateral soft-tissue impingement in the ankle: diagnosis using MR imaging. AJR Am J Roentgenol 1997; 169:829–35.

14. Liu SH, Nuccion SL, Finerman G. Diagnosis of anterolateral ankle impingement. Comparison between magnetic resonance imaging and clinical examination. Am J Sports Med 1997;25:389–93.

15. Cochet H, Pelé E, Amoretti N, et al. Anterolateral ankle impingement: diagnostic performance of MDCT arthrography and sonography. AJR Am J Roentgenol 2010;194:1575–80.

16. Donovan A, Rosenberg Z. MRI of ankle and lateral hindfoot impingement syndromes. AJR Am J Roentgenol 2010;195:595–604.

17. Linklater J. MR imaging of ankle impingement lesions. Magn Reson Imaging Clin N Am 2009;17: 775–800.

18. Wolin I, Glassman F, Sideman S, et al. Internal derangement of the talofibular component of the ankle. Surg Gynecol Obstet 1950;91:193–200.

19. Cerezal L, Abascal F, Canga A, et al. MR iimaging of ankle impingement syndromes. AJR Am J Roentgenol 2003;181:551–9.

20. Molloy S, Solan MC, Bendall SP. Synovial impingement in the ankle: a new physical sign. J Bone Joint Surg Br 2003;85:330–3.

21. Odak S, Ahluwalia R, Shivarathre DG, et al. Arthroscopic evaluation of impingement and osteochondral lesions in chronic lateral ankle instability. Foot Ankle Int 2015;36:1045–9.

22. Tol J, van Dijk C. Etiology of the anterior ankle impingement syndrome: a Ddescriptive anatomical study. Foot Ankle Int 2004;25:382–6.

23. Teh J, Suppiah R, Sharp R, et al. Imaging in the assessment and management of overuse injuries in the foot and ankle. Sem Musculoskelet Radiol 2011;15:101–14.

24. Vaseenon T, Amendola A. Update on anterior ankle impingement. Curr Rev Musculoskelet Med 2012;5: 145–50.

25. Hess G. Ankle impingement syndromes. Foot Ankle Spec 2011;4:290–7.

26. Talusan P, Toy J, Perez J, et al. Anterior ankle impingement. J Am Acad Orthop Surg 2014;22: 333–9.

27. Sanders T, Rathur S. Impingement syndromes of the ankle. Magn Reson Imaging Clin N Am 2008; 16:29–38.

28. Pesquer L, Guillo S, Meyer P, et al. US in ankle impingement syndrome. J Ultrasound 2013; 17:89–97.

29. Wong G, Tan T. MR imaging as a problem solving tool in posterior ankle pain: a review. Eur J Radiol 2016;85:2238–56.

30. Roche A, Calder J, Lloyd Williams R. Posterior ankle impingement in dancers and athletes. Foot Ankle Clin 2013;18:301–18.

31. Boonthathip M, Chen L, Trudell D, et al. Tibiofibular syndesmotic ligaments: MR arthrography in cadavers with anatomic correlation. Radiology 2010; 254:827–36.

32. Datir A, Connell D. Imaging of impingement lesions in the ankle. Tech Foot Ankle Surg 2008; 7:152–61.

33. Yasui Y, Hannon C, Hurley E, et al. Posterior ankle impingement syndrome: a systematic four-stage approach. World J Orthop 2016;7:657–63.

34. Sofka C. Posterior ankle impingement: clarification and confirmation of the pathoanatomy. HSS J 2009;6:99–101.

35. Lee J, Suh J, Huh Y, et al. Soft tissue impingement syndrome of the ankle: diagnostic efficacy of MRI and clinical results after arthroscopic treatment. Foot Ankle Int 2004;25:896–902.

36. Peace K, Hillier J, Hulme A, et al. MRI features of posterior ankle impingement syndrome in ballet dancers: a review of 25 cases. Clin Radiol 2004; 59:1025–33.

37. Robinson P. Impingement syndromes of the ankle. Eur Radiol 2007;17:3056–65.

38. Cheung Y. Normal variants. Magn Reson Imaging Clin N Am 2017;25:11–26.

39. Crim J. Medial-sided ankle pain. Magn Reson Imaging Clin N Am 2017;25:63–77.

40. Chhabra A, Subhawong T, Carrino J. MR imaging of deltoid ligament pathologic findings and associated impingement syndromes. Radiographics 2010;30: 751–61.

41. Koulouris G, Connell D, Schneider T, et al. Posterior tibiotalar ligament injury resulting in the posteromedial impingement. Foot Ankle Int 2003;24:575–83.

42. Jose J, Mirpuri T, Lesniak B, et al. Sonographically guided therapeutic injections in the meniscoid lesion in patients with anteromedial ankle impingement syndrome. Foot Ankle Spec 2014;7:409–13.

43. Paterson R, Brown J, Roberts S. The posteromedial impingement lesion of the ankle. Am J Sports Med 2001;29:550–7.

44. Robinson P, White L. Soft-tissue and osseous impingement syndromes of the ankle: role of imaging in diagnosis and management. RadioGraphics 2002;22:1457–69.

45. Messiou C, Robinson P, O'Connor P, et al. Subacute posteromedial impingement of the ankle in athletes: MR imaging evaluation and ultrasound guided therapy. Skeletal Radiol 2005;35:88–94.

46. Clair S, Monroe M, Manoli A. Medial impingement syndrome of the anterior tibiotalar fascicle of the deltoid ligament on the talus. Foot Ankle Int 2000;21:385–91.

47. van Dijk CN. Anterior and posterior ankle impingement. Foot Ankle Clin 2006;11:663–83.

Bone and Soft Tissue Tumors About the Foot and Ankle

Naoki O. Murai, MD[a], Oluwadamilola Teniola, MD[b],
Wei-Lien Wang, MD, MPH[c], Behrang Amini, MD, PhD[d],*

KEYWORDS

- Foot • Ankle • Neoplasm • Radiography • Computed tomography • MR imaging
- Nuclear medicine • PET/CT

KEY POINTS

- Most palpable masses about the foot and ankle are non-neoplastic. Of the neoplastic lesions, most are benign.
- Because of the complex anatomy of the foot and ankle, radiographs need to be augmented by cross-sectional imaging for diagnosis.
- Familiarity with the imaging appearance of bone and soft tissue neoplasms is necessary to ensure timely diagnosis and appropriate management.

INTRODUCTION

The foot and ankle delicately balance the need for support of the weight of the human body, with the need for flexibility. Palpable masses about the foot and ankle, therefore, are most commonly related to trauma or mechanical instability. Non-neoplastic causes, such as ganglia and callus, therefore, predominate. However, the radiologist must be aware of the imaging appearance of less common benign and malignant neoplasms that can involve the foot and ankle.

NORMAL ANATOMY AND IMAGING TECHNIQUE

Tumor imaging of the foot and ankle must allow the radiologist to confidently confine the lesion to the proper soft tissue compartment, which may provide clues as to the origin of the mass. These soft tissues include tendons, muscles, nerves, and fascia. At the same time, there must be adequate coverage of the surrounding structures to assess for local spread and satellite lesions. Therefore, it requires a wider field of view (FOV) than is typically used for assessment of internal derangement. The authors' institution's imaging protocols for the foot and ankle are summarized in **Table 1**. For the foot, wide FOV coverage is obtained from the toes to the heel with the option to narrow the FOV as needed based on radiographs, computed tomography (CT), or prereferral MR imaging. Long-axis and sagittal T2-weighted imaging (WI) with fat suppression (FS), sagittal T1-WI without FS, and short-axis T1-WI, T2-WI, and T1-WI postcontrast with FS are obtained. Imaging

Disclosure Statement: The authors have no relevant disclosures.
[a] Department of Diagnostic and Interventional Imaging, The University of Texas Health Science Center, 6431 Fannin Street, MSB 2.116, Houston, TX 77030, USA; [b] Department of Radiology, Baylor College of Medicine, 1 Baylor Plaza, Houston, TX 77030, USA; [c] Department of Pathology, The University of Texas, MD Anderson Cancer Center, 1515 Holcombe Boulevard, Houston, TX 77030, USA; [d] Department of Diagnostic Radiology, The University of Texas, MD Anderson Cancer Center, 1400 Pressler Street, Unit 1475, Houston, TX 77030, USA
* Corresponding author.
E-mail address: bamini@mdanderson.org

Radiol Clin N Am 56 (2018) 917–934
https://doi.org/10.1016/j.rcl.2018.06.010

Table 1
MD Anderson 2-dimensional imaging protocol for foot and ankle imaging on 1.5-T MR imaging

	Foot			Ankle		
Sequence	Max FOV (cm)	Thickness/Spacing (mm)	Sequence	Max FOV (cm)	Thickness/Spacing (mm)
Long-axis T2 FS	16	3–4/0	Coronal T2 FS	16	3–4/0
Sagittal T2 FS	16	3–4/0	Sagittal T2 FS	16	3–4/0
Sagittal T1	16	3–4/0	Sagittal T1	16	3–4/0
Short-axis T1	12–14	3.0/0.5	Axial T1	12–14	3.0/0.5
Short-axis T2 FS	12–14	3.0/0.5	Axial T2 FS	12–14	3.0/0.5
Short-axis T1 FS C+	12–14	3.0/0.5	Axial T1 FS C+	12–14	3.0/0.5

Abbreviations: C+, contrast enhanced; FS, fat suppression; Max, maximum.

of the ankle is typically more focused but allows the option of extending the FOV to cover the foot. Coronal and sagittal T2-WI with fat saturation, sagittal T1-WI without fat suppression, and axial T1-WI, T2-WI, and T1-WI postcontrast with fat saturation are acquired.

BONE TUMORS

Several benign and malignant bone neoplasms can affect the foot and ankle. Benign entities, such as giant cell tumor (GCT) of bone, osteoblastoma (OB), and chondroblastoma, predominate, whereas bone tissue sarcomas and metastases are much less common.

Giant Cell Tumor of Bone

GCT of bone is a relatively common, benign, locally aggressive, primary osseous neoplasm composed of osteoclastlike multinucleated giant cells.[1] GCT of bone is characteristically centered on the metaphyseal side of the growth plate. GCT of bone most commonly presents in the third decade, only 2% to 4% occur in children less than 14 years old.[2] GCT of bone is especially prevalent in China and southern India; women are probably more commonly affected than men.[3,4] GCT of bone most commonly arises in the metaphysis of a long bone; 2% to 5% are located in the distal tibia and 1% to 2% in the foot.[5–7] GCT of bone account for 4% of osseous neoplasms in the foot and ankle.[8] In the foot and ankle, GCT most commonly occurs in the talus and calcaneus and only rarely involves the metatarsals and phalanges.[9]

On radiography (**Fig. 1A**), most GCTs of bone present as geographic, lytic lesions with a well-defined, nonsclerotic margin. A minority of GCTs of bone feature ill-defined margins, cortical disruption, and even soft tissue masses, indicating more aggressive tumor behavior.[10]

Sclerotic margins are rarely seen radiographically; however, areas of peripheral sclerosis may be seen on CT in 20% of cases (**Fig. 1B**).[11] Most GCT of bone are eccentrically located.[4] In contradistinction to the typical radiographic appearance of GCT of bone, most GCTs of the foot exhibit an ill-defined, geographic pattern of osseous destruction. Nearly all GCTs of the foot are expansile and exhibit cortical breakthrough.[9] CT is more sensitive than MR imaging for the detection of cortical thinning, pathologic fracture, periosteal reaction, and evaluating remodeling. CT also has utility in excluding matrix mineralization that would point toward osteoid or chondroid lesions. MR imaging is superior to CT in identifying soft tissue extension.[12] On MR imaging (**Fig. 1C–F**), GCT of bone has low to intermediate signal intensity on T1-WI and high signal on fluid sensitive sequences and demonstrates avid enhancement.[4] Hemorrhage and hemosiderin deposition can be seen as low-signal areas on T2-WI.[11] On technetium-99m (Tc-99m) methylene diphosphonate (MDP) bone scan, GCT often demonstrates increased tracer uptake at the periphery of the lesion with a central photopenic defect due to central necrosis or osteolysis.[4,10]

The primary differential consideration for GCT in the foot and ankle is chondroblastoma, primary aneurysmal bone cyst, and, less commonly, OB. The age of patients can help narrow the list, because GCTs tend to occur in an older age group than the other entities. At times, GCT can have a very aggressive appearance and can mimic metastases and multiple myeloma.

Chondroblastoma

Chondroblastoma (CB) is a rare, benign, chondrogenic tumor with a predilection for the epiphyses or apophyses. CBs frequently develop secondary

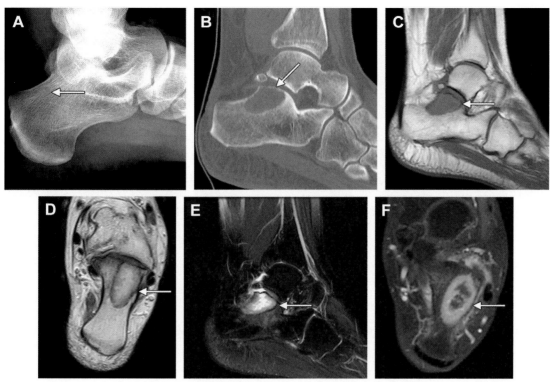

Fig. 1. GCT of bone in the calcaneus in a 29-year-old woman. (*A*) Lateral radiographs of the left foot show a very subtle lesion (*arrow*), which was not prospectively identified. CT and MR imaging were obtained 6 months later. (*B*) Sagittal reformation of a contrast-enhanced CT shows a lytic lesion with increased peripheral attenuation/ enhancement and a well-defined, mildly sclerotic margin. There is thinning of the cortex superiorly but no disruption. Note mild expansion of the cortex along the subtalar joint (*arrow*). (*C*) Coronal T1-WI shows a low to intermediate signal bone lesion (*arrow*). (*D*) Axial proton-density image shows a low to intermediate signal rim (*arrow*) and central high signal. (*E*) Sagittal T2-WI with FS shows a low to intermediate signal rim (*arrow*) and central high signal. Perilesional edema is also identified. (*F*) Postcontrast axial T1-WI with FS shows a thick enhancing rim (*arrow*) and central nonenhancement.

aneurysmal bone cysts.[13] Overall, CB has a 3:2 male preponderance with a peak incidence in the second decade.[14] Patients with CB in the foot tend to be older at the time of diagnosis. CB of the hand and foot has an average age at diagnosis of 24 years, and 80% occur in males.[15] The calcaneus and talus are the most commonly affected bones of the foot, collectively accounting for 72% of cases. The cuboid and metatarsals each accounted for 18% of cases.[15]

On radiographs (**Fig. 2**A), CB is typically a round, geographic, sharply demarcated lesion with a thin sclerotic rim situated at the epiphyses or apophyses. Endosteal scalloping is present in most lesions.[15] CT (**Fig. 2**B) is useful for detecting matrix mineralization, present radiographically in only 54% of lesions in the hand and foot.[15] MR imaging (**Fig. 2**C–E) is useful for detecting soft tissue extension, intraarticular involvement, and periosteal reaction. Peripheral lobulation is identifiable in most cases.[16] Owing to high cellularity, CB is low

to intermediate signal on T1. Most CBs of the hand and foot demonstrate aneurysmal bone cyst formation on MR imaging (see **Fig. 2**D).[15] Perilesional marrow edema (see **Fig. 2**E) is characteristic.[16] Most CBs demonstrate at least moderate uptake on Tc-99m MDP bone scan.[16]

The primary differential consideration for CB in the foot and ankle is GCT, primary aneurysmal bone cyst, and, less commonly, OB. GCT tends to occur in an older age group. There is, however, more overlap between the age range of CB and aneurysmal bone cyst and OB. Chondroid matrix, when present, can help narrow the differential to CB; however, differentiation can be difficult, especially when CB is associated with a secondary ABC.

Osteoblastoma

Osteoblastoma (OB) is a relatively uncommon, usually benign, bone-forming neoplasm that is occasionally locally aggressive and rarely behaves

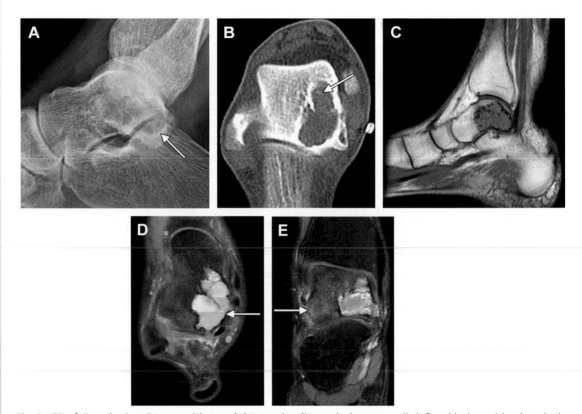

Fig. 2. CB of the talus in a 31-year-old man. (*A*) Lateral radiograph shows a well-defined lesion with sclerotic rim in the talus posteriorly (*arrow*). (*B*) CT obtained at the time of biopsy shows subtle arclike calcifications (*arrow*). (*C*) Sagittal T1-WI shows a lobulated lesion with a low-signal rim and intermediate central signal located in the posterior talus. (*D*) Axial proton-density-WI with FS shows several fluid-fluid levels (*arrow*) indicating secondary aneurysmal bone cyst formation. (*E*) Coronal postcontrast T1-WI with FS shows a peripherally enhancing lesion and extensive perilesional hyperemia (*arrow*). Note endosteal thinning along the articular surface of the talus.

malignantly.[17] Like osteoid osteomas, OBs most often present with pain. Although histologically similar to osteoid osteoma, OB is a distinct entity. Peak incidence is in the second and third decades, with a 2:1 male predominance. The foot and ankle is the third most common location for OB. OBs of the foot and ankle arise from the talus in 39% of cases, the forefoot in 34%, and the distal tibia in 15%.[18] A subperiosteal location at the dorsal surface of the talar head-neck junction is characteristic.[19]

On radiographs (**Fig. 3**A), most OBs of the foot and ankle are geographic, lytic lesions with variable borders. Radiographically detectable matrix is present in approximately half of lesions. An associated soft tissue mass is present in 24%. Surrounding reactive changes tend to be less exuberant than with osteoid osteoma.[18] CT (**Fig. 3**B) is useful for elucidating the degree of osseous destruction and the presence of matrix. MR imaging (**Fig. 3**C, D) aids in the identification of a soft tissue component. OBs demonstrate increased radiotracer uptake on Tc-99m MDP

bone scan.[20] A characteristic double density may be produced by exuberant tracer uptake centrally surrounded by moderate osseous uptake.[18] Because OB is uncommon, CB and primary ABC should be considered first when thinking about making a diagnosis of OB. Both OB and CB can be associated with significant perilesional edema.

Lymphoma

Osseous lymphoma may be primary lymphoma of bone (PLB) or secondary lymphoma. PLB is considered an osseous disease without evidence of a systemic disease for 6 months. Secondary lymphoma refers to the systemic spread of disease to bone. PLB has a better 5-year survival than secondary lymphoma.[21] PLB accounts for less than 5% of all malignant bone tumors.[22] PLB favors the appendicular skeleton, whereas secondary lymphoma favors the axial skeleton.[23] PLB involves the tarsal and/or metatarsal bones in 2% of cases.[24]

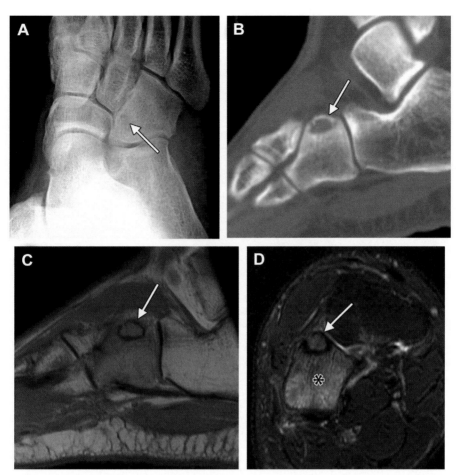

Fig. 3. OB of the cuboid in a 33-year-old man with midfoot pain. (*A*) Oblique radiograph of the foot shows a well-defined, subtle lucency (*arrow*) in the cuboid, which was not prospectively identified. (*B*) Sagittal reformation shows a well-defined lytic lesion (*arrow*) with increased attenuation of the adjacent marrow and focal cortical thinning. (*C*) Sagittal T1-WI shows an intermediate signal mass with low-signal margin (*arrow*) and subtle loss of signal in the adjacent marrow. (*D*) Long-axis T2-WI with FS of the midfoot shows an intermediate to low signal lesion in the cuboid with a low-signal rim (*arrow*) and adjacent marrow edema (*asterisk*).

Radiographically, PLB presents as a permeative metadiaphyseal lesion. This appearance is shared with other small round cell tumors, such as Ewing sarcoma and metastatic neuroblastoma. Periosteal reaction and soft tissue mass were seen radiographically in approximately one-half of cases in one series.[24] CT is useful for evaluating for visceral and nodal involvement. On magnetic resonance (MR), bone marrow replacement and soft tissue mass are characteristic of PLB. Marrow replacement is seen as enhancing foci of T1 hypointense and T2 hyperintense signal. Soft tissue mass is noted on MR in most lesions with a permeative pattern radiographically. There is a characteristic paucity of cortical destruction relative to the extent of soft tissue mass and marrow replacement (**Fig. 4**).[25] PLB shows increased uptake on Tc-99m MDP bone scan in 98% of cases.[24] The

positive predictive value of PET/CT for osseous lymphoma is superior to that of PET or CT alone.[26]

The primary differential consideration for lymphoma of bone is leukemia and other small round cell tumors (eg, Ewing sarcoma). Acral involvement with myeloma and metastases is rare.

Osteosarcoma

Osteosarcoma (OS) is the most common primary malignant tumor of bone in young adults and adolescents around the second decade of life. The lesion originates from the metaphysis of long bones.[27] OSs can be divided into intramedullary (osteoblastic, chrondroblastic, fibroblastic, telangiectatic, giant cell rich, and low-grade central) and surface (high-grade surface, periosteal, and parosteal) subtypes, with the most common being

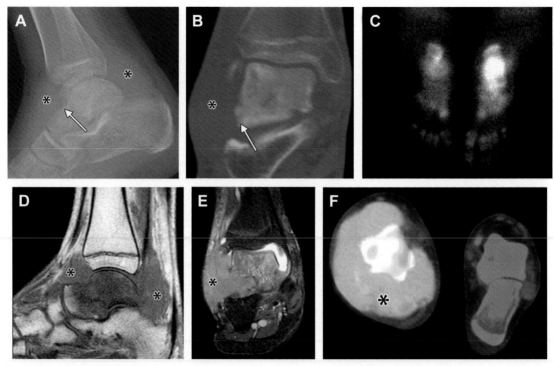

Fig. 4. Primary lymphoma of bone in a 14-year-old boy who presented with 1 year of right ankle pain. (*A*) Lateral radiograph of the ankle shows a sclerotic lesion in the talus, associated with cortical disruption (*arrow*) and soft tissue masses anteriorly and posteriorly (*asterisks*). (*B*) Coronal reformation of noncontrast CT shows a sclerotic lesion in the calcaneus with cortical disruption (*arrow*) and a soft tissue mass (*asterisk*). (*C*) Delayed image from a Tc-99m MDP bone scan shows increased uptake in the right ankle. (*D*) Sagittal T1-WI shows a heterogeneously low to intermediate signal lesion in the calcaneus, with areas of entrapped marrow fat and a large soft tissue mass (*asterisks*). (*E*) Coronal T2-WI shows an intermediate-signal lesion in the talus with a soft tissue mass (*asterisk*). (*F*) FDG-PET/CT shows avid uptake (standardized uptake value = 17) in the right talus and adjacent soft tissues (*asterisk*).

the conventional osteoblastic form.[28] Osteoblastic OS accounts for approximately 40% of all cases and produces an osteoid matrix leading to the sclerosis seen on imaging.[28,29] Subtypes of OS, such as chondroblastic, giant cell rich, and fibroblastic lesions, show destruction without a significant sclerotic component. OS in general is most common in adolescents and has a male predominance. Although a common primary malignancy of bone, the initial presentation in the foot is very rare, accounting for 1% to 2% of all OSs. OS of the foot often presents in the fourth decade, 1 to 2 decades after the classic OS presents. Because of a low index of suspicion, OS of the foot is often misdiagnosed as a benign foot lesion.[27]

On radiography (**Fig. 5**A), OS can present as a lytic or sclerotic lesion with a varying zone of transition and invasion into adjacent soft tissue.[27–29] There are also varying amounts of periosteal reaction, including sunburst pattern and Codman triangle. The predominating subtypes of OS in the foot are the low-grade lesions (42%), which often do

not exhibit the sunburst pattern or Codman triangle forms of periosteal reaction. In the ankle, the distal tibia is the most common location. The most common locations in the foot are the tarsal bones (56%–72%), followed by metatarsal (17%–33%) and phalanges (11%).[27] Tarsal lesions tend to be more sclerotic, whereas the others are mixed. CT (**Fig. 5**B) aids in the visualization of calcifications and subtle periosteal reactions not evident on radiographs.[27] On MR imaging (**Fig. 5**C, D), OS has intermediate signal on T1-WI. The mineralized portions are variable on T1-WI and low signal on T2-WI.[27] Avid contrast enhancement is noted, and fluid-fluid levels are also present when hemorrhagic portions are present. MR imaging aids in determining the extent of lesion invasion into the marrow, soft tissues, and joint space.[27] On diagnosis, metastatic workup is recommended with chest radiography for osseous metastasis, chest CT for pulmonary nodules, and skeletal scintigraphy for metachronous or distant metastasis.[27]

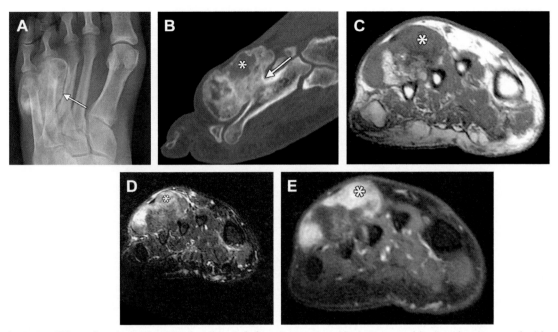

Fig. 5. Dedifferentiated parosteal OS from the left fourth metatarsal in a 63-year-old man who presented with a 20-year history of foot mass (*arrow*) with recent accelerated growth. (*A*) Oblique radiograph shows a mass in the region of the fourth and fifth metatarsals with amorphous central ossification and a thin rim of peripheral calcification. The origin of the mass could not be discerned from the radiographs. (*B*) Sagittal CT reconstruction along the long axis of the metatarsal shows the mass arises mid-diaphysis (*arrow*) with osteoid matrix and areas of soft tissue attenuation (*asterisk*). (*C*) Short-axis T1-WI shows normal medullary cavity of the fourth metatarsal with mature ossification arising from the surface of the bone and a low-signal soft tissue component (*asterisk*). (*D*) Short-axis short tau inversion recovery image shows normal medullary cavity of the fourth metatarsal with low-signal mature ossification arising from the surface of the bone and a high-signal soft tissue component (*asterisk*). (*E*) Short-axis axial postcontrast T1-WI with FS shows normal medullary cavity of the fourth metatarsal with low-signal mature ossification arising from the surface of the bone and an enhancing soft tissue component (*asterisk*).

The primary differential considerations for chondroblastic OS are bone lesions with chondroid matrix (chondrosarcoma, aggressive chondroblastoma). Fibroblastic OS can be purely lytic and nonspecific, in which case metastases should be considered.

Chondrosarcoma

Chondrosarcoma is the third most common malignant primary bone tumor. Patients often present with pain as chondrosarcomas grow exuberantly. Chondrosarcomas may be primary or arise secondarily within an enchondroma or osteochondroma. Conventional osteochondromas comprise 90% of all subtypes and are either central (medullary) or peripheral. Although enchondromas are common in the metatarsals, it is uncommon for secondary chondrosarcomas to arise within metatarsal enchondromas. Most chondrosarcomas in the feet are located in the calcaneus, followed by the metatarsals and phalanges.[30]

On radiographs (**Fig. 6**A), central chondrosarcomas are geographic, metaphyseal lesions with variable amounts of chondroid matrix. Deep (greater than two-thirds cortical width) endosteal scalloping is seen more commonly with chondrosarcomas and aids in differentiation from enchondromas, which typically exhibit shallow or no scalloping. Cortical thickening and pathologic fractures (see **Fig. 6**A) may occur. CT (**Fig. 6**B) is more sensitive than radiography for matrix mineralization, especially in anatomically complex areas, such as the foot. CT is also adequate for demonstrating both intraosseous and extraosseous soft tissue tumor components. On MR imaging (**Fig. 6**C–F), low-grade chondrosarcomas are lobulated. T2-hypointense septations and calcifications may be present. There is often T2 hyperintensity related to chondroid matrix in low-grade lesions and myxoid change in intermediate-grade lesions. High-grade lesions tend to be heterogenous in signal intensity with prominent associated soft tissue mass.[31] Chondrosarcoma of the foot is typically

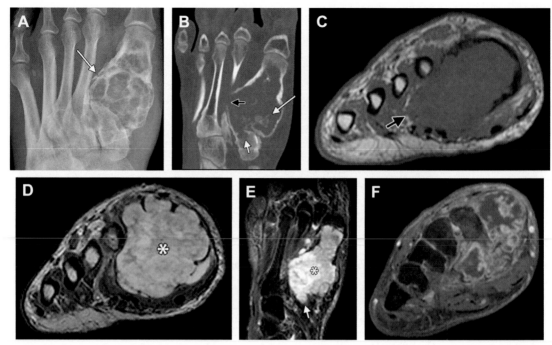

Fig. 6. Chondrosarcoma arising from an enchondroma of the first metatarsal in a 50-year-old man with an enlarging left foot mass over several months. (*A*) Oblique radiograph shows expansion of the first metatarsal bone, indicating a slowly growing lesion, such as an enchondroma. There is a focal area of cortical discontinuity (*arrow*) suggestive of a fracture. (*B*) Coronal reformation from a noncontrast CT shows internal areas of ring and arc calcification (*long arrow*), area of cortical disruption laterally (*short black arrow*) and extension into the medial cuneiform (*short white arrow*). (*C*) Short-axis T1-WI shows loss of cortical signal void laterally indicating soft tissue extension (*arrow*). (*D*) Short-axis T2-WI shows intense T2 signal within the mass (*asterisk*), concordant with cartilage composition. (*E*) Long-axis T2-WI with FS shows the mass in the first metatarsal (*asterisk*) with extension into the medial cuneiform (*short arrow*). (*F*) Short-axis axial postcontrast T1-WI with FS shows peripheral and septal enhancement seen with cartilage lesions.

a lobular, T2 hyperintense lesion with enhancing septations.

Differentiating low-grade chondrosarcomas from enchondromas can be difficult even on pathology. Cortical breakthrough can aid in differentiation from enchondroma.[32] Tc-99m MDP bone scan uptake in chondrosarcomas is greater than anterior superior iliac spine (ASIS) uptake in 82% of cases, whereas uptake in enchondromas is typically less than that of the ASIS.[31] ^{18}F-fluorodeoxyglucose (FDG)-PET may also have utility in differentiating benign from malignant cartilage forming tumors; however, there remains significant overlap in the degree of uptake between enchondromas and chondrosarcoma.[33]

Metastases

Metastasis to the foot and ankle is rare; 0.01% to 2.0% of patients with primary malignancies have metastasis to the foot or ankle.[34,35] The most common primary neoplasms metastasizing to the foot are colorectal, renal, lung, bladder, and breast cancers.[35,36] The tarsal bones, especially the talus and calcaneus, are the most commonly metastasized to in the foot.[35–37]

On radiographs (**Fig. 7**A), metastases to the foot are destructive lytic lesions in 80% of cases. Prostate metastases are typically sclerotic; breast, bladder, and colorectal primaries may yield mixed lytic-sclerotic metastases.[36,37] Periosteal reaction is present in only 4.5% of lesions and joint involvement (**Fig. 7**) is exceedingly uncommon, features that help differentiate metastases from infectious causes.[35] Foot metastases may be initially discovered on Tc-99m MDP bone scan as areas of increased uptake (see **Fig. 7**B). MR (see **Fig. 7**C–F) characteristics of foot metastases are variable. Lytic metastases tend to be low signal on T1-WI, high signal on T2-WI, and demonstrate enhancement, whereas blastic metastases have very low signal on all pulse sequences and minimal to no enhancement.[38] Metastases from thyroid and renal cell carcinoma (see **Fig. 7**D–F) may have visible flow voids indicating their highly vascular nature.

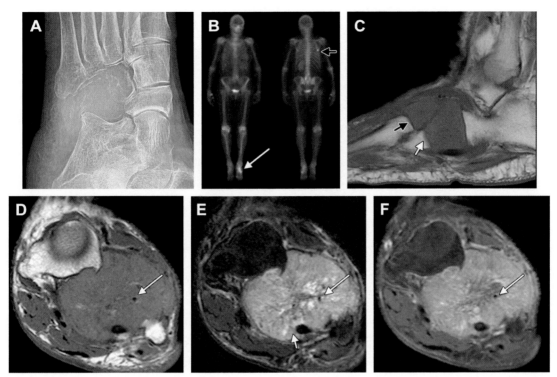

Fig. 7. Metastatic disease in the foot in a 71-year-old woman 9 years after right nephrectomy for renal cell carcinoma. (A) Oblique radiograph of the left foot shows destruction of the cuboid, lateral and middle cuneiforms. (B) Tc-99m MDP bone scan shows areas of increased uptake in the left foot (long arrow) and left scapula (short arrow). (C) Sagittal T1-WI shows lesions in the cuboid (white arrow) and lateral cuneiform (black arrow). (D) Short-axis T1-WI through the midfoot shows an intermediate-signal mass with small flow voids (arrow), concordant with vascular metastasis such as renal cell carcinoma. (E) Short-axis T2-WI with FS through the midfoot shows a high-signal mass (long arrow) with small flow voids (short arrow), concordant with vascular metastasis, such as renal cell carcinoma. (F) Short-axis postcontrast T1-WI with FS through the midfoot shows an enhancing mass with small flow voids (arrow), concordant with vascular metastasis, such as renal cell carcinoma.

The primary differential considerations for metastases are myeloma and lymphoma. All 3 entities are rare in the foot and ankle; patient history, laboratory workup, and ultimately biopsy are often needed.

SOFT TISSUE TUMORS

Several benign and malignant soft tissue neoplasms can affect the foot and ankle. Benign entities, such as fibromatosis and pigmented villonodular synovitis, predominate, whereas soft tissue sarcomas are much less common. The nonspecific imaging appearance of all but a few soft tissue lesions makes prospective diagnosis difficult.

Tenosynovial Giant Cell Tumor

Tenosynovial GCT (TGCT) is divided into 2 forms: localized and diffuse. The localized form is also known as localized GCT of tendon sheath, whereas the diffuse form is also known as pigmented villonodular synovitis (PVNS).[39] These two entities are histologically identical and represent uncommon benign neoplasm characterized by villous, nodular, or villonodular hyperplasia of synovial tissue. Pigmentation of the lesion is due to hemosiderin deposition. PVNS has a female to male ratio of 3:1. The incidence is highest in the third to fifth decades of life. Patients often present with a painful soft tissue mass.[40] The most common site for the localized, intraarticular form is the knee. The extra-articular form most commonly occurs in the hand and wrist. The foot/ankle is involved in less than 10% of cases.[41]

On radiography and CT (Fig. 8A, B), TGCT presents as a soft tissue density mass. The lesion may cause osseous erosion with characteristic well-defined sclerotic margins. Calcifications are exceedingly rare.[40] On ultrasound, TGCT is a solid, homogenously hypoechoic lesion with increased internal blood flow on Doppler. On MR imaging (Fig. 8C–E), TGCT demonstrates low to intermediate T1 and T2 signal. TGCT is often

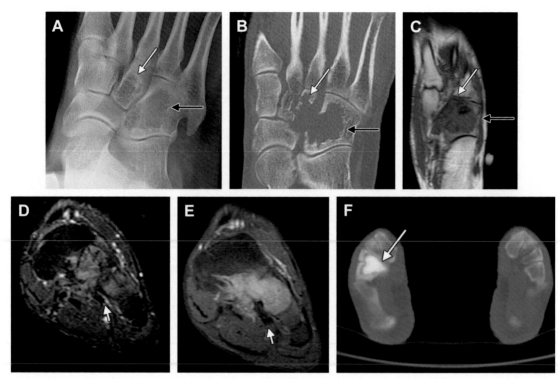

Fig. 8. Tenosynovial GCT in a 51-year-old woman with a 9-month history of foot pain. (*A*) Oblique radiograph shows well-defined lesions in the cuboid (*black arrow*) and lateral cuneiform (*white arrow*). (*B*) CT suggests that the lesions in the cuboid (*black arrow*) and lateral cuneiform (*white arrow*) are the result of extrinsic erosion by an articular or para-articular process. (*C*) Long-axis T1-WI shows a low-signal lesion involving the cuboid (*black arrow*) and lateral cuneiform (*white arrow*), related to hemorrhage. Short-axis inversion recovery (*D*) and post-contrast T1-WI with FS (*E*) images show the peroneus longus tendon (*arrows*) passing through the soft tissue lesion. The plantar aspect of the soft tissue mass has an infiltrative appearance. (*F*) Axial fused image from FDG PET/CT shows intense metabolic activity (*arrow*) in the right foot mass.

inhomogeneous, featuring hypointense fibrous septations on T1-WI and T2-WI. Blooming artifact on gradient echo sequences is due to hemosiderin's ferromagnetic properties and is nearly pathognomonic of GCT.[40] TGCT avidly enhances but lacks the perilesional edema of a more aggressive tumor. The ability of MR imaging to identify a synovial-based, plaquelike/nodular thickening with lack of surrounding edema and hemosiderin deposition makes it ideal for diagnosis and localization.[40,42] On FDG-PET, TGCT may mimic a more aggressive lesion because of its high tracer uptake (**Fig. 8**F). Clinically, FDG-PET can be used to evaluate the pretreatment appearance and posttreatment response.[43]

The primary feature of TGCT is its low T2 signal, which sets it apart from most soft tissue lesions and soft tissue sarcomas. Gouty tophi and amyloid can have a similar low T2-signal appearance. In these cases, radiographs can help if they demonstrate mineralization, which is rarely seen in TGCT but commonly seen in gout and sometimes in amyloid deposits.

Vascular Anomalies (Hemangiomas and Epithelioid Hemangioendothelioma)

There is much confusion in the terminology of vascular anomalies. The most widely accepted classification scheme is based on the degree of cellular proliferation and divides vascular anomalies into neoplasms and malformations.[44] Neoplasms include benign entities, such as congenital and infantile hemangiomas, and malignancies, such as angiosarcoma and epithelioid hemangioendothelioma. Vascular malformations, in turn, are classified as simple (capillary, lymphatic, venous, and arteriovenous malformations, and arteriovenous fistulas) or combined. The malformations may also be divided based on the rate of flow and low flow (capillary, lymphatic, venous malformations, and so forth) or high flow (arteriovenous malformations and fistulas).[44] Finally, the World Health Organization (WHO) has an entity known as intramuscular angioma, which is often used interchangeably with hemangioma.

Of these, venous malformations are the most common in the appendicular skeleton, accounting for more than 50% of lesions in the extremities.[45] Hyperemia can lead to bone demineralization, which may be visible on radiographs (**Fig. 9A**). There can also be involvement of the bone by mass effect or direct extension. Phleboliths can also be demonstrated on radiographs (see **Fig. 9A**). MR imaging (**Fig. 9B–E**) allows better characterization of these lesions, and T1-WI may show prominence of adjacent intramuscular and subcutaneous fat.[45] The lesion itself is lobulated and septated and often infiltrating and nonmasslike. Typically, there is extension from the skin through the subcutaneous tissue, with infiltration of various bone and soft tissue compartments (see **Fig. 9D**).[45] Somewhat counterintuitively, this infiltrative appearance helps to distinguish vascular malformations from more aggressive soft tissue neoplasms.[45] On T1-WI, lesions have low to intermediate signal intensity and may contain areas of internal fat.[45] On T2-WI, the masses have high signal intensity corresponding to venous lakes containing stagnant blood.[45] Because postcontrast images may underestimate the true extent of these lesions, optimization of the T2 FS technique (either through FS or inversion recovery) is key to accurate characterization of the extent of lesion.[45]

Epithelioid hemangioendothelioma (EHE) is a rare malignant, often indolent vascular neoplasm that may represent an intermediate grade between the benign epithelioid hemangioma and epithelioid sarcoma. It has a peak incidence during the second and third decades of life and tends to affect both sexes equally.[46] They more commonly involve the lung and liver and are multifocal about half the time.[47] When present in the extremity, they more commonly affect the lower limb. They can be multifocal often involve contiguous and dis-contiguous bone and soft tissue compartments.

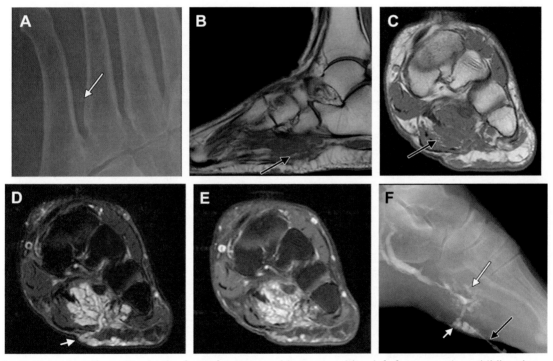

Fig. 9. Venous malformation in the foot of a 49-year-old woman with a left foot mass since childhood, now enlarging and painful. (*A*) Oblique radiograph shows mild demineralization of the bones and a small phlebolith (*arrow*). (*B*) Sagittal T1-WI shows atrophy of the plantar muscles with increased intramuscular fat (*arrow*). (*C*) Short-axis T1-WI shows atrophy of the plantar muscles with increased intramuscular fat (*arrow*). (*D*) Short-axis T2-WI with FS shows a large vein (*arrow*) draining into the lobulated, septated lesion. The lesion does not respect tissue planes and extends along the fascia, between tendons, and within muscle. (*E*) Short-axis delayed postcontrast T1-WI with FS shows pooling of contrast within the lobulated, septated mass. (*F*) Venogram obtained before sclerotherapy shows the injection needle (*black arrow*) in the vein indicated in panel (*D*) (*short white arrow*), accumulation of injected contrast into the mass (*long white arrow*), and subsequent drainage centrally.

On radiographs, bone erosions and lytic bone lesions may be evident (**Fig. 10**A). MR imaging (**Fig. 10**B) shows the lesions to better advantage, with intermediate signal on T1-WI, high signal on T2-WI, and moderate to avid enhancement on postcontrast sequences.

Depending on the specific imaging features, one may consider the following entities in the differential considerations. For vascular anomalies with large fatty components, angiolipoma, and well-differentiated liposarcoma may be considered.[48] For an avidly enhancing lesion, sarcoma should be in the differential. In the case of multifocal disease in the foot seen with EHE, one may consider metastases and myeloma but must also keep in mind how uncommonly there is multifocal metastatic or myelomatous involvement of the foot and ankle.

Fibromatosis

Fibromatosis is a benign soft tissue lesion of fibrous tissue that can be divided into superficial and deep fibromatosis.[49] Both are classified as intermediate, locally aggressive fibroblastic tumors by the WHO. Superficial fibromatosis has a strong predilection for males and affects mainly adult patients, with the incidence increasing with advancing age (almost 20% of the general population is affected by of 65 years of age).[49] In the foot and ankle, superficial fibromatosis is often multinodular and occurs along the medial or central band of the plantar fascia and has a nodular appearance.[50,51] A medial band lesion may overlie the digital branch of the nerve to the great toe and is often the cause of symptoms.[50] Fibromatosis is treated conservatively with antiinflammatory drugs, local steroid injection, or physical therapy.[52] Surgery is indicated for lesions refractory to conservative management and may include a fasciectomy with overlying skin excision, as recurrence is common.[52]

Because fibromatosis does not contain calcification, radiographs are helpful only to exclude the presence of a calcifying soft tissue mass. On ultrasound, plantar fibromatosis presents as discrete areas of fusiform thickening of the plantar aponeurosis. Most lesions are hypoechoic, well defined, and demonstrate no acoustic enhancement or vascularity.[53] However, there is a spectrum of activity; more hypercellular lesions can demonstrate vascularity and posterior acoustic enhancement (**Fig. 11**A). On MR imaging (**Fig. 11**B–E), plantar fibromas are well-defined nodules with abnormally low signal intensity on T1-WI and low to intermediate signal intensity on T2-WI. As with ultrasound, MR imaging reflects the spectrum of behavior of these lesions, with cellular components presenting as high signal on T2-WI and with varying degrees of enhancement on postcontrast images.[51]

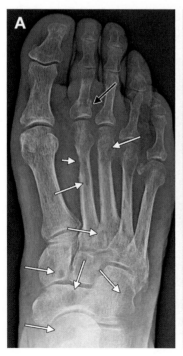
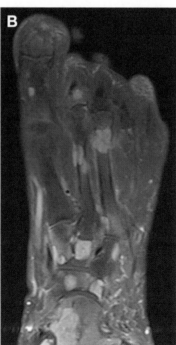

Fig. 10. EHE in a 77-year-old man. (*A*) Frontal radiograph shows multiple lytic lesions (*long white arrows*), one of which is associated with a pathologic fracture (*black arrow*). There is also an area of extrinsic bone erosion at the distal second metatarsal (*short arrow*). (*B*) Long-axis postcontrast T1-WI with FS shows multiple enhancing lesions corresponding to the lytic lesions seen on radiography.

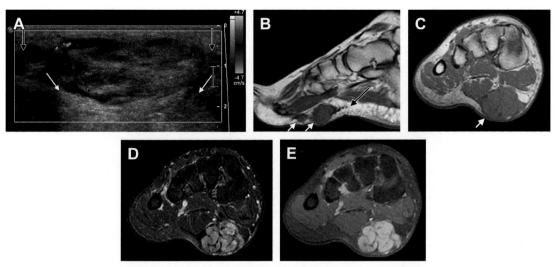

Fig. 11. Plantar fibromatosis in a 27-year-old man with a palpable plantar mass and aggressive imaging features. (*A*) Ultrasound shows a mass with flow on Doppler and posterior acoustic enhancement (*white arrows*) located within the plantar aponeurosis (*black arrows*). (*B*) Sagittal T1-WI shows 2 soft tissue masses with intermediate signal (*white arrows*) along the medial band of the plantar aponeurosis (*black arrow*). (*C*) Short-axis T1-WI at the level of the larger mass (*arrow*) shows the internal signal to better advantage. The mass is predominantly intermediate signal, with bands of low signal that correspond to collagenous components. Short-axis T2-WI with FS (*D*) and postcontrast T1-WI with FS (*E*) images at the level of the larger mass show a predominantly intermediate to high signal intensity, enhancing mass (corresponding to cellular components) with bands of low signal (corresponding to collagenous components).

The differential considerations for plantar fibromatosis are limited. Plantar fasciitis and injury to the plantar aponeurosis can cause focal thickening and mimic a mass. More cellular variants of plantar fibromatosis can mimic deep fibromatosis, but the typical location along the medial band of the plantar aponeurosis should be helpful. TGCT can have a low-signal appearance but will not arise from a nonsynovial connective tissue structure like the plantar aponeurosis. Other less common considerations include rheumatoid nodules.

Deep fibromatosis (DF) (also known as aggressive fibromatosis and desmoid) has been reported in patients with familial adenomatous polyposis syndromes with an incidence of 3.5% to 32.0%.[54,55] On ultrasound, lesions of superficial and DF are often hypoechoic, oval, and lack intrinsic vascularity.[50,54] DF typically presents as a poorly defined, hypoechoic soft tissue mass. Large lesions may demonstrate posterior acoustic shadowing and demonstrate hypervascularity on Doppler ultrasound.[56] On MR imaging (**Fig. 12A–C**), single or multiple lesions may be present. They can be hypointense to hyperintense to muscle with varying degrees of signal due to different amounts of collagen and cellularity.[57,58] MR imaging is used to determine the extent of these lesions with relation to the dermis, neurovascular

structures, and other structures like tendons and ligaments for surgical planning.[54,58] Because DF can have extensive tails that spread from the main part of the lesion, a large FOV and careful attention to the edges of all images is required to accurately delineate the extent of the lesion. Sometimes other sites of disease can be remote from the area of imaging (**Fig. 12D**).

The infiltrative appearance of DF with internal bands of low signal is seen in very few entities, and usually the diagnosis can be made relatively confidently. Occasionally, DF presents as a well-defined, round or oval mass, with high T2 signal and avid enhancement.[59] In such cases, differentiation from soft tissue sarcoma may be difficult.

Peripheral Nerve Sheath Tumor

Peripheral nerve sheath tumors (PNSTs) are soft tissue neoplasms that originate peripheral nerves and can be benign or malignant. The two main classes of benign PNSTs are schwannomas and neurofibromas (NFs). Schwannomas are encapsulated masses composed entirely of benign neoplastic Schwann cells and are the more common of the two entities. NFs, on the other hand, are unencapsulated masses that contain a mixture of Schwann cells, perineurial-like cells, and

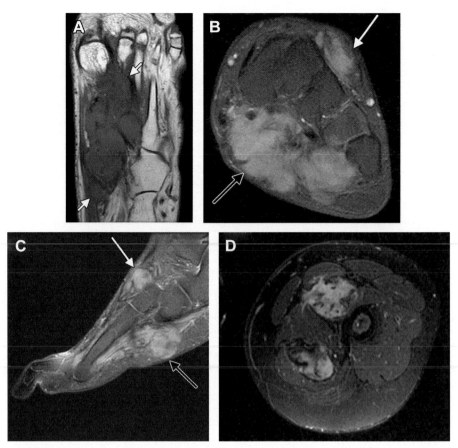

Fig. 12. Desmoid fibromatosis in a 25-year-old man with an enlarging mass of the left foot and thigh. (*A*) Long-axis axial T1-WI shows an intermediate signal mass (*arrows*) in the plantar compartment with bands of low signal. (*B*) Short-axis proton density-FS image through the metatarsals shows intermediate to high signal masses occupying the plantar (*black arrow*) and dorsal (*white arrow*) compartments. No connection between the masses was discerned on imaging, characteristic of microscopic spread of DF along fascial planes. (*C*) Sagittal postcontrast T1-WI with FS shows avid lesion enhancement in both the plantar (*black arrow*) and dorsal (*white arrow*) compartments. (*D*) Axial T2-WI with FS through the left thigh shows additional sites of disease.

fibroblasts interspersed with nerve fibers, wirelike strands of collagen, and myxoid matrix.[60] Foot and ankle involvement is uncommon and accounts for only about 2% to 3% of cases.[61] The tarsal tunnel is the most common location in the foot, and space constraints in the foot and ankle typically bring these lesions to medical attention when they are small.[61]

On ultrasound, PNSTs are round or oval, well-confined lesions that are predominantly hypoechoic.[62] Color Doppler reveals minimal to absent flow in these lesions. On MR imaging (**Fig. 13**), PNSTs have intermediate to high signal on T1-WI, high signal on T2-WI, and diffuse enhance.[63] The target sign of peripheral high signal and central low signal on T2-WI is seen in most PNSTs.[63] A cap of fat surrounding the lesion (**Fig. 13C**), although not specific to PNSTs, indicates slow growth.

The primary differential consideration is a soft tissue sarcoma that has either originated from or secondarily involved a peripheral nerve or a small intramuscular soft tissue sarcoma.[64]

Soft Tissue Sarcomas

Soft tissue sarcomas that have a predilection for the foot and ankle include undifferentiated pleomorphic sarcoma (UPS), synovial sarcoma (SS), and dermatofibrosarcoma protuberans (DFSP). UPS is the most common soft tissue sarcoma in adults. Up to 5% of these tumors will present as a fluctuant hemorrhagic mass and may be misdiagnosed as a hematoma. Approximately 3.5% of undifferentiated pleomorphic sarcomas are located in the foot and ankle.[65] SS is a soft tissue sarcoma commonly found in the lower extremities of young adults and often

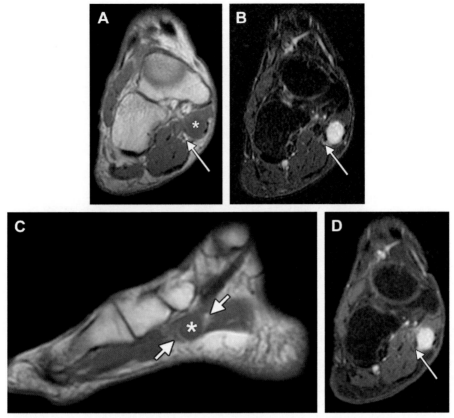

Fig. 13. Schwannoma in a 56-year-old woman with a 6-month history of medial foot pain. Short-axis T1-WI (*A*) and short tau inversion recovery (*B*) images through the midfoot show a low to intermediate T1-weighted and intensely hyperintense T2-weighted mass (*asterisk*) located within the abductor hallucis muscle. The medial plantar nerve (*arrows*) is not involved, and no target sign is identified. (*C*) Sagittal T1-WI shows the low to intermediate signal mass (*asterisk*) surrounded by caps of fat (*arrows*), indicating slow growth. (*D*) Short-axis post-contrast T1-WI with FS shows avid lesion enhancement mass and no involvement of medial plantar nerve (*arrow*).

located near joints. SS is the sixth most common soft tissue malignancy and involves the foot and ankle in 18% of cases. DFSP presents in early adulthood as a firm subcutaneous nodule protruding from the skin, a feature that, when present, can be used to make a prospective diagnosis on imaging.[66] DFSP is the fifth most common soft tissue malignancy and involves the foot and ankle in 5% of cases and the foot alone in 2%.[65,66]

Radiographs and CT are useful for detecting periosteal reaction and extrinsic cortical erosion and detecting and characterizing soft tissue calcifications (**Fig. 14**A), because between 20% and 30% of SS will be associated with calcifications. Ultrasound is useful for differentiating solid sarcomatous lesions from cysts.[67] On ultrasound, soft tissue sarcomas are large, usually subfascial, heterogeneously hypoechoic masses.

On MR imaging (**Fig. 14**B–D), soft tissue sarcomas can have nonspecific imaging features and can be difficult to differentiate from one another. Soft tissue sarcomas can have variable T1 and T2 characteristics owing to frequent hemorrhage and necrosis.[67] When large, these lesions commonly have marked heterogeneity on T2-WI sequences, with hemorrhage and necrosis mixed with solid components. The so-called triple sign is seen frequently with SS and is described as areas of low, intermediate, and high signal intensity on long repetition time sequences.[68] However, this finding is not specific for SS and can be seen with other soft tissue sarcomas as well.[68] Finally, the radiologist must be aware that small soft tissue sarcomas can have deceptively low-grade appearances on imaging because of their homogeneous appearance. The sensitivity of FDG uptake for soft tissue sarcomas is 80% to 90%.[69]

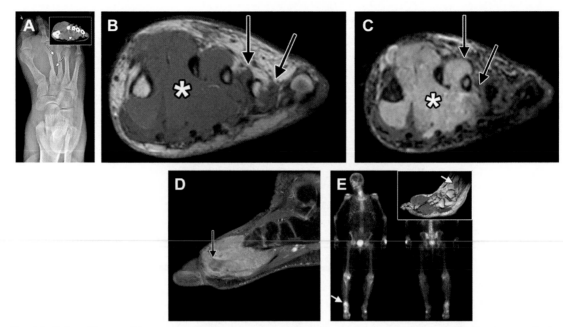

Fig. 14. SS in a 55-year-old woman with right foot mass and pain. (*A*) Frontal radiograph demonstrates splaying of the first and second metatarsals with extrinsic erosion of the medial cortex of the second metatarsal. Soft tissue calcifications (*arrows*) project between the second and third metatarsals and should not be mistaken for athero-sclerotic calcifications. *Inset:* CT image from PET/CT confirms calcifications within the lesion (*arrow*). (*B*) Short-axis T1-WI shows an intermediate to high signal mass (*asterisk*) centered between the first and second metatarsals that erodes the second metatarsal, involves both the dorsal and plantar compartments, and extends laterally (*arrows*). (*C*) Short-axis short tau inversion recovery image shows an intermediate to high signal mass (*asterisk*) centered between the first and second metatarsals, eroding the second metatarsal, involving both the dorsal and plantar compartments, and extending laterally (*arrows*). (*D*) Sagittal postcontrast T1-WI with FS shows the complexity of the mass, with a dominant enhancing component and a necrotic area anteriorly (*arrow*). (*E*) Tc-99m MDP bone scan shows uptake in the ankle and in the distal tibia (*arrow*). The distal tibia was not imaged on initial imaging performed at an outside facility. *Inset:* Repeat imaging with a wide FOV shows the distal tibial lesion (*arrow*). The lesion in the contralateral midfoot was mechanical in cause and related to altered weight bearing by the patient because of the large right foot mass.

SUMMARY

Lesions about the foot and ankle are most commonly non-neoplastic masses or benign neoplasms. Appropriate care of patients presenting with palpable masses about the foot and ankle requires awareness of the often nonspecific imaging features of bone and soft tissue neoplasms and knowledge of the cases when specific features allow for a prospective diagnosis to be made.

REFERENCES

1. Wulling M, Engels C, Jesse N, et al. The nature of gi-ant cell tumor of bone. J Cancer Res Clin Oncol 2001;127:467–74.
2. Frassica FJ, Sanjay BK, Unni KK, et al. Benign giant cell tumor. Orthopedics 1993;16:1179–83.
3. Reddy CR, Rao PS, Rajakumari K. Giant-cell tumors of bone in South India. J Bone Joint Surg Am 1974; 56:617–9.
4. Chakarun CJ, Forrester DM, Gottsegen CJ, et al. Gi-ant cell tumor of bone: review, mimics, and new de-velopments in treatment. Radiographics 2013;33: 197–211.
5. Burns TP, Weiss M, Snyder M, et al. Giant cell tumor of the metatarsal. Foot Ankle 1988;8:223–6.
6. Wold LE, Swee RG. Giant cell tumor of the small bones of the hands and feet. Semin Diagn Pathol 1984;1:173–84.
7. Dahlin DC, Cupps RE, Johnson EW Jr. Giant-cell tu-mor: a study of 195 cases. Cancer 1970;25:1061–70.
8. Ozdemir HM, Yildiz Y, Yilmaz C, et al. Tumors of the foot and ankle: analysis of 196 cases. J Foot Ankle Surg 1997;36:403–8.
9. Biscaglia R, Bacchini P, Bertoni F. Giant cell tumor of the bones of the hand and foot. Cancer 2000;88: 2022–32.
10. Hudson TM, Schiebler M, Springfield DS, et al. Radi-ology of giant cell tumors of bone: computed tomog-raphy, arthro-tomography, and scintigraphy. Skeletal Radiol 1984;11:85–95.

11. Murphey MD. Giant cell tumor. In: Davies M, editor. Imaging of bone tumors and tumor-like lesions. Berlin (Germany): Springer; 2009. p. 321–36.

12. Murphey MD, Nomikos GC, Flemming DJ, et al. From the archives of AFIP. Imaging of giant cell tumor and giant cell reparative granuloma of bone: radiologic-pathologic correlation. Radiographics 2001;21:1283–309.

13. Kyriakos M, Land VJ, Penning HL, et al. Metastatic chondroblastoma. Report of a fatal case with a review of the literature on atypical, aggressive, and malignant chondroblastoma. Cancer 1985;55: 1770–89.

14. McLeod RA, Beabout JW. The roentgenographic features of chondroblastoma. Am J Roentgenol Radium Ther Nucl Med 1973;118:464–71.

15. Davila JA, Amrami KK, Sundaram M, et al. Chondroblastoma of the hands and feet. Skeletal Radiol 2004;33:582–7.

16. Weatherall PT, Maale GE, Mendelsohn DB, et al. Chondroblastoma: classic and confusing appearance at MR imaging. Radiology 1994;190:467–74.

17. Miyayama H, Sakamoto K, Ide M, et al. Aggressive osteoblastoma of the calcaneus. Cancer 1993;71: 346–53.

18. Temple HT, Mizel MS, Murphey MD, et al. Osteoblastoma of the foot and ankle. Foot Ankle Int 1998;19: 698–704.

19. Giannestras NJ, Diamond JR. Benign osteoblastoma of the talus: a review of the literature and report of a case. J Bone Joint Surg Am 1958;40-A:469–78.

20. Martin NL, Preston DF, Robinson RG. Osteoblastomas of the axial skeleton shown by skeletal scanning: case report. J Nucl Med 1976;17:187–9.

21. Kirsch J, Ilaslan H, Bauer TW, et al. The incidence of imaging findings, and the distribution of skeletal lymphoma in a consecutive patient population seen over 5 years. Skeletal Radiol 2006;35:590–4.

22. Ruzek KA, Wenger DE. The multiple faces of lymphoma of the musculoskeletal system. Skeletal Radiol 2004;33:1–8.

23. Braunstein EM, White SJ. Non-Hodgkin lymphoma of bone. Radiology 1980;135:59–63.

24. Mulligan ME, McRae GA, Murphey MD. Imaging features of primary lymphoma of bone. AJR Am J Roentgenol 1999;173:1691–7.

25. Krishnan A, Shirkhoda A, Tehranzadeh J, et al. Primary bone lymphoma: radiographic-MR imaging correlation. Radiographics 2003;23:1371–83.

26. Taira AV, Herfkens RJ, Gambhir SS, et al. Detection of bone metastases: assessment of integrated FDG PET/CT imaging. Radiology 2007;243:204–11.

27. Sanchez E, Martin-Carreras T, Bornstein G, et al. Osteosarcoma of the foot. Orthopedics 2015;38:656, 708–11.

28. Clayer M. Many faces of osteosarcoma on plain radiographs. ANZ J Surg 2015;85:22–6.

29. Murphey MD, Robbin MR, McRae GA, et al. The many faces of osteosarcoma. Radiographics 1997; 17:1205–31.

30. Dahlin DC, Henderson ED. Chondrosarcoma, a surgical and pathological problem; review of 212 cases. J Bone Joint Surg Am 1956;38-A:1025–38.

31. Soldatos T, McCarthy EF, Attar S, et al. Imaging features of chondrosarcoma. J Comput Assist Tomogr 2011;35:504–11.

32. Hottya GA, Steinbach LS, Johnston JO, et al. Chondrosarcoma of the foot: imaging, surgical and pathological correlation of three new cases. Skeletal Radiol 1999;28:153–8.

33. Aoki J, Watanabe H, Shinozaki T, et al. FDG-PET in differential diagnosis and grading of chondrosarcomas. J Comput Assist Tomogr 1999;23:603–8.

34. Hattrup SJ, Amadio PC, Sim FH, et al. Metastatic tumors of the foot and ankle. Foot Ankle 1988;8: 243–7.

35. Maheshwari AV, Chiappetta G, Kugler CD, et al. Metastatic skeletal disease of the foot: case reports and literature review. Foot Ankle Int 2008;29:699–710.

36. Libson E, Bloom RA, Husband JE, et al. Metastatic tumours of bones of the hand and foot. A comparative review and report of 43 additional cases. Skeletal Radiol 1987;16:387–92.

37. Zindrick MR, Young MP, Daley RJ, et al. Metastatic tumors of the foot: case report and literature review. Clin Orthop Relat Res 1982;170:219–25.

38. Schwartz ED, Donahue FI, Bromson MS, et al. Metastatic prostate carcinoma to the foot with magnetic resonance imaging and pathologic correlation. Foot Ankle Int 1998;19:594–7.

39. Nielsen GP, O'Connell JX. Tumors of synovial tissue. In: Folpe AL, Inwards CY, editors. Bone and soft tissue pathology. Philadelphia: Saunders/Elsevier; 2010. p. 255–61.

40. Murphey MD, Rhee JH, Lewis RB, et al. Pigmented villonodular synovitis: radiologic-pathologic correlation. Radiographics 2008;28:1493–518.

41. Brien EW, Sacoman DM, Mirra JM. Pigmented villonodular synovitis of the foot and ankle. Foot Ankle Int 2004;25:908–13.

42. Cheng XG, You YH, Liu W, et al. MRI features of pigmented villonodular synovitis (PVNS). Clin Rheumatol 2004;23:31–4.

43. Amber IB, Clark BJ, Greene GS. Pigmented villonodular synovitis: dedicated PET imaging findings. BMJ Case Rep 2013;2013:3.

44. International Society for the Study of Vascular Anomalies. ISSVA classification of vascular anomalies. 2014. Available at: issva.org/classification. Accessed January 28, 2018.

45. Moukaddam H, Pollak J, Haims AH. MRI characteristics and classification of peripheral vascular malformations and tumors. Skeletal Radiol 2009;38: 535–47.

46. Folpe AL. Vascular tumors of soft tissue. In: Folpe AL, Inwards CY, editors. Bone and soft tissue pathology. Philadelphia: Saunders/Elsevier; 2010. p. 164–92.

47. Bruegel M, Waldt S, Weirich G, et al. Multifocal epithelioid hemangioendothelioma of the phalanges of the hand. Skeletal Radiol 2006;35:787–92.

48. Teniola O, Wang KY, Wang WL, et al. Imaging of liposarcomas for clinicians: characteristic features and differential considerations. J Surg Oncol 2018;117:1195–203.

49. Guillou L, Folpe AL. Fibroblastic and fibrohistiocytic tumors. In: Folpe AL, Inwards CY, editors. Bone and soft tissue pathology. Philadelphia: Saunders/Elsevier; 2010. p. 53–8.

50. Zgonis T, Jolly GP, Polyzois V, et al. Plantar fibromatosis. Clin Podiatr Med Surg 2005;22:11–8.

51. Theodorou DJ, Theodorou SJ, Farooki S, et al. Disorders of the plantar aponeurosis: a spectrum of MR imaging findings. AJR Am J Roentgenol 2001;176:97–104.

52. Veith NT, Tschernig T, Histing T, et al. Plantar fibromatosis–topical review. Foot Ankle Int 2013;34:1742–6.

53. Griffith JF, Wong TY, Wong SM, et al. Sonography of plantar fibromatosis. AJR Am J Roentgenol 2002;179:1167–72.

54. Hosalkar HS, Fox EJ, Delaney T, et al. Desmoid tumors and current status of management. Orthop Clin North Am 2006;37:53–63.

55. Saleem O, Sayres S, O'Malley M. Extra-abdominal periosteal desmoid tumor of the third toe. Orthopedics 2013;36:e1209–12.

56. Murphey MD, Ruble CM, Tyszko SM, et al. From the archives of the AFIP: musculoskeletal fibromatoses: radiologic-pathologic correlation. Radiographics 2009;29:2143–73.

57. Llauger J, Palmer J, Monill JM, et al. MR imaging of benign soft-tissue masses of the foot and ankle. Radiographics 1998;18:1481–98.

58. English C, Coughlan R, Carey J, et al. Plantar and palmar fibromatosis: characteristic imaging features and role of MRI in clinical management. Rheumatology (Oxford) 2012;51:1134–6.

59. Kamali F, Wang WL, Guadagnolo BA, et al. MRI may be used as a prognostic indicator in patients with extra-abdominal desmoid tumours. Br J Radiol 2016;89(1058):20150308.

60. Gilchrist JH, Donahue JE. Peripheral nerve tumors. In: Shefner JM, Maki R, editors. UpToDate. 2018. Available at: https://www.uptodate.com/contents/peripheral-nerve-tumors. Accessed January 28, 2018.

61. Kwon JH, Yoon JR, Kim TS, et al. Peripheral nerve sheath tumor of the medial plantar nerve without tarsal tunnel syndrome: a case report. J Foot Ankle Surg 2009;48:477–82.

62. Winter N, Rattay TW, Axer H, et al. Ultrasound assessment of peripheral nerve pathology in neurofibromatosis type 1 and 2. Clin Neurophysiol 2017;128:702–6.

63. Varma DG, Moulopoulos A, Sara AS, et al. MR imaging of extracranial nerve sheath tumors. J Comput Assist Tomogr 1992;16:448–53.

64. Chrisinger JSA, Salem UI, Kindblom LG, et al. Synovial sarcoma of peripheral nerves: analysis of 15 cases. Am J Surg Pathol 2017;41:1087–96.

65. Kransdorf MJ. Malignant soft-tissue tumors in a large referral population: distribution of diagnoses by age, sex, and location. AJR Am J Roentgenol 1995;164:129–34.

66. McPeak CJ, Cruz T, Nicastri AD. Dermatofibrosarcoma protuberans: an analysis of 86 cases–five with metastasis. Ann Surg 1967;166:803–16.

67. Robinson E, Bleakney RR, Ferguson PC, et al. Oncodiagnosis panel: 2007: multidisciplinary management of soft-tissue sarcoma. Radiographics 2008;28:2069–86.

68. Murphey MD, Gibson MS, Jennings BT, et al. From the archives of the AFIP: imaging of synovial sarcoma with radiologic-pathologic correlation. Radiographics 2006;26:1543–65.

69. Mettler FA, Guiberteau MJ. Essentials of nuclear medicine imaging. 5th edition. Philadelphia: Saunders/Elsevier; 2006.

An Update and Comprehensive Review of the Posterolateral Corner of the Knee

Jack Porrino, MD[a,*], Jake W. Sharp, MD[b],
Tolu Ashimolowo, MD[b], Gregor Dunham, MD[b]

KEYWORDS

- Posterolateral corner • Fibular collateral ligament • Lateral collateral ligament • Biceps femoris
- Popliteus • Arcuate ligament • Fabellofibular ligament • Popliteofibular ligament

KEY POINTS

- Isolated injuries to the posterolateral corner (PLC) of the knee are rare, and usually occur in conjunction with injury to a cruciate ligament.
- If unrecognized, PLC injuries can result in posterolateral instability, and may contribute to cruciate ligament graft failure.
- The anatomy of the PLC is confusing as a result of the number of structures that have been described, variability in nomenclature, and variability in identification of said structures.
- A recognition of the variations in anatomy and of the limitations of MR imaging with regard to evaluation of the PLC is necessary in the imaging assessment.
- Low-grade injuries of the PLC are often managed nonoperatively, whereas more significant PLC injuries, or those involving the biceps femoris, fibular collateral ligament, and/or popliteus, may require operative intervention.

INTRODUCTION

The lateral compartment of the knee is composed of numerous ligamentous and tendinous structures, providing primary restraint against varus angulation, external-internal rotation, and anterior-posterior translation.[1] Lateral knee instability, whether acute or chronic, is not as common as medial, and posterolateral instability is considerably less common than anterolateral.[1–3] The lateral ligaments are under extreme tension when the knee is at or near full extension during standing and walking. This results in considerable distraction of the lateral compartment, and may explain why instability in the lateral compartment causes significantly more disability than an equivalent amount in the medial compartment.[1,2]

Isolated injury to the lateral knee structures is rare, instead, typically combined with cruciate ligament tears or damage to the medial stabilizing structures.[1,4–11] Injuries to the posterolateral corner (PLC) structures of the knee can easily be overlooked on knee examination, in particular when there is a concomitant tear of the anterior cruciate ligament.[1,3,5,7,12–14] Injury to the PLC can be misdiagnosed as a tear of the lateral meniscus or posterior cruciate ligament.[2]

Disclosures: The authors report no commercial or financial conflicts of interest, nor any funding sources.
[a] Radiology and Biomedical Imaging, Yale School of Medicine, 20 York Street, New Haven, CT 06510, USA;
[b] Department of Radiology, University of Washington, 1959 Northeast Pacific Street, Seattle, WA 98195-7117, USA
* Corresponding author.
E-mail address: rhees27@yahoo.com

Radiol Clin N Am 56 (2018) 935–951
https://doi.org/10.1016/j.rcl.2018.06.006
0033-8389/18/© 2018 Elsevier Inc. All rights reserved.

The injury can result in posterolateral rotary instability, with resultant pain and functional impairment, including reduced activity and a sense of knee disability and instability. Acutely, pain over the joint line, ecchymosis, swelling, sequela of peroneal nerve injury, and an inability to walk are the main complaints, whereas in chronic cases, instability with side-to-side activities, inadvertent hyperextension or a varus thrust, difficulty maintaining full extension, and limited ability to resume sports activities are common complaints. The varied mechanisms of injury that have been described in the literature include a posterolateral/varus force applied to the proximal anteromedial tibia of an extended knee, noncontact injury causing hyperextension and external rotation or severe tibial external rotation in a partially flexed knee, contact hyperextension, external tibial rotation over a fixed foot, direct varus force with the tibia in external rotation, twisting, and a valgus force on a flexed knee.[3–7,9–11,13,15–17]

Various clinical tests are used to assess for posterolateral instability. These have numerous names and descriptions in the literature, and include the external rotation-recurvatum test, reverse pivot shift test, posterolateral external rotation test with the knee at 30° of flexion, adduction test at 30° of flexion, posterolateral draw test both with and without internal tibial rotation, lateral joint opening at 20° under varus stress, external rotation at 30° and at 90° (dial test), hyperextension/recurvatum test, and the external rotation drawer test.[5,8,9,15,18] In addition to posterolateral instability, it has been recognized and demonstrated that failure of a reconstructed cruciate ligament may be due to associated, and unaddressed, damage of the PLC.[1,3,6,8–10,12,14,16,17,19–22]

NORMAL ANATOMY AND IMAGING TECHNIQUE

The anatomy of the PLC can be described as both complex and poorly understood. This is related to the sheer number of structures that have been described, their variability in visibility on imaging, as well as their variability in nomenclature and presence from person to person.[5,7,16,20,21,23] For decades, there have been numerous attempts made to divide the lateral knee, and the posterolateral aspect specifically, into separate structures to assist with mitigating this confusion.

In 1976, Hughston and colleagues[2] divided the lateral compartment ligaments into anterior, middle, and posterior thirds. In this description, the anterior third of the lateral compartment of the knee is composed of the capsular ligament,

extending posteriorly from the lateral aspect of the patella, to the anterior border of the iliotibial band. This ligament is reinforced by the lateral extension, or retinaculum, of the quadriceps tendon.[2] The middle third of the lateral ligaments is composed of the iliotibial band and the capsular ligament deep to it, extending posteriorly to the fibular collateral ligament. The middle third of the lateral capsular ligament, or more recently the anterolateral ligament, attaches proximally to the lateral epicondyle of the femur and distally at the tibial joint margin.[2,24] The posterior third of the lateral compartment of the knee is a single functional unit, dubbed the arcuate complex, and composed of both capsular and noncapsular ligaments. Hughston and colleagues[2] defined these components as the fibular collateral ligament, arcuate ligament, and the tendoaponeurotic unit formed by the popliteus muscle.

Later, in 1982, Seebacher and colleagues[25] divided the lateral structures into 3 layers, from superficial to deep. The superficial layer, or layer 1, is composed of the iliotibial tract, and its expansion anteriorly, as well as the biceps femoris, and its expansion posteriorly. Layer 2 is composed of the retinaculum of the quadriceps, 2 patellofemoral ligaments, and a patellomeniscal ligament. Layer 3, or the deepest layer, is the lateral part of the joint capsule. The capsular attachment to the outer periphery of the lateral meniscus is termed the coronary ligament, with the popliteus tendon coursing through a hiatus in the coronary ligament to attach to the femur. The capsule is divided into 2 laminae, the superficial of which is composed of the fibular collateral ligament and fabellofibular ligament, whereas the deeper lamina is composed of the coronary ligament and Y-shaped arcuate ligament. The investigators noted variability in the presence and size of the fabellofibular (absent when the fabella is not present, and supplemented by a robust arcuate ligament) and arcuate ligaments on cadaveric dissection.[25]

Robert LaPrade has authored numerous studies that have described a detailed portrayal of the PLC. In the late 1990s, LaPrade and Terry[15] provided an in-depth review of the PLC through varied works. In these descriptions, a variety of structures, with elaborate divisions, comprise the PLC. These structures include superficial, capsulo-osseous, and deep layers of the iliotibial tract; long head of the biceps femoris muscle (anterior, direct, and reflected arms; anterior and lateral aponeuroses); short head of the biceps femoris muscle (proximal attachment to the biceps tendon, capsular arm, biceps-capsulo-osseous layer of the iliotibial tract confluens, anterior and direct arms, and lateral aponeurotic expansion); fibular collateral ligament; midthird lateral capsular ligament; fabellofibular ligament; posterior arcuate ligament (medial and lateral limbs); popliteus complex (muscle; tendon; anteroinferior, posterosuperior, and posteroinferior popliteomeniscal fascicles; and popliteofibular ligament); coronary ligament; posterior capsule; and lateral gastrocnemius tendon.[26] This level of detail is not perceptible on a routine MR imaging study of the knee.

Numerous other investigators, through a variety of other studies and reviews, have described the PLC structures throughout the 1990s and early 2000s. These structures and names have included, but are not limited to, the iliotibial band, biceps femoris, lateral collateral ligament or fibular collateral ligament, popliteus muscle and tendon, arcuate ligament, fabellofibular ligament, popliteal origin from the fibular head or popliteal fibular ligament or popliteofibular ligament, popliteal meniscal ligament or popliteomeniscal fibers or popliteomeniscal fascicles, popliteotibial fibers, popliteocapsular fibers, lateral head of the gastrocnemius, oblique popliteal ligament, and posterolateral joint capsule.[1,3–5,7,8,11,20,27]

Notably, some of the defined structures of the PLC have only variably been present on prior anatomic dissections, as well as on MR imaging–based studies. For instance, although the superior and inferior popliteomeniscal fascicles are reportedly apparent on MR imaging most of the time, Johnson and De Smet[28] identified 2 cases in which both fascicles were not apparent in one knee, and the superior not apparent in another, without an arthroscopic explanation in either case. In a study comparing anatomic dissection with MRI, De Maeseneer and colleagues[14] reviewed 122 MR examinations of knees, using standard imaging planes, without PLC symptomatology, and found the fabellofibular ligament identifiable in 33%, the medial limb of the arcuate ligament in 25%, the lateral limb of the arcuate ligament in 23%, the popliteofibular ligament in 38%, and the fabella in 26% (18% of knees with a bony fabella, and 8% with a cartilaginous fabella) of knees. Munshi and colleagues[21] reported variable identification of the arcuate ligament, or components thereof, on 7 cadaveric knees that were sectioned, as well as imaged with MR imaging. The investigators were unable to identify the fabellofibular ligament on section or MR imaging. The popliteofibular ligament was visualized in 57% (4 of 7) of the specimens. Rajeswaran and co-authors[6] nicely summarized the literature regarding the ability to identify the popliteofibular ligament on MR imaging, with a range of 8% to 69% using varied routine, as well as optimized protocol

techniques to evaluate the PLC. In a recent review of those with documented PLC pathology, Collins and colleagues[9] concluded that the arcuate ligament and fabellofibular ligament could not be confidently visualized in any of 22 MR images reviewed, but noted that abundant signal abnormality in the region of the posterior capsule, which was present in all cases, suggests an injury of the arcuate ligament.

As Temponi and colleagues[22] reported, the major confusion about PLC anatomy in the orthopedic literature lies with the structures that course from the fibular head and attach the popliteus complex and the joint capsule of the posterolateral aspect of the knee. All of these structures are difficult to identify separately in cadaveric and clinical evaluations. We detail the more commonly described structures of the PLC (**Fig. 1**).

COMMON STRUCTURES
Iliotibial Band

The iliotibial band is a combination of the tendon of the tensor fascia lata and the deep and superficial fibers of the fascia lata.[1,16] The structure originates from the anterior superior iliac spine and the anterior aspect of the iliac crest, and inserts primarily onto the anterolateral tibial plateau.[17] It has been divided into superficial, deep, and capsulo-osseous layers at its distal attachment. The superficial layer inserts distally onto the Gerdy tubercle at the anterolateral tibia, and is rarely injured, serving as a useful reference point for lateral knee structures (see **Fig. 1**).[1,13,16,17] The deep layer of the iliotibial band attaches the superficial layer to the lateral supracondylar tubercle of the femur, blending into the intermuscular septum at the distal femur, and is reportedly susceptible to avulsion injury and interstitial-type tears.[13,16,17,23] The capsulo-osseous layer is situated deep and posterior to the deep layer, and forms a sling over the lateral femoral condyle, inserting onto the tibial tuberosity posterior and proximal to Gerdy tubercle. The deep and capsulo-osseous layers of the iliotibial band are commonly known as "Kaplan fibers."[17,23]

Biceps femoris muscle

The biceps femoris muscle is fusiform, with 2 heads: long and short.[17] The biceps femoris tendon descends behind the iliotibial tract.[1] LaPrade and colleagues[13] provided the most detailed description of the biceps femoris muscle and tendon at the level of the knee. They divide the long head into 2 tendinous components (a direct and anterior arm) and either 3 or 4 fascial components: reflected arm, anterior and lateral

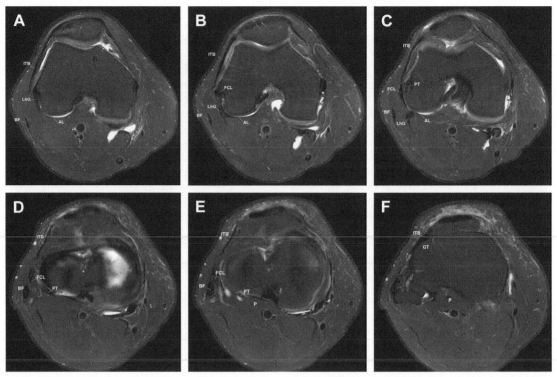

Fig. 1. Normal anatomy of the posterolateral corner in a 45-year-old man with recent hyperextension injury. Sequential axial T2 fat-suppressed images from cranial to caudal (*A-F*) show the relationships of the iliotibial band (*ITB*), fibular collateral ligament (*FCL*), lateral head of the gastrocnemius (*LhG*), biceps femoris (*BF*), arcuate ligament (*AL*), and popliteus muscle (*P*) and tendon (*PT*). The ITB inserts onto Gerdy tubercle (*GT*) on the antero-lateral tibia. The LhG, FCL, and PT all have posterolateral attachments on the femur. Note, the LhG arises most proximal, followed by the FCL, then the PT. This relationship is universally maintained in all patients. The BF joins the FCL distally to form a conjoined tendon that attaches to the fibular head.

aponeurotic expansions, and a distal expansion to the lateral gastrocnemius complex (the distal expansion is not mentioned in all of the LaPrade descriptions). The direct arm inserts onto the posterolateral edge of the fibular head, whereas the anterior arm attaches to the lateral edge of the fibular head or the lateral tibial plateau (this description varies among LaPrade publications and descriptions). The reflected arm attaches to the posterior edge of the iliotibial tract, just proximal to the fibular head, whereas the lateral aponeurotic expansion connects the long and short heads of the biceps femoris to the posterolateral fibular collateral ligament.[17,23,26] LaPrade and colleagues[13] found that the direct and anterior arms were reliably identifiable on MR imaging.

Terry and LaPrade divide the short head of the biceps femoris into 6 components, with attachments to the long head biceps femoris muscle, posterolateral joint capsule, capsule-osseous layer of the iliotibial tract, 2 sites on the fibular head, and to the fibular collateral ligament.[26] The 2 tendinous components (the direct and anterior

arms) are reportedly readily apparent on MR imaging. The direct arm inserts onto the posterolateral fibular head, just lateral to the tip of the styloid process and medial to the direct arm attachment of the long head of the biceps femoris, whereas the anterior arm passes medial to the fibular collateral ligament, inserting onto the posterolateral tibial tuberosity, posterior to Gerdy tubercle (the same attachment site as the midthird lateral capsular ligament).[13] A capsular arm inserts just lateral to the tip of the fibular styloid or the posterolateral joint capsule and lateral gastrocnemius complex depending on the reference.[17,23]

Munshi and co-authors[21] divided the long head of the biceps femoris into a direct arm, attaching to the anterior and posterolateral aspects of the fibular head, and an anterior arm, attaching anteriorly relative to the direct arm onto the anterolateral edge of the fibular head, and continuing distally and terminating as the anterior aponeurosis around the leg. The investigators divided the short head of the biceps femoris into 2 tendinous components, with the direct arm inserting onto the fibular head and the anterior arm onto the supero-lateral edge of the lateral tibial condyle, continuing anteriorly as far as 1 cm posterior to the Gerdy tubercle.[21]

In more simplistic terms, the biceps femoris tendon consists of different portions, including tendinous and fascial components, most of which attach to the fibular head, although an attachment to the tibia also may be present.[14] In a cadaveric dissection, Lee and colleagues[5] demonstrated the distal tendon of the biceps femoris merging with the fibular collateral ligament 1 cm above the fibular head, and inserting as a single band, or "conjoined tendon," onto the lateral aspect of the fibular head. This conjoined attachment of the biceps femoris and fibular collateral ligament is how we conceptualize the fibular attachment of these structures as well (**Fig. 2**).

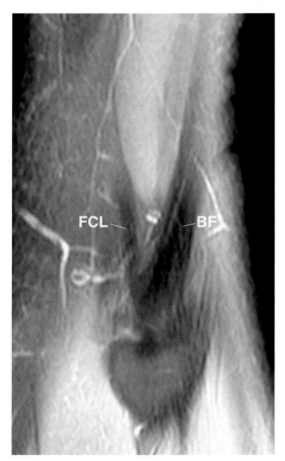

Fig. 2. Normal conjoined tendon in a 21-year-old man with pain following basketball injury. Sagittal proton density fat-suppressed image shows the normal fibular collateral ligament (*FCL*) and biceps femoris (*BF*) tendon as they blend into a conjoined tendon at their insertion onto the fibular head.

Fibular/lateral collateral ligament The fibular collateral ligament, or lateral collateral ligament, originates from the distal femur in a fanlike fashion between the lateral epicondyle and supracondylar process (attaching just proximal and posterior to the lateral epicondyle), and directly anterior to the lateral head of the gastrocnemius muscle. Distally, the medial fibers attach to the lateral edge of the fibular head, most commonly joining with the biceps femoris tendon as a "conjoined tendon," as described previously, whereas the lateral fibers continue distally, and blend with the superficial fascia of the lateral compartment of the leg (see **Fig. 2**). The insertion of the fibular collateral ligament on the fibular head is anterior and lateral relative to the fabellofibular and arcuate ligaments, and distal to the tip of the fibular styloid process.[1,4,7,13,14,16,17,21,23,26,29] The ligament is extracapsular and has no meniscal attachment.[7,17]

Popliteus, popliteofibular ligament, and popliteomeniscal fascicles

The popliteus muscle has a wide attachment onto the posteromedial tibia proximal to the soleal line, and is composed of anterior and posterior fibers, or deep and superficial layers.[1,17,20,26] The tendon, which is intracapsular, but extra-articular and extrasynovial, ascends around the posterolateral aspect of the knee, deep to the arcuate and fabellofibular ligaments (which form the "arcuate roof" of the popliteal hiatus per Munshi and colleagues[21]), through the popliteal hiatus, passes under the fibular collateral ligament, with its tendon attaching to the lateral surface of the lateral femoral condyle at the popliteal groove or sulcus (see **Fig. 1**).[1,7,13,14,17,27,29]

The presence of a fibular attachment of the popliteus, or popliteofibular ligament, was described as early as 1894, but largely ignored until 1950, when the structure was termed the "short external lateral ligament" by Last RJ.[20] De Maeseneer and colleagues[14] reported that this ligament is present in "most" knees. In the early description of the deep PLC soft tissues by Watanabe and colleagues,[27] the popliteus demonstrates an attachment to the fibular head, present in 93% of cadaveric knees evaluated. The investigators named this attachment the "popliteus muscle with origin from the fibular head," or OFH. LaPrade and colleagues[29] provided a very thorough description of the popliteofibular ligament. The investigators reported a popliteofibular ligament inserting onto the fibular head in an inverted Y-shaped configuration, anterior to the styloid, and therefore anterior to the 2 structures that attach to the styloid: lateral limb of the arcuate ligament and fabellofibular ligament. The popliteofibular ligament is separated from these 2 structures by the inferior lateral geniculate artery. The investigators reported 2 divisions of the popliteofibular ligament (anterior and posterior), with fibers extending to the fibula and lateral tibia.[17,23,26]

There have been numerous descriptions of the popliteofibular ligament in the literature. In these descriptions, the popliteofibular ligament originates within the region of the musculotendinous junction of the popliteus, descending and attaching to the fibular head. In contrast to the description of the fibular attachment being anterior to the arcuate and fabellofibular ligament by LaPrade and colleagues,[13,29] others have reported an insertion onto the upper facet of the apex of the fibular head, just medial and posterior to the insertions of the arcuate and fabellofibular ligaments (**Fig. 3**).[1,3,5,7,10,19–21]

The popliteomeniscal fascicles are the synovial attachments of the lateral meniscus that form the popliteus bursa, through which the popliteus tendon passes. These 2 structures, superior and inferior, serve as struts, stabilizing the posterior horn of the lateral meniscus. The superior arises from the medial fibers of the aponeurosis of the popliteus tendon, whereas the inferior extends from the meniscus to the tibia. Disruption of the fascicles may lead to subluxation or tear of the meniscus.[28] Numerous investigators support this description, and explain that these 2 fascicles form the superior and inferior boundaries of the popliteal hiatus, and that well-defined fluid surrounding the popliteus muscle and tendon is said to be within the popliteus bursa (**Fig. 4**).[7,21,30]

Others have presented variations to this description. For instance, LaPrade and colleagues reported attachment of the posterior horn of the lateral meniscus with the aponeurosis of the popliteus and to the tibia by way of the posteroinferior popliteomeniscal fascicle, and attachment of the posterior horn of the lateral meniscus with the popliteal tendon by way of the posterosuperior popliteomeniscal fascicle. The investigators also reported an anteroinferior popliteomeniscal fascicle, arising along the anterior edge of the popliteal tendon, forming the anterior boundary of the popliteal hiatus. The medial boundary of the popliteal hiatus is reportedly formed by the coronary ligament, which connects lateral meniscus to tibia.[17,23,26] Recondo and colleagues[1] described attachment of the popliteus muscle to the lateral meniscus via a popliteal meniscal ligament.

Fabellofibular ligament
Based on numerous prior reports, the fabellofibular ligament is a potentially variably present

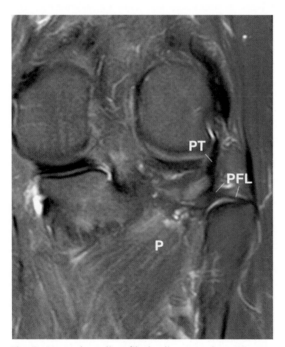

Fig. 3. Normal popliteofibular ligament in a 53-year-old man undergoing surveillance of soft tissue sarcoma. Coronal short tau inversion recovery image shows the popliteofibular ligament (*PFL*) arising from the musculotendinous junction of the popliteus muscle (*P*) and tendon (*PT*) and attaching onto the fibular head.

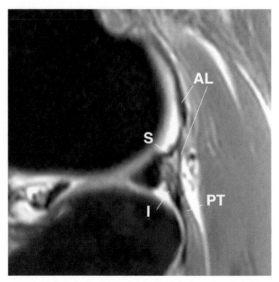

Fig. 4. Normal popliteomeniscal fascicles in a 54-year-old woman with knee pain. Sagittal proton density fat-suppressed image shows the borders of the popliteal hiatus derived from the superior (*S*) and inferior (*I*) popliteomeniscal fascicles. The popliteus tendon (*PT*) enters through the hiatus. AL, arcuate ligament.

structure within the PLC of the knee (**Figs. 5** and **6**). For instance, Lee and co-authors could not identify the fabellofibular ligament during anatomic dissection of 3 cadaveric specimens.[5] However, LaPrade and colleagues[23] have reported that the structure is always present, but more substantial in knees with a bony fabella, is difficult to identify when the knee is flexed and the ligament lax, and is particularly difficult to identify in formalin-preserved knees.

LaPrade and colleagues[13] described the ligament as a thickening of the distal edge of the capsular arm of the short head of the biceps femoris muscle.[17,23] The ligament reportedly runs from the fabella, or fabella-analog, inserting just lateral to the tip of the fibular styloid process, posterior to the arcuate ligament, anterolateral or posterior to the popliteofibular ligament depending on the reference, and medial to the direct arm of the short head of the biceps femoris muscle.[3,13,17,21,25,27]

Although some investigators have reported that the ligament is absent if there is no fabella, others have contradicted this statement.[25] LaPrade and colleagues[17,26] reported the ligament is indeed present regardless of the presence of a fabella: when the fabella is absent, the ligament runs from the posterior aspect of the supracondylar process of the femur, blending with the lateral

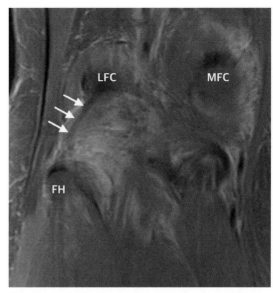

Fig. 6. Fabellofibular ligament in a 34-year-old man following trauma. Coronal proton density fat-suppressed image shows edema within the posterior soft tissues, which helps outline the fabellofibular ligament (*arrows*). FH, fibular head; LFC, lateral femoral condyle; MFC, medial femoral condyle.

gastrocnemius tendon, to the fibular styloid process just posterior to the lateral arm of the arcuate. Recondo and colleagues[1] reported a fabella present in 20% of the population, and when present, the fabellofibular ligament extends from the styloid process of the fibula to the fabella. When the fabella is absent, the fabellofibular ligament attaches to the lateral femoral condyle. De Maeseneer and colleagues[14] stated the fabellofibular ligament is present in 24% to 80% of knees, with the ligament extending from fabella to fibular styloid. When the fabella is absent, the ligament may still be present, extending from the posterolateral aspect of the external femoral condyle. In a recent report, Jadhav and colleagues[7] reported the fabella, a sesamoid bone in the lateral head of the gastrocnemius, as being present in approximately 20% of the population. When present, the fabella anchors the fabellofibular ligament, which runs from the fabella to the styloid process of the fibular head. If the fabella is absent, the ligament attaches to the lateral femoral condyle. In their description, this ligament is usually not a discrete structure, instead blending into the fibrous tissue.

Arcuate ligament
The arcuate ligament has also been reported as a variably present structure, and even when present, is difficult to visualize on MR imaging.[5,7,9,14,21] Early descriptions of the arcuate ligament are

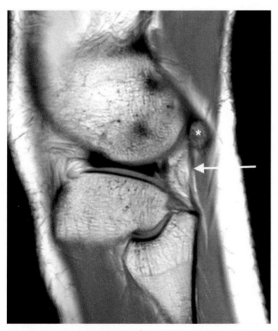

Fig. 5. Normal fabellofibular ligament in a 20-year-old woman following a volleyball injury. Sagittal proton density image shows the fabellofibular ligament (*arrow*) originating from the fabella (*asterisk*) and inserting distally onto the fibular head.

contradictory in several respects. The arcuate ligament is a thin, triangular band of capsular fibers in what Watanabe and co-authors[27] described as the middle layer of the PLC in 1993, originating from the posterior apex of the fibula styloid process, coursing superior and medial over the popliteus tendon, and spreading out over the posterior capsule. Although Seebacher and colleagues[25] described a firmly adherent ligament to the underlying musculotendinous junction of the popliteus, Watanabe and colleagues[27] found no strong fibrous connections to the adjacent popliteus on cadaveric dissection. Watanabe and colleagues[27] described the arcuate ligament as a condensation of fibers, as opposed to a separate ligament. Alternatively, Seebacher and colleagues[25] described a discrete structure composed of a vertical limb (from the fibula to the condensation of fibers at the lateral head of the gastrocnemius) and a medial limb that joins the fibers of the oblique popliteal ligament of Winslow.

In usual fashion, LaPrade and colleagues provided a detailed description of the ligament in the late 1990s. The authors reported the ligament as "several structures" that combine to form an arched or arcuate appearance, with medial and lateral limbs crossing over the popliteus musculotendinous junction. The lateral limb inserts just anterior to the fabellofibular ligament on the fibular styloid. The medial limb was said to be formed by the oblique popliteal ligament, or ligament of Winslow, which itself is formed by a coalescence of the oblique popliteal expansion of the semimembranosus and the capsular arm of the posterior oblique ligament at the medial knee.[26] Ironically in 2005, Moorman and LaPrade[23] reported that the arcuate ligament is not a distinct structure, having most likely been described in older articles and texts that failed to recognize the popliteofibular ligament, falsely referring to this structure as the arcuate ligament instead. The investigators recommended that the term arcuate ligament no longer be used to describe posterolateral knee anatomy to prevent further confusion.[23]

There have been numerous reports describing the arcuate ligament as a Y-shaped thickening of the capsule, with the medial limb running over the popliteus muscle and tendon joining the oblique popliteal ligament, and with the lateral limb ascending to blend with the capsule near the lateral gastrocnemius muscle at its condylar insertion (**Figs. 7** and **8**).[1,4,5,7,14,21]

Midthird lateral capsular ligament
The midthird lateral capsular ligament is a thickening of the lateral capsule of the knee, divided into 2 components: meniscofemoral and

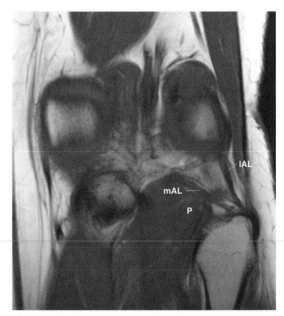

Fig. 7. Normal arcuate ligament in a 48-year-old woman with chronic knee pain. Coronal proton density image shows the arms of the arcuate ligament in its commonly described "Y formation," emanating from the posterior fibular head to the oblique popliteal ligament of the posterior capsule and lateral femoral condyle. IAL, lateral arm of the arcuate ligament; mAL, medial arm of the arcuate ligament; P, popliteus muscle.

mensicotibial. This structure has recently been referred to as the anterolateral ligament, drawing renewed attention, attaching anterior and proximal to the lateral femoral epicondyle proximally, and to

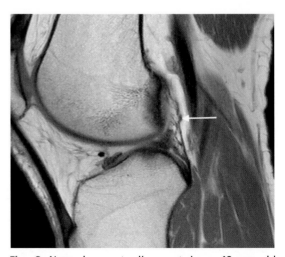

Fig. 8. Normal arcuate ligament in a 48-year-old woman with knee pain. Sagittal proton density image shows the arcuate ligament (*arrow*) as a thickening of the lateral aspect of the posterior capsule.

the tibia just distal to the articular cartilage margin, posterior to Gerdy tubercle. The ligament has a capsular attachment to the lateral meniscus by way of its discrete meniscofemoral and meniscotibial subcomponents (**Fig. 9**).[13,16,17,23,24,26] Specifically, the lateral tibial attachment for the lateral meniscus is provided by the meniscotibial portion of the midthird lateral capsular ligament.[17,26] Notably, LaPrade and colleagues[17,23] differentiated this structure from the coronary ligament in some reports, stating that the coronary ligament is situated posterior to the midthird lateral capsular ligament.

Lateral gastrocnemius

The lateral gastrocnemius tendon becomes adherent to the posterior capsule of the knee at the level of the fabella, and inserts onto the distal femur at the supracondylar process, just posterior to the fibular collateral ligament attachment.[13,16,17,23,29]

IMAGING PROTOCOLS

Initial radiographs acquired for isolated injury to the PLC may be normal, or demonstrate an avulsion fracture of the fibular head, the so-called arcuate sign. This sign is believed to be pathognomonic of an injury to 1 or more of the structures of the PLC.[3–5] A standing long-leg anterior-posterior (AP) radiograph may be obtained in chronic cases

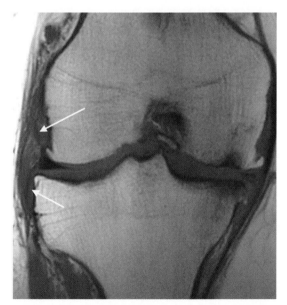

Fig. 9. Normal midthird lateral capsular ligament in a 54-year-old woman with knee pain. Coronal proton density image shows the midthird lateral capsular ligament (*arrows*). The meniscofemoral and meniscotibial components are depicted by the superior and inferior arrows, respectively.

of posterolateral instability, as limb alignment can be corrected using an osteotomy before, or at the same time of, the reconstruction procedure. Varus and posterior cruciate ligament (PCL) stress radiographs can be obtained to quantify the amount of lateral compartment varus gapping and a combined PLC and PCL injury, respectively.[8]

Bilateral fluoroscopic varus stress views may be obtained to compare lateral joint space opening.[9]

MR imaging can be very useful in the diagnosis of injuries to the lateral knee, but require knowledge of the complex anatomy of this area. Routine spin-echo MR imaging performed in 3 planes provides detailed visualization of the lateral knee structures. Some have advocated the acquisition of a coronal oblique sequence, with a coronal plane slanted parallel to the direction of the popliteus tendon, providing improved visualization of the arcuate, fabellofibular, and popliteofibular ligament.[1,8] Our routine knee protocol is presented in **Table 1**.

IMAGING FINDINGS/PATHOLOGY

As with all ligaments and tendons, the PLC structures are susceptible to variable degrees of tear, ranging from low-grade partial tear, high-grade partial tear, and fully torn (**Table 2**). Unique pathologic features to individual structures are described in the following sections.

Iliotibial Band

The deep layer of the iliotibial band is reportedly susceptible to avulsion and interstitial-type tears in the context of posterolateral knee injury.[13] Tears of the iliotibial band are seen best on axial and coronal images as an interruption distally near the tibial attachment, or avulsion fracture at the Gerdy tubercle (**Fig. 10**).[1]

Biceps Femoris

Avulsions of the direct or anterior arm of the long head of the biceps femoris tendon, as LaPrade and colleagues[13] have described, off the fibular styloid result in focal discontinuity, nonvisualization, increased signal intensity, or proximal retraction, on occasion with an osseous avulsion, on MR imaging. Injuries of the short-head biceps femoris include avulsion of LaPrade's direct arm from its fibular styloid attachment, and avulsion of LaPrade's anterior arm from its insertion onto the tibia posterior to Gerdy tubercle. MR imaging demonstrates focal discontinuity, thickening, increased/altered signal intensity, nonvisualization, and osseous avulsions (**Fig. 11**).[14]

Table 1
Knee MR imaging routine protocol

Pulse Sequences	Field of View, mm; Frequency × Phase	Slice Thickness, mm	Slice Gap, mm	Acquisition Matrix, Frequency × Phase	Parallel Imaging Factor	TR/TE	Echo Train Length	Bandwidth, Hz/Pixel
Axial T2 spectral fat suppression	150 × 150	3.5	0.3	272 × 260	1.7	7446/65	17	353
Sagittal PD spectral fat suppression	138 × 160	3.5	0	364 × 374	2	2921/17	12	361
Sagittal PD	138 × 160	3.5	0	396 × 447	1.9	1621/17	12	332
Coronal T1	130 × 130	3	0.5	212 × 204	1.7	615/20	5	333
Coronal PD spectral fat suppression	130 × 130	3	0.5	252 × 232	1.7	1934/17	11	335

Abbreviations: PD, proton density; TE, echo time; TR, repetition time.

Table 2 Diagnostic criteria for posterolateral corner ligament and tendon injury		
Low-Grade Partial Tear	**High-Grade Partial Tear**	**Full-Thickness Tear**
Periligamentous or peritendinous edema	Periligamentous or peritendinous edema	Full-thickness disruption of the involved structure
Abnormal attenuation or thickening	Abnormal attenuation or thickening	
Abnormal intrasubstance signal but without frank fiber discontinuity	Abnormal intrasubstance signal with frank, but only partial fiber discontinuity	

It is worth noting that there is controversy over the ability to distinguish individual divisions of the biceps femoris at the level of its fibular insertion. For instance, the fibular insertions of the short and long head of the biceps femoris tendon cannot be reliably distinguished on MR imaging per Haims and co-authors.[16] Conversely, Munshi and co-authors[21] reliably separated the short and long head of the biceps femoris into 3 separate arms at the tendinous attachment to the fibular head in most MR images reviewed (71%).

Fibular/Lateral Collateral Ligament

Most common injury patterns of the fibular collateral ligament include soft tissue avulsion from the attachment on the femur or as an osseous avulsion from the fibular head.[1,13] At MR imaging, complete disruption of the ligament appears as interruption of its normal contour with possible nonvisualization, whereas features of partial tear have been described as thickening, high signal intensity within its substance, and possible peri-ligamentous edema.[1,14] Juhng and co-authors[4] stated that avulsion of the fibular collateral ligament usually occurs at its distal attachment from the head of the fibula, as opposed to its proximal femoral attachment (see **Fig. 11; Fig. 12**).

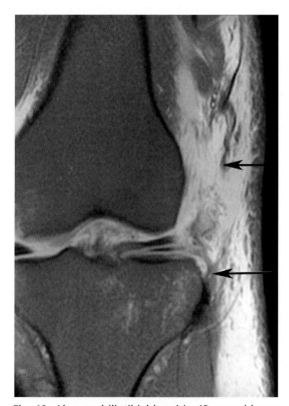

Fig. 10. Abnormal iliotibial band in 43-year-old man following a motorcycle accident. Coronal proton density fat-suppressed image delineates the distally torn and retracted iliotibial band, with large resultant gap (*arrows*).

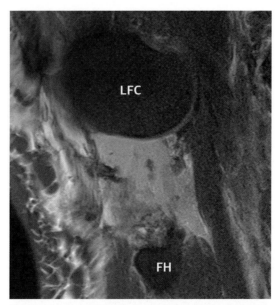

Fig. 11. Abnormal biceps femoris tendon in a 23-year-old woman following sports-related injury. Sagittal proton density fat-suppressed image shows avulsion of the conjoined attachment of the biceps tendon and fibular collateral ligament from the fibular head (*FH*), with concomitant opening of the lateral joint space and marked soft tissue edema. LFC, lateral femoral condyle.

Popliteus, Popliteofibular Ligament, and Popliteomeniscal Fascicles

Most popliteus tears are extra-articular, involving the muscle or myotendinous portion. Less commonly, injuries occur at the tendon, within the region of the popliteal hiatus or near its femoral insertion.[1,14] Injuries to the popliteus musculotendinous junction or femoral insertion are common in high-grade injuries to the PLC, with isolated injuries less common, representing less than 10% of popliteus injuries.[1,7,16]

At MR imaging, injuries of the popliteus vary based on location of injury and severity/grade. Abnormal signal may be present within the popliteus muscle, there may be irregular contour and signal of the tendon with peritendinous edema, or the tendon may be avulsed from its femoral attachment.[1] Muscle and tendon injuries have been classified as first degree (stretch injury resulting in interstitial edema and hemorrhage at the myotendinous junction and feathery appearance on MR imaging), second degree (partial tear), or third degree (complete rupture). With popliteus tears, it is important to note the site of tear (intra-articular or extra-articular), extent of tear (partial or full-thickness), presence of a bone fragment if there has been tendon avulsion, and degree of tendon retraction (see **Fig. 12**).[7]

Identifying injury to the popliteofibular ligament on MR imaging has been reported. For instance, Collins and colleagues[9] examined 22 knees with a PLC injury, and reported 19 with an injury of the popliteofibular ligament; 16 with a complete tear, and 3 with a partial tear. We feel identifying injury to this structure can be challenging (**Fig. 13**).

An abnormal appearance of the superior popliteomeniscal fascicle has been reported to be associated with tear of the posterior horn of the lateral meniscus. However, this finding is not specific for a lateral meniscal tear.[30] Variability in the appearance of the fascicles makes diagnosing injury challenging (**Fig. 14**).

Fabellofibular Ligament

On MR imaging, LaPrade and colleagues[13] reported the varied appearance of injuries to the fabellofibular ligament, including distal avulsion, thickening of the ligament, increased signal intensity, or nonvisualization. Avulsion of the fabellofibular ligament from the fibular head reportedly often occurs in conjunction with avulsion of LaPrade's direct arm of the short head of the biceps femoris muscle.[13] Conversely, while reviewing 22 knees with a PLC injury, Collins and colleagues[9] were

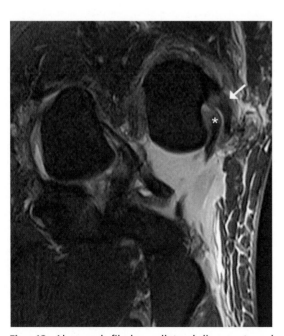

Fig. 12. Abnormal fibular collateral ligament and popliteus in a 23-year-old woman following a sports-related injury. Coronal proton density fat-suppressed image shows complete tear of the fibular collateral ligament (*arrow*) and popliteus (*asterisk*), with concomitant opening of the lateral joint space.

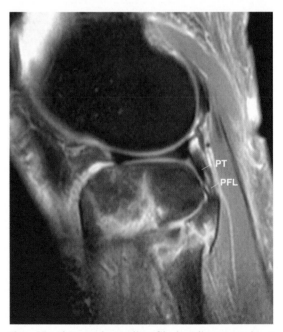

Fig. 13. Abnormal popliteofibular ligament in a 54-year-old woman following a fall from a ladder. Sagittal proton density fat-suppressed image shows the popliteus tendon (*PT*) as it enters the popliteal hiatus. The popliteofibular ligament (*PFL*) is thickened with abnormal intrasubstance signal compatible with partial tear. Notably, there are fractures of the tibia and fibula.

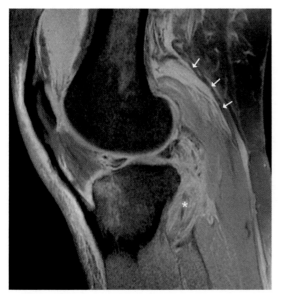

Fig. 14. Abnormal popliteomeniscal fascicles in an 18-year-old woman following a soccer injury. Sagittal proton density fat-suppressed image shows no demonstrable popliteomeniscal fascicles along the posterior periphery of the lateral meniscus, compatible with tear. In addition, there is a high-grade tear of the popliteus, which has a macerated and edematous appearance (*asterisk*), as well as a high-grade tear of the lateral head of the gastrocnemius (*arrows*). Notably, there is no perceptible posterior capsule superficial to the popliteus tendon, implying disruption of the arcuate and/or fabellofibular ligament.

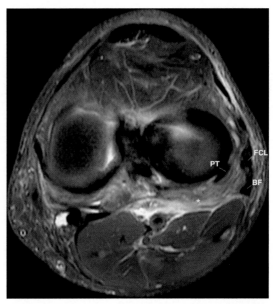

Fig. 15. Abnormal arcuate and fabellofibular ligament in a 42-year-old man with acute chronic knee pain. Axial T2 fat-suppressed image shows intact dominant structures of the posterolateral corner (biceps femoris, fibular collateral ligament, and popliteus tendon). However, there is edema localizing to the posterolateral capsule at the expected level of the arcuate and fabellofibular ligaments, (*asterisk*) raising concern for injury to these structures. BF, biceps femoris; FCL, fibular collateral ligament, PT, popliteus tendon.

unable to identify the fabellofibular ligament in any of the cases. In keeping with the description of the "arcuate roof" by Munshi and colleagues,[21] in which the arcuate and fabellofibular ligaments form the roof of the popliteal hiatus through which the popliteus tendon runs, when we identify edema localizing to this region, we report possible injury to the fabellofibular and arcuate ligaments (see **Fig. 14; Fig. 15**).

Arcuate Ligament

Identifying injury to the arcuate ligament is largely based on secondary signs in the literature, and in our practice. For instance, Recondo and co-authors[1] explained that only fat should be apparent behind the popliteus tendon; therefore, the presence of fluid posterior to the tendon should suggest a capsular, or more specifically arcuate, tear. Lee and colleagues[5] based injury to the popliteofibular and arcuate ligaments on MR imaging by the presence of an arcuate sign (fibular head avulsion fracture) or marrow edema in the fibular head on MR imaging, or both, with an otherwise intact fibular collateral ligament and biceps femoris tendon; the investigators could not directly

visualize the injuries to the popliteofibular or arcuate ligaments. Collins and colleagues[9] reported that abundant signal abnormality within the region of the posterior capsule suggests injury to the arcuate ligament (see **Figs. 14 and 15**).

Midthird Lateral Capsular Ligament

LaPrade and colleagues found that the meniscotibial component of the midthird lateral capsular ligament could be readily visualized on MR imaging, with injuries manifest as focal discontinuity, increased signal intensity and thickening, or nonvisualization of the normal low signal structure. Porrino and co-authors[24] reliably visualized the meniscofemoral arm on MR imaging as well. Osseous avulsion of the lateral tibia at the mensicotibial attachment is termed a Segond fracture, and is best depicted on radiographs (**Fig. 16**).[13,24]

Lateral Gastrocnemius

Injuries of the lateral head of the gastrocnemius are rare.[13] When lateral gastrocnemius injury does occur, severity varies from low-grade partial-thickness tear to full-thickness tear/avulsion (see **Fig. 14; Fig. 17**).

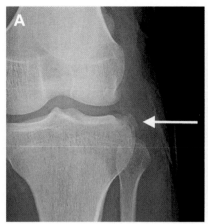
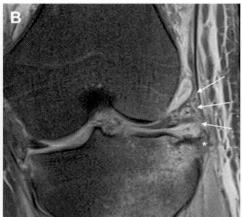

Fig. 16. Abnormal midthird lateral capsular ligament in a 19-year-old man struck by a motor vehicle. (*A*) Frontal radiograph demonstrates an avulsion fracture (*arrow*) at the lateral tibial plateau (Segond fracture). (*B*) Coronal proton density fat-suppressed MR image demonstrates the midthird lateral capsular ligament (*arrows*) attaching to the avulsed fragment (*asterisk*).

DIFFERENTIAL DIAGNOSIS

In our experience, identifying and appropriately reporting an injury to what Collins and colleagues[9] described as the large structures of the PLC (biceps femoris, fibular collateral ligament, popliteus) is relatively straightforward and without much ambiguity on MR imaging. However, evaluating the

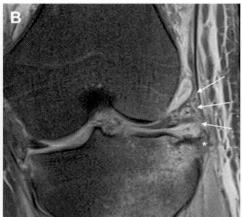

Fig. 17. Abnormal lateral head gastrocnemius in a 31-year-old man following a crush injury to the lower extremity. Axial T2 fat-suppressed image shows an intramuscular hematoma (*asterisk*) within the myotendinous junction of the lateral head of the gastrocnemius. The tendon of the lateral head of the gastrocnemius (*arrow*) is intact.

smaller structures (arcuate ligament, fabellofibular ligament, popliteofibular ligament, and popliteomeniscal fascicles) can be more challenging as a result of their varied visibility, warranting reliance on secondary signs of injury.

A differential diagnosis is often provided when an avulsion fracture of the fibular head is identified on radiographs (**Table 3**). An avulsion of the fibular head and styloid at the fibular attachment of the PLC tendinous and ligamentous structures is termed an arcuate fracture or arcuate sign. On radiographs, the differential diagnosis includes injury to any of the following soft tissue structures, better defined by MR imaging: biceps femoris, fibular collateral ligament, fabellofibular ligament, arcuate ligament, and popliteofibular ligament.[4,5,13]

The location of a fibular head avulsion fracture, and size of the fracture fragment can help predict the underlying soft tissue structure attached. Those with an arcuate or popliteofibular ligament injury demonstrate a small, 1-mm to 8-mm fragment, displaced just medial and superior to the

Table 3	
Summary of the differential diagnosis for avulsion fracture of the fibular head	
Fibular Head Fracture	**Structures Involved**
Small (<1 cm) fragment from the medial fibular head	Arcuate, fabellofibular, and/or popliteofibular ligament
Large (>1 cm) fragment from the lateral fibular head	Fibular collateral ligament and/or biceps femoris tendon

styloid process of the fibula, whereas those with an injury of the fibular collateral ligament and/or biceps femoris tendon exhibit a fragment arising from the lateral aspect of the fibular head, which is much larger: 1.5 to 2.5 cm. Similarly, marrow edema is reportedly more diffuse, involving the entire fibular head or the lateral aspect of the fibular head in those with an injury of the fibular collateral ligament or biceps femoris tendon, whereas a smaller focus of edema localized to the styloid process of the fibular head is reportedly evidence of injury to the popliteofibular or arcuate ligaments.[5]

Huang and colleagues[3] also emphasized the different types of potential avulsion fractures that can occur at the fibular head. The investigators state that an avulsion of the arcuate complex, that being the arcuate, fabellofibular, and popliteofibular ligaments, involves the apex of the fibular head (styloid process), exhibiting a characteristic elliptical fragment of bone with long axis oriented horizontal on an AP radiograph of the knee. This avulsion is in contrast to that caused by an avulsion of the fibular collateral ligament and/or biceps femoris tendon, which occurs at the lateral margin of the fibular head.

PEARLS, PITFALLS, VARIANTS

MR imaging is a useful tool to evaluate the PLC of the knee. Although all structures may not always be evident, the modality provides important information with regard to injury of this complex area of the knee.[14] A recognition of the variations in anatomy and of the limitations of MRI with regard to evaluation of the PLC of the knee is important in the imaging assessment of this region.[21] The radiologist must take into account the variability in identifying, in particular, the smaller structures of the PLC (arcuate ligament, fabellofibular ligament, popliteofibular ligament, and popliteomeniscal fascicles). If edema localizes to the soft tissues of the knee within the PLC, in particular along the superficial aspect of the popliteus, with an otherwise intact biceps femoris, fibular collateral ligament, and popliteus, an injury to the arcuate, fabellofibular, or popliteofibular ligament may be present, especially if these structures cannot be reliably visualized and cleared (**Box 1**).

WHAT THE REFERRING PHYSICIAN NEEDS TO KNOW

Low-grade injuries of the PLC are often managed nonoperatively, whereas more significant PLC injuries often require operative intervention to avoid poor outcome. From a clinical perspective, the need for surgical repair/reconstruction is based

---

> **Box 1**
> **Pearls, pitfalls, variants**
>
> - A recognition of the variations in anatomy and of the limitations of MR imaging with regard to evaluation of the posterolateral corner (PLC) of the knee is important in the imaging assessment.
> - The arcuate ligament, fabellofibular ligament, popliteofibular ligament, and popliteomeniscal fascicles are not always perceptible on MR imaging.
> - Abnormal signal within the region of the posterolateral capsule may imply injury to a smaller structure of the PLC (arcuate ligament, fabellofibular ligament, and popliteofibular ligament).

---

on the grade of instability on examination and stress radiography.[9]

In a review of 22 knees with a PLC injury requiring surgical intervention, all 22 knees exhibited injury to at least 2 of the dominant 3 PLC structures (biceps femoris, fibular collateral ligament, popliteus) on preoperative MR imaging. In all 22 knees, the fibular collateral ligament was abnormal. The popliteofibular ligament was injured in 19 knees; neither the arcuate ligament nor the fabellofibular ligament were confidently identified in a single knee. The investigators concluded that although MR imaging assessment of the PLC injury is challenging due to anatomic complexity, the larger structures are easy to evaluate with standard MR technique, and direct visualization of small structure involvement on MRI is not necessary to report a clinically unstable PLC injury.[9] We agree with this conclusion, and approach the PLC using a similar perspective (**Box 2**).

> **Box 2**
> **What the referring physician needs to know**
>
> - Is there injury to the biceps femoris, fibular collateral ligament, or popliteus? If so, is this injury a low-grade partial tear, high-grade partial tear, or full-thickness tear?
> - Is there injury, or suggestion of injury (such as edema localizing to the posterolateral capsule), to a small structure of the PLC (arcuate ligament, fabellofibular ligament, and popliteofibular ligament)?
> - Are there additional injuries present involving a cruciate ligament, collateral ligament, the hyaline cartilage, or bone?

SUMMARY

Although the anatomy of the PLC can be confusing as a result of the number of structures that have been described, variability in nomenclature, and variability in identification of said structures, MR imaging still has the ability to provide valuable information with regard to injury within this region. Low-grade injuries of the PLC are often managed nonoperatively, whereas more significant PLC injuries, or those involving the biceps femoris, fibular collateral ligament, and/or popliteus, are easy to identify on MR imaging, and will more likely require operative intervention.

REFERENCES

1. Recondo JA, Salvador E, Villanúa JA, et al. Lateral stabilizing structures of the knee: functional anatomy and injuries assessed with MR imaging. Radiographics 2000;20(Spec No):S91–102.
2. Hughston JC, Andrews JR, Cross MJ, et al. Classification of knee ligament instabilities. Part II. The lateral compartment. J Bone Joint Surg Am 1976; 58:173–9.
3. Huang GS, Yu JS, Munshi M, et al. Avulsion fracture of the head of the fibula (the "arcuate" sign): MR imaging findings predictive of injuries to the posterolateral ligaments and posterior cruciate ligament. AJR Am J Roentgenol 2003;180:381–7.
4. Juhng S-K, Lee JK, Choi S-S, et al. MR evaluation of the "arcuate" sign of posterolateral knee instability. AJR Am J Roentgenol 2002;178:583–8.
5. Lee J, Papakonstantinou O, Brookenthal KR, et al. Arcuate sign of posterolateral knee injuries: anatomic, radiographic, and MR imaging data related to patterns of injury. Skeletal Radiol 2003;32:619–27.
6. Rajeswaran G, Lee JC, Healy JC. MRI of the popliteofibular ligament: isotropic 3D WE-DESS versus coronal oblique fat-suppressed T2W MRI. Skeletal Radiol 2007;36:1141–6.
7. Jadhav SP, More SR, Riascos RF, et al. Comprehensive review of the anatomy, function, and imaging of the popliteus and associated pathologic conditions. Radiographics 2014;34:496–513.
8. Crespo B, James EW, Metsavaht L, et al. Injuries to posterolateral corner of the knee: a comprehensive review from anatomy to surgical treatment. Rev Bras Ortop 2015;50:363–70.
9. Collins MS, Bond JR, Crush AB, et al. MRI injury patterns in surgically confirmed and reconstructed posterolateral corner knee injuries. Knee Surg Sports Traumatol Arthrosc 2015;23:2943–9.
10. McKean D, Yoong P, Yanny S, et al. The popliteal fibular ligament in acute knee trauma: patterns of injury on MR imaging. Skeletal Radiol 2015;44: 1413–9.
11. Domnick C, Frosch K-H, Raschke MJ, et al. Kinematics of different components of the posterolateral corner of the knee in the lateral collateral ligament-intact state: a human cadaveric study. Arthroscopy 2017;33:1821–30.
12. LaPrade RF, Resig S, Wentorf F, et al. The effects of grade III posterolateral knee complex injuries on anterior cruciate ligament graft force. A biomechanical analysis. Am J Sports Med 1999;27: 469–75.
13. LaPrade RF, Gilbert TJ, Bollom TS, et al. The magnetic resonance imaging appearance of individual structures of the posterolateral knee. A prospective study of normal knees and knees with surgically verified grade III injuries. Am J Sports Med 2000; 28:191–9.
14. De Maeseneer M, Shahabpour M, Vanderdood K, et al. Posterolateral supporting structures of the knee: findings on anatomic dissection, anatomic slices and MR images. Eur Radiol 2001;11: 2170–7.
15. LaPrade RF, Terry GC. Injuries to the posterolateral aspect of the knee. Association of anatomic injury patterns with clinical instability. Am J Sports Med 1997;25:433–8.
16. Haims AH, Medvecky MJ, Pavlovich R, et al. MR imaging of the anatomy of and injuries to the lateral and posterolateral aspects of the knee. AJR Am J Roentgenol 2003;180:647–53.
17. Sanchez AR, Sugalski MT, LaPrade RF. Anatomy and biomechanics of the lateral side of the knee. Sports Med Arthrosc Rev 2006;14:2–11.
18. Geeslin AG, LaPrade RF. Outcomes of treatment of acute grade-III isolated and combined posterolateral knee injuries: a prospective case series and surgical technique. J Bone Joint Surg Am 2011;93: 1672–83.
19. Veltri DM, Deng XH, Torzilli PA, et al. The role of the popliteofibular ligament in stability of the human knee. A biomechanical study. Am J Sports Med 1996;24:19–27.
20. Shahane SA, Ibbotson C, Strachan R, et al. The popliteofibular ligament. An anatomical study of the posterolateral corner of the knee. J Bone Joint Surg Br 1999;81:636–42.
21. Munshi M, Pretterklieber ML, Kwak S, et al. MR imaging, MR arthrography, and specimen correlation of the posterolateral corner of the knee: an anatomic study. AJR Am J Roentgenol 2003;180:1095–101.
22. Temponi EF, de Carvalho Júnior LH, Saithna A, et al. Incidence and MRI characterization of the spectrum of posterolateral corner injuries occurring in association with ACL rupture. Skeletal Radiol 2017;46: 1063–70.
23. Moorman CT, LaPrade RF. Anatomy and biomechanics of the posterolateral corner of the knee. J Knee Surg 2005;18:137–45.

24. Porrino J, Maloney E, Richardson M, et al. The antero-lateral ligament of the knee: MRI appearance, association with the Segond fracture, and historical perspective. AJR Am J Roentgenol 2015;204:367–73.

25. Seebacher JR, Inglis AE, Marshall JL, et al. The structure of the posterolateral aspect of the knee. J Bone Joint Surg Am 1982;64:536–41.

26. Terry GC, LaPrade RF. The posterolateral aspect of the knee. Anatomy and surgical approach. Am J Sports Med 1996;24:732–9.

27. Watanabe Y, Moriya H, Takahashi K, et al. Functional anatomy of the posterolateral structures of the knee. Arthroscopy 1993;9:57–62.

28. Johnson RL, De Smet AA. MR visualization of the popliteomeniscal fascicles. Skeletal Radiol 1999; 28:561–6.

29. LaPrade RF, Ly TV, Wentorf FA, et al. The posterolateral attachments of the knee: a qualitative and quantitative morphologic analysis of the fibular collateral ligament, popliteus tendon, popliteofibular ligament, and lateral gastrocnemius tendon. Am J Sports Med 2003;31:854–60.

30. Blankenbaker DG, De Smet AA, Smith JD. Usefulness of two indirect MR imaging signs to diagnose lateral meniscal tears. AJR Am J Roentgenol 2002; 178:579–82.

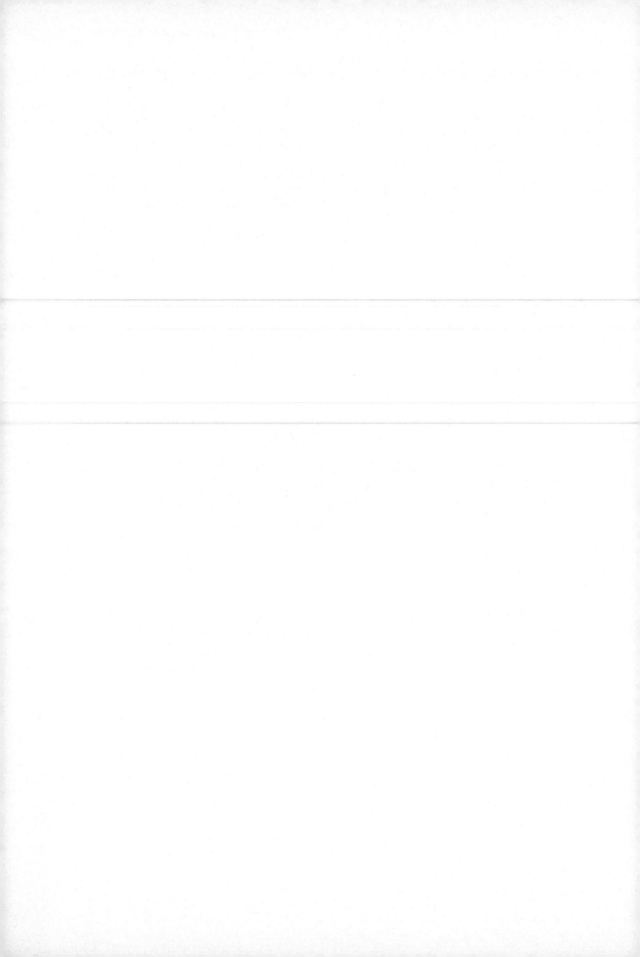

Imaging of the Postoperative Meniscus

Russell Chapin, MD

KEYWORDS

- Postoperative knee • Meniscectomy • Meniscal repair • MR imaging • MR arthrography

KEY POINTS

- The expected appearance of a meniscus after meniscectomy includes smooth regular margins with a variably decreased size.
- MR imaging criteria for meniscal re-tear are high T2-weighted signal reaching the articular surface, abnormal meniscal morphology, a displaced fragment, or tear at a different meniscal site.
- Data indicate that the diagnostic criteria and accuracy of routine nonarthrographic MR imaging for meniscal re-tear after low-grade meniscal excision are the same as for nonoperative menisci.
- When a detailed history is available, nonarthrographic MR imaging is reasonable after partial meniscectomy.
- MR arthrography may be helpful after higher grade meniscectomies and meniscal repair.

INTRODUCTION

As of 2011, approximately 580,000 meniscectomies, 38,000 meniscal repairs, and 700 meniscal allograft transplant procedures were performed annually in the United States.[1,2] Success rates for meniscectomy and meniscal repair are high, but evaluation of the postoperative meniscus with MR imaging can be difficult. Clinical management, imaging protocol selection, and accurate diagnosis in these patients require thoughtful consideration because expected postoperative change can meet criteria used to diagnose meniscal tear in the nonoperative knee, particularly increased T1-weighted or proton density (PD) signal contacting the articular surface. Reviewing the decision process that guides treatment of meniscal tears as well as literature on the appearance of the normal and failed postoperative meniscus allows for a rational approach to protocol selection and image interpretation.

MENISCAL STRUCTURE AND FUNCTION

The appropriate treatment for a meniscal tear or re-tear is based on an understanding of the function of the meniscus, the morphology of the tear, and its potential for healing. The function of the menisci is primarily to distribute weight at the knee and protect the hyaline articular cartilage, while contributing to knee stability and likely proprioception and cartilage nourishment.[3] All meniscal tears can be broadly classified as horizontal cleavage tears, radial vertical tears, longitudinal vertical tears, or a combination thereof, with or without a displaced fragment. As they extend from the inner to the peripheral portion of the C-shaped menisci, radial vertical meniscal tears disrupt circumferentially oriented collagen fibers and cause incrementally increased loss of hoop strength and meniscal function. To maintain function, some outer hoop fibers must remain intact. Horizontal and longitudinal vertical tears do not compromise the function of the

The author has nothing to disclose.
Department of Radiology, Medical University of South Carolina, 96 Jonathan Lucas Street, MSC 323, Charleston, SC 29425, USA
E-mail address: chapinrw@musc.edu

Radiol Clin N Am 56 (2018) 953–964
https://doi.org/10.1016/j.rcl.2018.06.007

meniscus as significantly but may cause pain and mechanical symptoms.[3] Because of an intact blood supply, the outer vascularized one-third of the meniscus is referred to as the red zone and is considered capable of healing. In contrast, the inner one-third of the meniscus is avascular, known as the white zone, and traditionally considered to be incapable of healing.[4] In children and adolescents, some blood supply may persist in the inner and middle portions of the meniscus.[1]

FUNDAMENTALS OF MENISCAL TEAR TREATMENT

The tenets of treating a meniscal tear are stability of the meniscal tissue and preservation of a maximal amount of the meniscus, particularly the peripheral circumferentially oriented collagen fibers responsible for hoop strength. With increasing loss of meniscal tissue, there is an increased degree of cartilage damage and joint destruction.[5] Therefore, emphasis in the development of surgical techniques and physician education is on minimization of the degree of meniscectomy and on meniscal repair rather than meniscectomy when possible. Based on a sample of United States insurance data, the rate of meniscal repair increased by 11% from 2005 to 2011, although there was no significant change in the rate of meniscectomy.[1] One study found that 60% of meniscectomy patients had radiographically progressive arthritis at an average follow-up of 9 years, whereas only 19% of meniscal repair patients showed evidence of arthritis.[6] However, a large percentage of meniscal injuries remain unamendable to repair, as reflected in the persistent greater than 10:1 ratio between meniscectomy and meniscal repair.

As well as location in the periphery of the meniscus, factors associated with improved meniscal healing include being in the lateral meniscus, tear length of less than 25 mm, acute tears, patient age less than 30 years, and accompanying anterior cruciate ligament (ACL) reconstruction.[7,8] The favorable effect of ACL reconstruction on meniscal healing is attributed to biologic stimulation. In contrast, persistently unstable ACL-deficient knees have a higher rate of repair failure. Because the lateral meniscus is more mobile, medial meniscal tears are more subject to strain forces and susceptible to tear propagation.[8] Vertical longitudinal tears of less than 10 mm in length tend to be stable. It is interesting to note that, based on these factors, there is increasing awareness that some meniscal tears

may be left to heal on their own without performing repair or resection. In such cases, healing may be augmented with trephination, synovial abrasion, fibrin clot, or platelet-rich plasma.[4,9]

The ideal meniscal tear to leave in situ, with or without stimulation, is a peripheral red zone less than 10 mm vertical longitudinal nondisplaced tear in the posterior horn, particularly of the lateral meniscus, in the setting of ACL reconstruction.[9] Similarly, the ideal tear for suture repair is vertical, longitudinal, in the red zone of the posterior horn, and 10 to 25 mm in length.[8] The portion of these tears that extend into the body of the meniscus, particularly the medial meniscus, benefit most from repair. For longer tears that bucket-handle, the central portion of the tear may be excised while the peripheral portion is repaired.[8] As a general rule, horizontal cleavage tears, inner one-third flap or radial tears, and chronic degenerative tears should be treated with partial meniscectomy rather than repair.[8] Horizontal cleavage degenerative tears in the posterior horn of the medial meniscus of patients over age 50 years are frequently asymptomatic and, as such, may not require treatment.[9] In properly selected cases using the modern techniques of all-inside or inside out meniscal repair, the success rate of meniscal repair is approximately 90%.[1]

CONSIDERATIONS FOR MENISCAL ALLOGRAFT

Although orders of magnitude less common than partial meniscectomy or meniscal repair, meniscal allograft transplantation is reported to have good outcomes in more than 80% of patients.[5] Synthetic grafts or augmentation with polyurethane or collagen are currently not approved by the US Food and Drug Administration and only performed within trials in the United States.[4] Candidates for meniscal transplant are younger patients (<50 years) with symptoms referable to a high-grade meniscectomy or irreparable meniscal injury. Patients must fail to respond to conservative measures and must not have significant radiographic arthritis. The knee joint should be stable and well-aligned with no high-grade (Outerbridge grade III or IV) cartilage lesions. Simultaneous or staged treatment of cartilage injury, instability, or malalignment to allow for meniscal transplant is also described. Obesity (body mass index of >35) is a contraindication (**Box 1**).[5]

IMAGING CRITERIA FOR MENISCAL TEAR

Criteria for meniscal tear in the nonpostoperative knee include abnormal signal on PD or

<table>
<tr><td>

Box 1
Principles of meniscal tear treatment

- Minimize degree of meniscal tissue loss
- Repair, rather than resect, when appropriate
- Tears that heal well
  - Peripheral location in the outer third
  - Lateral meniscal tear
  - Tear length less than 10 mm
  - Acute tear less than 8 weeks
  - Patient age less than 25 years of age
  - Accompanying anterior cruciate ligament reconstruction
- Tears that do not heal well (may be left alone if stable and asymptomatic; otherwise require partial meniscectomy)
  - Horizontal cleavage tears
  - Inner third flap tear
  - Inner third radial tear
  - Chronic degenerative tears
- Indications for meniscal allograft transplant
  - Age less than 50 years and body mass index less than 35
  - Prior high-grade meniscectomy or irreparable meniscal injury
  - Symptoms referable to the joint space of meniscal deficiency
  - Failure to respond to conservative measures
  - No significant radiographic arthritis
  - No Outerbridge grade III or IV cartilage lesions
  - Stable and well-aligned knee joint

</td></tr>
</table>

T1-weighted images that contacts the articular surface on 2 or more images, abnormal meniscal morphology, or displaced flaps of meniscal tissue. There is a particular emphasis on the 2-touch rule for abnormal signal reaching the articular surface. Based on these criteria, accuracy of MR imaging for diagnosing meniscal tear in the virgin knee exceeds 90% with a sensitivity of 85% to 90% and a specificity of 90% to 95%.[10] However, altered morphology is expected after meniscectomy and abnormal signal contacting the meniscus surface on short echo time (TE) images is common after both meniscectomy and meniscal repair (**Fig. 1**).[7]

NORMAL POSTOPERATIVE MENISCAL MORPHOLOGY

When meniscal repair is performed without resection, the postoperative meniscal morphology is essentially normal, in contrast with the MR imaging appearance after partial meniscectomy. From a pragmatic perspective, the most important starting point for evaluating a postoperative meniscus is recognizing that surgery has been performed, particularly to avoid describing expected changes as a tear. Although the full patient chart is increasingly available to interpreting radiologists owing to the proliferation of electronic medical records, the history of prior surgery is unfortunately often not reported or not detailed. Clues to prior arthroscopic surgery on MR imaging include low signal primarily linear areas of scar in Hoffa's fat pad, focal thickening of the patellar tendon, and foci of magnetic susceptibility artifact from microscopic metallic fragments (**Fig. 2**).[11] The meniscal morphology after being partially resected is characterized by some diminution of meniscal tissue with a smooth regular appearance and often a slightly blunted free edge.[12] In a large majority of cases, this finding will be localized in the posterior horn of the medial meniscus. In all cases where a deficiency of meniscal tissue is noted with uncertain surgical history, an accompanying displaced fragment should be carefully sought. The most common location for displaced meniscal fragments from the medial meniscus is adjacent to the posterior cruciate ligament or stacked adjacent to the body in the medial recess. The most common location for a displaced fragment of the lateral meniscus is stacked in the lateral recess adjacent to the meniscal body or posterior to the meniscus, often in the popliteal hiatus.[10] Comparison with any prior examinations is essential and, in the case of known partial meniscectomy, review of the operative report detailing the exact location and extent of resection is helpful if that is available.

MR IMAGING FINDINGS AFTER MENISCAL REPAIR

After meniscal repair, increased signal contacting the articular surface is consistent with fibrovascular or granulation tissue.[7,13] Intrameniscal signal is particularly increased within the first 12 weeks postoperatively and has been shown to persist beyond 10 years (**Fig. 3**).[7,13] In studies of meniscal repair, Farley and colleagues[14] reported increased signal on short TE images

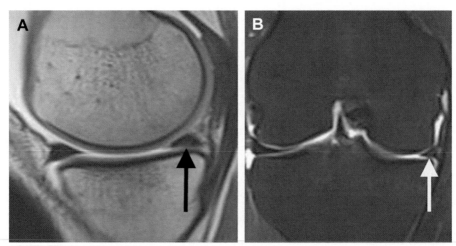

Fig. 1. Expected findings after partial meniscectomy in 34-year-old man status post partial medial meniscectomy 7 months prior for a horizontal cleavage tear at the junction of the posterior horn and body. (*A*) Sagittal proton density image shows mild blunting of the inner edge and faint increased signal contacting the inferior articular surface of the posterior horn of the medial meniscus (*arrow*). (*B*) Coronal T2-weighted fat-saturated image shows slightly diminutive body of the medial meniscus with increased signal that does not contact the articular surface (*arrow*). Both findings are consistent with an expected appearance after meniscectomy, without definite imaging findings of tear. The patient subsequently underwent arthroscopy coinciding with myotendinous hamstring release, which demonstrated no tear or meniscal instability.

contacting the articular surface in more than 60% of untorn menisci. Miao and colleagues[15] found a specificity of approximately 50% to 60% for PD surfacing signal, once again reflecting that 40% to 50% of patients without meniscal re-tear have this finding. For this reason, the presence of high T2-weighted signal (greater than that of hyaline cartilage or equal to fluid signal) is more helpful in evaluating for re-tear of a meniscal repair on conventional nonarthrographic MR imaging. Surfacing high T2-weighted signal was reported to have a sensitivity and specificity of approximately 60% and 90% by Farley and colleagues[14] and Miao and colleagues[15] for meniscal re-tear. When present more than 3 months postoperatively, definitively surfacing fluidlike high T2-weighted signal is specific for tear of a repaired meniscus, but the sensitivity of this finding on MR imaging is limited. The additional criteria of abnormal meniscal morphology not concordant with prior surgery, a displaced flap, or a tear at another location increase the accuracy of MR imaging for evaluation of the postoperative meniscus, but are less commonly seen (**Box 2**).[16] In postmeniscectomy knees, Kijowski and colleagues[12] found that the presence of a displaced fragment had a sensitivity of 28% and specificity of 100% for re-tear. In another study, Magee and co-authors[17] reported that performing direct MR arthrography after conventional MR imaging was necessary for the

diagnosis of meniscal tear in all cases of prior meniscal repair.

MR IMAGING FINDINGS AFTER MENISCECTOMY

Because meniscectomy is more frequent than repair, more data are available regarding the performance of conventional MR imaging after partial meniscectomy. As for meniscal repair, surfacing high T2-weighted signal on MR imaging is the most accurate finding for meniscal re-tear after meniscectomy (**Fig. 4**).[18] In the study by White and colleagues,[18] 93 of 104 menisci had been treated with meniscectomy. Based on the presence of contacting high T2-weighted signal and meniscal morphologic changes beyond those expected postoperatively, the sensitivity and specificity of MR imaging for re-tear were found to be 86% and 67%, respectively.[18] More recently, Kijowski and colleagues[12] found a sensitivity and specificity of 40% and 96%, respectively, for surfacing high T2-weighted signal in the diagnosis of re-tear after meniscectomy. Similar to the post repair meniscus, the postmeniscectomy meniscus frequently is found to have increased short TE signal reaching the articular surface.[7,12,18] This is likely because otherwise degenerative intrasubstance signal has been debrided back to a stable base in these cases. This finding of surfacing short TE signal was present in 50% of the untorn menisci

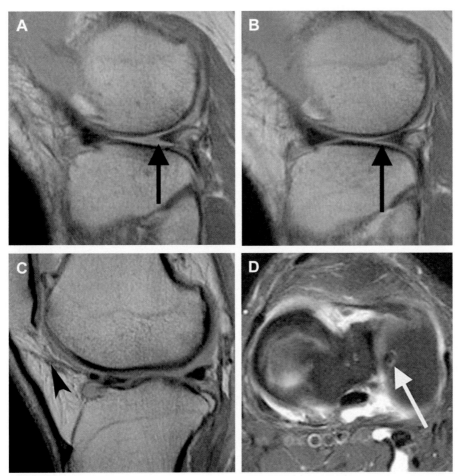

Fig. 2. Expected findings after partial meniscectomy in 57-year-old woman. When sagittal proton density post-operative image (*A*) is compared with preoperative MR imaging 8 months prior (*B*), subtle interval truncation of the inner margin of the posterior horn of the lateral meniscus (*arrow*) is noted. (*C*) Additionally, a linear low signal scope scar is seen in Hoffa's fat pad (*arrowhead*). (*D*) Axial proton density fat-saturated image shows magnetic susceptibility artifact (*arrow*) at the medial femoral condyle where chondroplasty was performed.

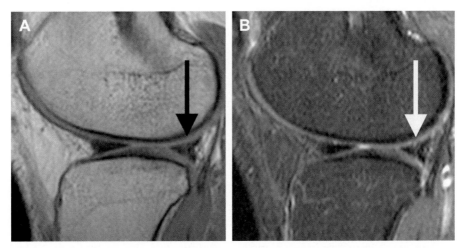

Fig. 3. Expected findings after suture repair of posterior horn lateral meniscus in 34-year-old woman. Sagittal proton density (*A*) and T2-weighted fat-saturated (*B*) images demonstrate thin incomplete increased signal (*arrows*) contacting the superior and inferior articular surface. The signal is isointense to hyaline cartilage and not as intense as joint fluid, consistent with expected postoperative appearance. Patient had no lateral joint line pain and a negative McMurray test.

in the study by White and co-authors,[18] and more than 50% of untorn menisci in the study by Kijowski and colleagues.[12]

INFLUENCE OF THE DEGREE OF MENISCECTOMY ON ACCURACY

Several studies have shown MR imaging to have high diagnostic accuracy for meniscal re-tears in the setting of low-grade (<25%) meniscectomy but to perform less adequately when greater than 25% of meniscal tissue has been resected.[18,19] In fact, the criteria for diagnosing a re-tear after meniscectomy of less than 25% have been stated to be identical to those for the nonoperative meniscus, particularly with respect to the 2-touch rule for short TE sequences.[16] As a caveat to this, improvements in signal and resolution of MR imaging sequences will make subtle changes in meniscal morphology and signal more evident after meniscectomy, and the presence of T2-weighted signal contacting the articular surface in addition to T1-weighted or PD signal will increase specificity. White and colleagues[18] found an accuracy of MR imaging of 100% in patients with less than 25% meniscectomy versus an accuracy of 78% with greater than 25% meniscectomy. Applegate and colleagues[19] found an accuracy of MR imaging of 89% for less than 25% meniscectomy cases versus 65% for greater than 25% meniscectomy cases. The reason for this discrepancy in accuracy based on increased meniscal resection is less clear, but it is hypothesized to be due to increased irregularity of residual tissue accompanying greater degrees of tissue resection.

MR IMAGING VERSUS MR ARTHROGRAPHY FOR MENISCECTOMY OF MORE THAN 25%

Based on this finding, MR arthrography has been advocated as an alternative to MR imaging in patients with greater than 25% meniscectomy. Similar to prior authors, Magee and colleagues[17] reported that nonarthrographic MR imaging was accurate for the diagnosis of tear in all patients with less than 25% prior meniscectomy, but that MR arthrography was necessary to diagnose tear in 16 of 61 patients with prior meniscectomy of more than 25%. However, in this group of 61 patients, 32 had alternate diagnoses including concomitant severe degenerative change, chondral defects, or avascular necrosis, which obviated any additional benefit for MR arthrography.[17] Therefore, in 79% of cases (48 of 61) where a greater than 25% meniscectomy was performed in this series, MR imaging without arthrography was adequate for guiding patient treatment (Fig. 5).

MR ARTHROGRAPHY CRITERIA FOR MENISCAL TEAR

Direct MR arthrography is performed by obtaining mostly T1-weighted fat-saturated sequences after the imaging-guided intraarticular injection of dilute (1:200) gadolinium-based contrast agents at volumes of 20 to 40 mL. Although gadolinium-based contrast agents remain unapproved by the US Food and Drug Administration for intraarticular injection, this practice is widely accepted. Reported complication rates are exceedingly low and are essentially never related to the use of gadolinium contrast. The diagnosis of meniscal tear at MR arthrography is primarily based on linear signal equal in T1-weighted intensity to the injected contrast contacting or communicating with the meniscal surface (see Box 2; Figs. 6 and 7).[7,16,19] Increased detection of meniscal tears using MR arthrography is attributed to joint distention, a lower viscosity of injectate compared with synovial fluid (allowing for insinuation into meniscal tears), and the use of short TE images as opposed to T2-weighted images, with a resultant increase in the signal-to-noise ratio (Fig. 8).[16] However, several authors have noted that the increased T1-weighted signal contacting the meniscal surface in cases of re-tear is not as intense as the intraarticular contrast.[20,21] This occurred in 41% of recurrent tears in 1 series and has been hypothesized to be due to volume averaging or imbibition of the intraarticular gadolinium into the tear without a free-flowing defect.[20] Other authors recommend

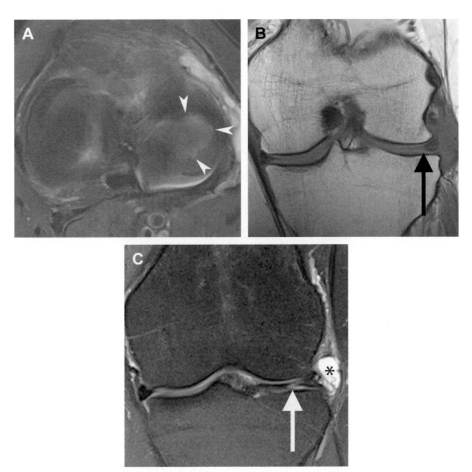

Fig. 4. Meniscectomy with re-tear. A 44-year-old woman imaged 11 months after meniscectomy of 50% of the lateral meniscus who had increased pain after a mud run. (*A*) Axial proton density fat-saturated image shows the expected appearance after a biter and shaver were used along the inner margin of the lateral meniscus (*arrowheads*). (*B*) Coronal proton density image shows horizontal signal and blunted inner margin (*arrow*) of the meniscal body that, in isolation, would not be specific for a meniscal tear in the setting of meniscectomy of greater than 50%. (*C*) However, coronal T2-weighted fat-saturated image shows thin but definite fluid signal contacting the inferior surface of the anterior horn (*arrow*) and communication with a moderate sized parameniscal cyst (*arrowhead*). Both findings are highly specific for meniscal re-tear.

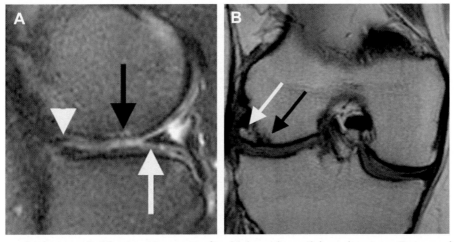

Fig. 5. No meniscal re-tear in 37-year-old woman after high-grade partial meniscectomy 2 years prior. (*A*) The anterior (*arrowhead*) and posterior (*white arrow*) horns of the lateral meniscus are diminutive, without evidence of re-tear. There is a full-thickness Outerbridge grade 4 chondral loss in the adjacent lateral femoral condyle (*black arrow*). (*B*) Coronal T1-weighted image shows cortical changes consistent with severe chondral injury (*black arrow*) and adjacent osteophytes (*white arrow*), felt to be the etiology of the patient's pain.

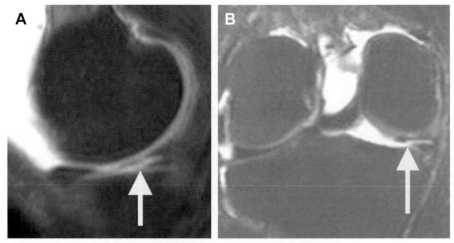

Fig. 6. Meniscal re-tear on MR arthrography in 40-year-old man with prior medial meniscectomy. (*A*) Sagittal T1-weighted fat-saturated image shows surfacing/communicating T1-weighted signal (*arrow*) equal to that of intraarticular gadolinium. (*B*) Coronal T2-weighted fat-saturated image shows horizontal fluid-equivalent signal (*arrow*) extending to the inferior articular surface.

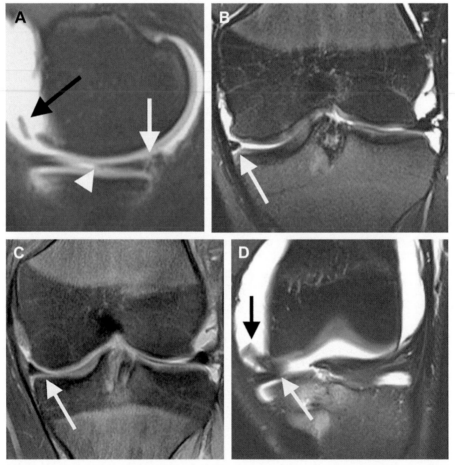

Fig. 7. Combined criteria for MR arthrography diagnosis of meniscal re-tear in 19-year-old man status post posterior horn medial meniscal repair and anterior cruciate ligament reconstruction 3 years prior. (*A*) Sagittal MR arthrogram shows longitudinal signal (*white arrow*) in the peripheral posterior horn of the medial meniscus that contacts both articular surfaces but is not as intense as contrast. No tear was found at this location on arthroscopy. However, there is irregularity of the free edge (*arrowhead*) of the body, with a fragment noted anterior to the medial femoral condyle (*black arrow*). Coronal T2-weighted fat-saturated postoperative image (*B*) shows diminutive anterior body of the medial meniscus, which is new since preoperative MR imaging (*C*) and there was not an interval meniscectomy. (*D*) Far anterior coronal T2-weighted fat-saturated image shows the large displaced meniscal fragment (*black arrow*) arising from the anterior horn (*white arrow*) and body of the medial meniscus.

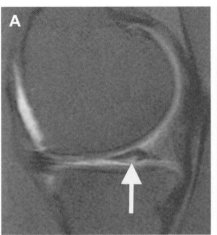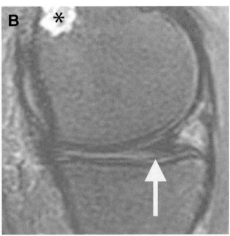

Fig. 8. Advantage of demonstrating meniscal re-tear on T1-weighted images with MR arthrography in 56-year-old woman after partial medial meniscectomy. (A) Sagittal T1-weighted fat-saturated image shows slightly complex, horizontal intrameniscal T1-weighted signal (*arrow*) extending to the inferior articular surface that is not as intense as contrast, but slightly greater than hyaline cartilage. (B) Because of poorer signal-to-noise ratio on sagittal short T1 inversion recovery image, the tear was not seen. Arthroscopy performed 1 month later showed re-tear. Incidental note made of enchondroma (*asterisk*).

comparison of the postarthrogram T1-weighted images with prearthrogram T1-weighted images performed with the same imaging parameters for detection of subtle increases in signal at the site of tear.[21] Most important, these studies have emphasized that surfacing T2-weighted signal otherwise diagnostic of a meniscal tear should also be interpreted as a tear to increase the accuracy of MR arthrography.[21] Including T2-weighted fat-saturated images in the MR arthrography protocol is also helpful to evaluate for nonmeniscal pathology, particularly of the subchondral bone, ligaments, and extraarticular tendons.

DIAGNOSTIC PERFORMANCE OF DIRECT MR ARTHROGRAPHY

Overall, Applegate and colleagues[19] found a significantly improved performance of MR arthrography compared with MR imaging, with a sensitivity and specificity of 69% and 60% for MR imaging and 89% and 86% for MR arthrography, respectively. Magee also reported a sensitivity and specificity of 78% and 75% for MR imaging and 88% and 100% for MR arthrography, respectively, in a large group of patients after meniscectomy.[21] In contrast, the study by White and colleagues[18] found no significant difference between the performance of nonarthrographic MR imaging and MR arthrography. The sensitivity, specificity, and combined accuracy of MR imaging was 86%, 67%, and 80% versus 90%, 78%, and 85%, respectively, for

MR arthrography. However, other authors found MR arthrography to be superior to MR imaging, with a sensitivity, specificity, and combined accuracy of 58%, 80%, and 63% for MR imaging versus 92%, 100%, and 93%, respectively, for MR arthrography.[22] Another study found that accuracy was increased from 77% to 92% when MR arthrography was performed rather than MR imaging.[23]

INDIRECT MR ARTHROGRAPHY

Because of the invasive nature of direct joint arthrography as well as the logistical challenge of coordinating patient arrival with physician and equipment availability, indirect MR arthrography has been suggested as an alternative to MR arthrography. After intravenous injection of gadolinium-based contrast agents, the contrast diffuses through synovial tissues and preferentially localizes to areas of pathology secondary to hyperemia.[22] Some of the enthusiasm for indirect arthrography may be dampened by accumulating literature on the significance of the long-term deposition of gadolinium in the brain as well as other tissues after intravenous administration.[24] In a series of 94 patients randomized to MR imaging, MR arthrography, and indirect MR arthrography, the overall accuracy for tear of the postoperative meniscus was 80%, 85%, and 81%, respectively.[18] In another series of 41 patients, the accuracy for meniscal re-tear was 63%, 93%, and 94% for MR imaging, MR arthrography, and indirect MR arthrography, respectively.[22] Notably, some degree of enhancement in stable healed granulation tissue is an expected finding in the postoperative meniscus after intravenous contrast administration, which results in a potential false-positive examination.[16] Despite some promise, there is an overall paucity of data on indirect MR arthrography for meniscal re-tears, which should temper recommendations for routine implementation.

NORMAL AND ABNORMAL MR IMAGING FINDINGS IN THE MENISCAL ALLOGRAFT

The anterior and posterior roots of a meniscal allograft may be affixed with bone anchors, allograft bone plugs in a tunnel, or a recessed beveled longitudinal block of bone slotted into the intercondylar eminence.[5] Peripherally, the graft is affixed to any small residual rim of meniscal tissue with numerous sutures (Fig. 9). In addition to resolving changes at the bone–graft and suture interfaces, diffuse increased signal of the graft meniscus, meniscal shrinkage, and mild graft extrusion are considered expected findings (Fig. 10).[4,7] Additionally, surfacing signal has been reported in almost 60% of grafts, but is often stable.[7] The primary usefulness of MR imaging after allograft placement is to evaluate for graft displacement and progressive cartilage damage, which can be done without arthrography.[4]

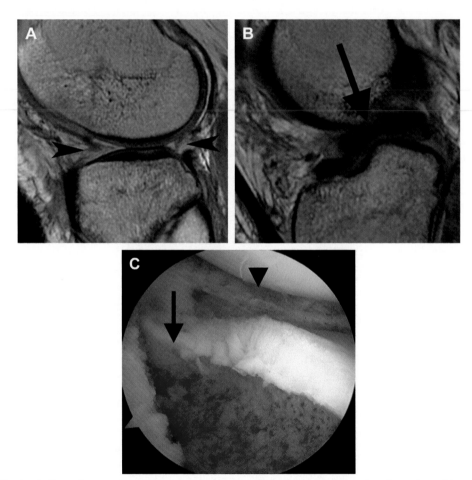

Fig. 9. Meniscal allograft procedure in 28-year-old woman who presented 7 months after subtotal lateral meniscectomy. (A) Sagittal proton density images at the time of the initial injury demonstrated no significant residual lateral meniscal tissue (arrowheads). (B) All fibrocartilage signal tissue seen in the intercondylar notch (arrow) consisted of the displaced lateral meniscus. Subtotal lateral meniscectomy was performed. (C) Arthroscopy image facing laterally during the meniscal allografting shows a prepared bony trough (arrow) at the lateral edge of the intercondylar eminence where the bone block was placed. Further laterally, the rim of meniscocapsular tissue (arrowhead) was rasped in preparation for inside out suture fixation to the outer margin of the meniscal transplant.

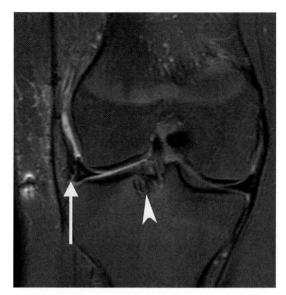

Fig. 10. Expected MR imaging findings of meniscal allograft in 16-year-old girl imaged 4 months after lateral meniscal allograft placement. Coronal proton density fat-saturated image shows a bone anchor (*arrowhead*) for the anterior root of the meniscus at the lateral margin of the intercondylar eminence. There is mild increased signal at the sutured interface of the meniscus allograft (*arrow*) as well as very mild extrusion. All findings are an expected postoperative appearance.

SUMMARY

Postmeniscectomy menisci are expected to have smooth regular margins accompanying a somewhat diminutive meniscus. Linear high signal on short TE sequences is common in postmeniscectomy and repaired menisci that are not retorn. In contrast, high T2-weighted signal touching the meniscal surface has high specificity (90%) but low sensitivity (60%) for meniscal re-tear. On MR arthrography, surfacing signal as bright as the intraarticular gadolinium should be used as the primary criterion for re-tear, but tears may not exhibit signal intensity equal to the contrast agent. Even when not filling with contrast, high T2-weighted signal areas reaching the meniscal surface on MR arthrography likely represent tears.

The pooled sensitivity, specificity, and accuracy of nonarthrographic MR imaging for re-tear of the postoperative meniscus are approximately 70%, 80%, and 80%, respectively. Performing direct MR arthrography in some cases is estimated to improve these performance measures by approximately 10%. Conventional MR imaging performs well for meniscectomy patients in whom less than 25% meniscal excision has been performed. In these patients, the diagnostic criteria and diagnostic accuracy of routine nonarthrographic MR imaging for meniscal re-tear are the same as for nonoperative menisci. Particularly for patients with greater degrees of meniscal resection, the criteria for meniscal re-tear after partial meniscectomy are high T2-weighted signal reaching the articular surface, abnormal meniscal morphology not explained by the prior surgery, a displaced fragment, or tear at a different meniscal site.

Partial meniscectomy is performed far more commonly than meniscal repair, but there is a continuing trend toward more limited meniscectomy and more frequent meniscal repair. If a detailed history is available delineating prior meniscal surgery as meniscal repair or the precise degree of meniscectomy, the imaging protocol can be tailored. Patients with meniscectomy of less than 25% of meniscal tissue should be imaged with nonarthrographic MR imaging (**Box 3**). Although accuracy for diagnosing meniscal tears is decreased in the setting of prior meniscectomy of greater than 25%, the accuracy remains reasonable, and there is a significant prevalence of alternative symptomatic pathology evident on conventional MR imaging to select that as the initial advanced imaging modality. For patients who have had prior meniscal repair, proceeding directly to MR arthrography should be strongly considered. MR imaging of symptoms related to prior meniscal transplant primarily serves to detect cartilage injury or graft displacement and should also be performed without arthrography. Finally, based on these recommendations and the lesser prevalence of meniscal

---

Box 3
Protocol for imaging the postoperative meniscus

- History of meniscectomy: recommend nonarthrogram MR imaging
  - Include T2-weighted FS sequences in the sagittal and coronal planes
  - Sagittal PD, sagittal T2-weighted FS, coronal T1-weighted, coronal T2-weighted FS, axial PD FS
- History of meniscal repair: MR arthrogram
  - May also consider when meniscectomy is greater than 25%
  - Sagittal T1-weighted FS, sagittal T2-weighted FS, sagittal PD, coronal T1-weighted, coronal T2-weighted FS, axial PD FS

Abbreviations: FS, fat-saturated; PD, proton density.

repair relative to meniscectomy, a patient with prior meniscal surgery that is not further detailed should be evaluated with conventional nonarthrographic MR imaging.

REFERENCES

1. Abrams GD, Frank RM, Gupta AK, et al. Trends in meniscus repair and meniscectomy in the United States, 2005-2011. Am J Sports Med 2013;41: 2333–9.

2. Cvetanovich GL, Yanke AB, McCormick F, et al. Trends in meniscal allograft transplantation in the United States, 2007 to 2011. Arthroscopy 2015;31: 1123–7.

3. McDermott ID, Amis AA. The consequences of meniscectomy. Bone Joint J 2006;88:1549–56.

4. Boutin RD, Fritz RC, Marder RA. Magnetic resonance imaging of the postoperative meniscus: resection, repair, and replacement. Magn Reson Imaging Clin N Am 2014;22:517–55.

5. Lee AS, Kang RW, Kroin E, et al. Allograft meniscus transplantation. Sports Med Arthrosc Rev 2012;20: 106–14.

6. Stein T, Mehling AP, Welsch F, et al. Long-term outcome after arthroscopic meniscal repair versus arthroscopic partial meniscectomy for traumatic meniscal tears. Am J Sports Med 2010;38:1542–8.

7. Fox MG. MR imaging of the meniscus: review, current trends, and clinical implications. Radiol Clin North Am 2007;45:1033–53.

8. Johnson D, Weiss WM. Meniscal repair using the inside-out suture technique. Sports Med Arthrosc Rev 2012;20:68–76.

9. Shelbourne KD, Gray T. Meniscus tears that can be left in situ, with or without trephination or synovial abrasion to stimulate healing. Sports Med Arthrosc Rev 2012;20:62–7.

10. De Smet AA. How I diagnose meniscal tears on knee MRI. AJR Am J Roentgenol 2012;199:481–99.

11. Morrison WB, Sanders TG. Imaging of the knee. In: Morrison WB, Sanders TG, editors. Problem solving in musculoskeletal imaging. Philadelphia: Mosby/Elsevier; 2008. p. 634.

12. Kijowski R, Rosas H, Williams A, et al. MRI characteristics of torn and untorn post-operative menisci. Skeletal Radiol 2017;46:1353–60.

13. Muellner T, Egkher A, Nikolic A, et al. Open meniscal repair: clinical and magnetic resonance imaging findings after twelve years. Am J Sports Med 1999; 27:16–20.

14. Farley TE, Howell SM, Love KF, et al. Meniscal tears: MR and arthrographic findings after arthroscopic repair. Radiology 1991;180:517–22.

15. Miao Y, Yu JK, Ao YF, et al. Diagnostic values of 3 methods for evaluating meniscal healing status after meniscal repair: comparison among second-look arthroscopy, clinical assessment, and magnetic resonance imaging. Am J Sports Med 2011;39: 735–42.

16. Sanders TG. Imaging of the postoperative knee. Semin Musculoskelet Radiol 2011;15:383–407.

17. Magee T, Shapiro M, Rodriguez J, et al. MR arthrography of postoperative knee: for which patients is it useful? Radiology 2003;229:159–63.

18. White LM, Schweitzer ME, Weishaupt D, et al. Diagnosis of recurrent meniscal tears: prospective evaluation of conventional MR imaging, indirect MR arthrography, and direct MR arthrography. Radiology 2002;222:421–9.

19. Applegate GR, Flannigan BD, Tolin BS, et al. MR diagnosis of recurrent tears in the knee: value of intraarticular contrast material. AJR Am J Roentgenol 1993;161:821–5.

20. De Smet AA, Horak DM, Davis KW, et al. Intensity of signal contacting meniscal surface in recurrent tears on MR arthrography compared with that of contrast material. AJR Am J Roentgenol 2006;187:W565–8.

21. Magee T. Accuracy of 3-Tesla MR and MR arthrography in diagnosis of meniscal retear in the postoperative knee. Skeletal Radiol 2014;43:1057–64.

22. Vives MJ, Homesley D, Ciccotti MG, et al. Evaluation of recurring meniscal tears with gadolinium-enhanced magnetic resonance imaging. Am J Sports Med 2003;31:868–73.

23. Sciulli RL, Boutin RD, Brown RR, et al. Evaluation of the postoperative meniscus of the knee: a study comparing conventional arthrography, conventional MR imaging, MR arthrography with iodinated contrast material, and MR arthrography with gadolinium-based contrast material. Skeletal Radiol 1999;28:508–14.

24. McDonald RJ, McDonald JS, Kallmes DF, et al. Intracranial gadolinium deposition after contrast-enhanced MR imaging. Radiology 2015;275: 772–82.

Current Concepts of Femoroacetabular Impingement

Aria Ghaffari, MD[a], Ivan Davis, MD[a],*, Troy Storey, MD[a], Michael Moser, MD[b]

KEYWORDS

- Femoroacetabular impingement • Cam • Pincer • Mixed-type • Hip • Cartilage • Labrum

KEY POINTS

- Femoroacetabular impingement (FAI) is a syndrome caused by osseous pathomorphology that alters normal hip biomechanics, causing characteristic patterns of chondral and labral injuries.
- FAI eventually causes osteoarthritis and may be a primary contributor to idiopathic hip osteoarthritis.
- Imaging findings of FAI are subtle, requiring the use of a routine checklist during imaging interpretation.
- Patients can benefit from intervention early in the disease process, making early recognition and efficient comprehensive reporting essential to advancing clinical decision-making.

INTRODUCTION

Femoroacetabular impingement (FAI) is a clinical syndrome characterized by osseous pathomorphology of the acetabulum and/or femoral head-neck junction (FHNJ) leading to abutment between the acetabulum and femur during hip motion.[1,2] FAI usually presents in active young and middle-aged adults with hip or groin pain, often exacerbated by activity or prolonged sitting.[3,4] Clinically, the differential diagnosis is wide (Box 1).

FAI pathomorphology is categorized into cam and pincer deformities.[1,2] Mixed-type FAI, where both cam and pincer morphologies are present, is the most common form of FAI.[5] Cam and pincer deformities are each present in approximately one in three asymptomatic men and approximately one in six asymptomatic women in the general population.[6] In adult athletes, the prevalence of cam and mixed FAI morphology is considerably higher, present in 66% and 57%, respectively.[7]

FAI leads to hip osteoarthritis and is likely the primary contributor to idiopathic hip osteoarthritis.[2,8–11] It also causes soft tissue abnormalities, such as focal cartilage defects, cartilage delamination, chondrolabral separation, and labral tears.[1,2,12] At this time, preventative treatment in asymptomatic patients with FAI morphology is controversial.[13] Conversely, patients with symptomatic FAI can benefit from early noninvasive and surgical interventions. Positive treatment outcome is inversely correlated with the degree of soft tissue injury and osteoarthritis present in the affected hip. Thus, early recognition of FAI and appropriate characterization of associated abnormalities is vital to clinical outcome.[4]

The imaging findings of FAI are frequently subtle and overlooked. A checklist approach based on

Disclosure Statement: The authors have nothing to disclose.
[a] Department of Radiology, College of Medicine, University of Florida, Post Office Box 100374, Gainesville, FL 32610-0374, USA; [b] Department of Orthopaedics and Rehabilitation, UF Orthopaedics and Sports Medicine Institute, University of Florida, 3450 Hull Road, Gainesville, FL 32607, USA
* Corresponding author.
E-mail address: davivc@radiology.ufl.edu

Radiol Clin N Am 56 (2018) 965–982
https://doi.org/10.1016/j.rcl.2018.06.009

current concepts of FAI improves diagnostic performance, allowing the radiologist to efficiently generate comprehensive reports that advance clinical decision-making (**Box 2**).[14] In this article, we detail our approach to the imaging assessment of FAI.

FEMOROACETABULAR IMPINGEMENT: NORMAL ANATOMY

The hip joint is a tightly congruent ball-in-socket joint.[15] Normal range of motion is limited by the osseous structures and requires a spherical femoral head, normal femoral head neck offset,

and normal containment of the femoral head by the acetabulum (**Fig. 1**).[16]

The fibrocartilaginous labrum arises from the acetabular margin and continues across the acetabular notch inferiorly as the histologically identical transverse ligament.[17] The labrum expands the acetabular articular surface and assists in joint stability.[15] The labrum also induces a seal effect that maintains pressurized fluid between the femoral head and acetabular cartilage layers, decreasing cartilage wear and enhancing joint lubrication.[18]

Both the femoral head and acetabulum are largely covered by a 1- to 3-mm-thick layer of hyaline cartilage.[19] The bone immediately underlying the cartilage is termed the subchondral bone plate. The chondrolabral junction is a histologic 1- to 2-mm transition zone between the hyaline cartilage of the acetabulum and the labrum.[17] Knowledge of hyaline cartilage histology fosters understanding of compositional cartilage MR imaging (cMRI), discussed later. The hyaline cartilage is largely composed of an extracellular matrix with a small concentration of chondrocytes. The extracellular matrix is primarily water interspersed among a highly organized cross-linked matrix composed of proteoglycans and collagen fibers.[20] This matrix serves as the structural framework and provides much of the tensile and shear strength of cartilage.[21] Glycosaminoglycan molecules are attached to the proteoglycans, possess considerable negative charge, and confer compressive strength to cartilage.[21]

FEMOROACETABULAR IMPINGEMENT: PATHOLOGY

In FAI, osseous pathomorphology leads to repetitive abutment between the acetabulum and proximal femur during hip motion, leading to soft tissue injury and accelerated hip osteoarthritis. In a small subset of patients, FAI can occur with normal osseous anatomy, typically in those with joint hypermobility and excessive use, such as in gymnasts.[22] There are two types of osseous pathomorphology in FAI: cam and pincer.[12] Each type induces a characteristic pattern of biomechanical perturbation and consequent predictable pattern of soft tissue injury. Recall that mixed-type FAI is most common, with these patients exhibiting a hybrid injury pattern. Knowledge of these patterns fosters an accurate and efficient search pattern, aiding the radiologist in generation of a clinically useful report.[14] The following section describe the pathomorphology, pathomechanics, and expected soft tissue injury patterns of pincer and cam FAI.

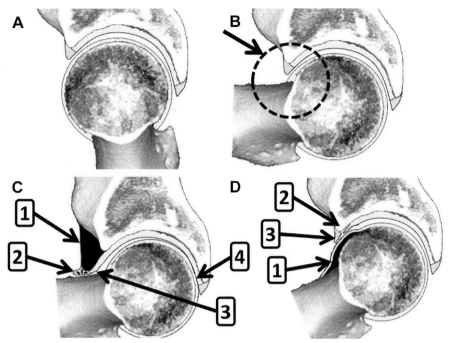

Fig. 1. Patterns of soft tissue damage in isolated cam and pincer-type FAI. (*A*) Normal sagittal illustration of hip in extension. (*B*) Normal hip in flexion shows normal femoral head sphericity and femoral head-neck offset, allowing femur to clear the acetabulum in flexion (*arrow/circle*). (*C*) Hip with pincer morphology in flexion shows: (1) anterior osseous acetabular overcoverage, (2) primary labral damage with intrasubstance fissuring, (3) load is transferred to thin rim of adjacent acetabular cartilage, and (4) contrecoup FAI with posterior femoral head and acetabular cartilage injury. (*D*) Hip with cam-type morphology in flexion shows: (1) osseous prominence at the anterior FHNJ; (2) chondrolabral separation with adjacent cartilage delamination; and (3) mildly displaced labrum, but otherwise intact and still fixed to the underlying bone.

Pincer Femoroacetabular Impingement

Pincer FAI is defined by osseous acetabular overcoverage, of which there are four patterns (**Box 3**, **Fig. 2**). Distinguishing between these patterns informs clinical decision-making. The cause is usually idiopathic but can be post-traumatic or iatrogenic from overcorrection of hip dysplasia.[13] With hip flexion and internal rotation, the FHNJ compresses the labrum against the subchondral bone plate of the acetabulum, causing labral tears and degeneration (see **Fig. 1**).[12] This force is then transmitted to a thin rim of neighboring acetabular cartilage, causing a narrow band of chondral injury along the acetabular rim (**Fig. 3**).[12]

> **Box 3**
> **Patterns of pincer FAI morphology**
>
> - Global acetabular overcoverage
> - Focal anterior rim overcoverage
> - Acetabular retroversion
> - Focal posterior rim overcoverage

With continued hip flexion, the anterior rim leverages the femoral head, causing transient posterior hip subluxation. The posteromedial femoral head then abuts the posteroinferior acetabulum, causing focal femoral and/or acetabular cartilage injury, termed contrecoup injury (see **Fig. 1**).[12] Multiple forms of abnormal mineralization occur at the superolateral acetabulum in the setting of FAI, particularly when a pincer component is present (**Table 1**).[22]

Cam-Type Femoroacetabular Impingement

The cam-type deformity is characterized by asphericity of the femoral head and/or insufficient concavity at the FHNJ, most commonly occurring anterolaterally.[12] Participation in high-impact sporting activities during skeletal maturation is associated with an increased risk of developing cam morphology.[23] Other potential causes include malunited femoral neck fracture, prior femoral head osteotomy, Perthes disease, and slipped capital femoral epiphysis.[13]

During hip flexion, the anterior femoral neck protuberance contacts the 12:00 through 2:00

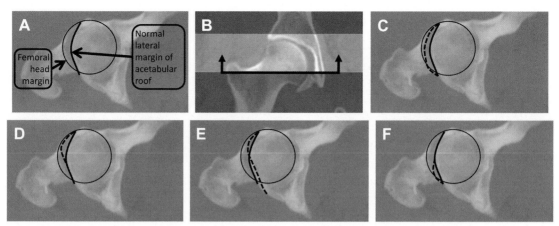

Fig. 2. Patterns of pincer morphology. (*A*) Three-dimensional (3D) maximum intensity projection image from CT slab demarcates normal landmarks. (*B*) Coronal CT image highlights the slab (*arrows*) corresponding to **Fig. 1**A. (*C*) 3D maximum intensity projection in the axial projection shows global acetabular overcoverage of the femoral head (*circle*) by the acetabulum (*dashed lines*) (*normal acetabular margin = curved solid line*). (*D*) Focal anterior rim overcoverage (*dashed line*), with normal posterior rim. (*E*) Acetabular retroversion (*dashed line*), with anterior rim overcoverage and posterior rim deficiency. (*F*) Focal posterior rim overcoverage (*dashed line*), with normal anterior rim.

positions of the anterosuperior articular cartilage. This pathologic contact drives the underlying acetabular cartilage centrally and the adjacent labrum peripherally, inducing a large tensile load at the chondrolabral junction, causing chondrolabral separation (see **Fig. 1**).[12] Shear stresses generated between the deep layer of the acetabular cartilage and the subchondral bone plate cause cartilage delamination. Delaminating injury communicating with the cartilage surface is termed a cartilage flap. Surgeons can probe deep to this flap during arthroscopy.[24] Delamination without surface communication is termed carpet phenomenon. At arthroscopy, the surgeon can mobilize the cartilage with respect to the underlying bone plate but no surface injury is visible.[24] In isolated cam-type FAI, the labrum is spared until advanced cartilage damage is already established (see **Fig. 3**).[2,5,12] Femoral retrotorsion and coxa vara are additional morphologic abnormalities that can result in cam-type impingement.[22]

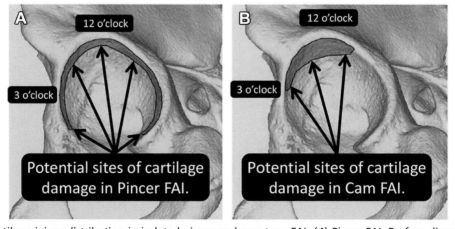

Fig. 3. Cartilage injury distribution in isolated pincer and cam-type FAI. (*A*) Pincer FAI. En face diagram of the acetabulum shows cartilage damage along a thin strip adjacent to the labrum with mean transverse width of 4 mm. Much of the acetabular circumference can be involved (*arrows*). (*B*) Cam FAI. Cartilage damage is confined to the 3:00 (anterior) through 11:00 (anterosuperior) clock face positions, with mean transverse width of 11 mm (*arrows*).

Table 1		
Types of abnormal mineralization occurring about hip in FAI		
Type	**Morphology**	**Etiology/comment**
Labral mineralization	Amorphous mineralization	Response to chronic labral irritation
Os acetabuli	Triangular fragment; corticomedullary architecture	Chronic fracture of the lateral acetabular roof
Acetabular reactive change	Bone apposition adjacent to or thickening of lateral acetabular roof	Chronic stress response; leads to further deepening of the acetabulum and worsening pincer FAI

FEMOROACETABULAR IMPINGEMENT: IMAGING ASSESSMENT

FAI is typically assessed with radiography, MR imaging, and direct magnetic resonance arthrography (MRA). Radiography depicts the osseous abnormality of FAI in symptomatic and asymptomatic patients. Given the prevalence of FAI in asymptomatic patients and the potential benefits of early intervention, the radiologist should routinely assess for FAI morphology on all adult pelvic and hip radiographs without evidence of moderate-to-advanced hip osteoarthritis. MR imaging/MRA plays two roles: multiplanar visualization of osseous anatomy and soft tissue injury staging. We find a checklist approach for both modalities essential because findings of FAI are frequently subtle.

Other modalities are less useful to characterize FAI. Computed tomography accurately visualizes the osseous morphology but does not depict the cartilage or labrum. Ultrasound is reliable in detecting cam morphology, although its role in FAI is not yet established.[25] In the following section, we detail our technique and checklist to the radiographic and MR evaluation of FAI. Included are descriptions of normal imaging anatomy and findings of FAI.

RADIOGRAPHIC IMAGING TECHNIQUE

The imaging assessment of FAI begins with a high-quality anteroposterior pelvic radiograph. Radiographic technique is well described in the literature.[22,26] To avoid potential false-positive findings of pincer FAI, the anteroposterior radiograph should be upright and must be centered on the patient's midline rather than the hip.[2,22,27] A complete radiographic examination also includes a lateral view, of which multiple types exist.[26] We find the frog-leg lateral radiograph to be sufficient in our practice.

Radiographic Checklist, Anatomy, and Imaging Findings of Femoroacetabular Impingement

We ensure a comprehensive radiographic assessment of FAI by systematically following a checklist (**Box 4, Figs. 4–9**).[28–30] We recognize suboptimal radiographic positioning, which degrades multiple signs of FAI (see **Fig. 4; Fig. 10**). We not only identify pincer FAI, but further classify it (see **Figs. 5–7; Fig. 11, Table 2**). We detect obvious and subtle cam deformities (**Box 5**; see **Figs. 8 and 9; Fig. 12**). Finally, we recognize common associated findings of FAI, such as abnormal labral mineralization, synovial herniation pits, and osteoarthritis (**Figs. 13 and 14**).

Box 4
Checklist of radiographic imaging findings in the assessment of FAI
1. Radiographic positioning (see **Fig. 4**)
2. Coxa profunda and coxa protrusio (protrusio acetabuli) (see **Fig. 5**)
3. Center-edge angle of Wiberg (see **Fig. 6**)
4. Acetabular index (see **Fig. 6**)
5. Crossover sign (see **Fig. 7**)
6. Posterior wall sign (see **Fig. 7**)
7. Ischial spine sign (see **Fig. 7**)
8. Femoral head sphericity on all views (see **Fig. 8**)
9. FHNJ waisting on all views (see **Fig. 8**)
10. If indicated, measurement of alpha angle and femoral head-neck offset distance (see **Fig. 9**)
11. Presence of abnormal acetabular mineralization, synovial herniation pits, or osteoarthritis

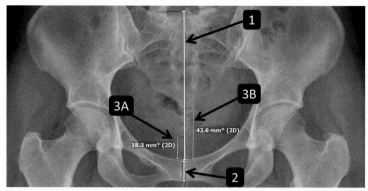

Fig. 4. Assessment of radiographic positioning on anteroposterior pelvic radiograph. Lateral rotation and pelvic tilt must be assessed by: (1) drawing a line bisecting the sacrum and (2) drawing a line bisecting the pubic symphysis. Lines (1) and (2) should be coincident or less than 1.0 cm apart. Next, measure the distance between the superior margin of the pubic symphysis and the tip of the coccyx (3A) (normal = 1–3 cm) or sacrococcygeal joint (3B) (normal = 3–5 cm). Measurements above normal ranges indicate pelvic inclination. Measurements below normal ranges indicate pelvic reclination.

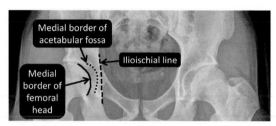

Fig. 5. Qualitative assessment of global acetabular depth. Assessment for pincer morphology begins with qualitative assessment of the global acetabular depth. Three normal landmarks are the medial border of femoral head, medial border of acetabular fossa, and ilioischial line. Coxa profunda occurs when the medial border of acetabular fossa contacts or is medial to the ilioischial line, and coxa protrusio or protrusio acetabuli occurs when the medial border of the femoral head contacts or is medial to the ilioischial line.

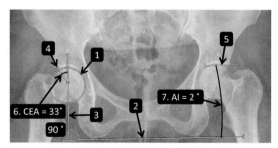

Fig. 6. Normal center-edge angle (CEA) and acetabular index (AI). Global acetabular overcoverage can also be assessed quantitatively using the CEA and AI (Tonnis angle) by: (1) drawing a circle approximating the femoral head, (2) drawing a line connecting the inferior pubic rami, (3) drawing a perpendicular line through the femoral head center, (4) drawing a line from femoral head center to lateral edge of acetabular sourcil, and (5) drawing a line between medial and lateral margins of the acetabular sourcil. (6) CEA is the angle between lines 3 and 4 (normal = 25°–39°; acetabular overcoverage >39°). (7) AI is the angle between lines 2 and 5 (normal is between 0° and 10°).

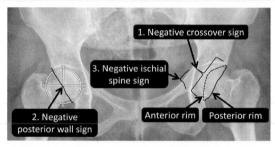

Fig. 7. Crossover, posterior wall, and ischial spine signs are associated with pincer FAI. (1) Crossover sign. The anterior rim normally remains medial to the posterior rim. If the anterior rim extends lateral to the posterior rim superiorly, a crossover sign is present. (2) Posterior wall sign. The posterior rim should cross at or near the femoral head center. If posterior rim is lateral, then posterior wall overcoverage is present. If posterior rim is medial, then a deficient posterior wall is present. (3) Ischial spine sign. The ischial spine is normally largely obscured by the medial acetabulum. If prominent, acetabular retroversion may be present.

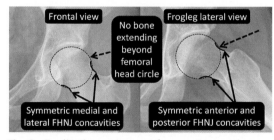

Fig. 8. Qualitative assessment for cam-type pathomorphology in a normal hip. Cam morphology can result from femoral head asphericity and/or abnormal waisting at the FHNJ. Qualitative assessment is usually sufficient, performed by approximating the femoral head with a circle by visual assessment or with a PACS tool. The FHNJ contours should be compared on the frontal and lateral views (*arrows*). Cam morphology typically has increased radius of curvature of the anterior to lateral FHNJ. Any bone extending beyond the circle, particularly anterolaterally (*dashed arrows*), is suspicious for cam pathomorphology.

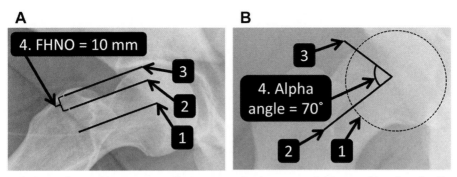

Fig. 9. Quantitative radiographic assessment for cam-type impingement. (*A*) Femoral head-neck offset (FHNO) is assessed on lateral view by: (1) drawing a line bisecting the femoral neck, (2) drawing a parallel line along the femoral neck's anterior margin, and (3) drawing a parallel line tangential to femoral head's anterior margin. (4) FHNO is distance between 2 and 3 (FHNO <10 mm indicates cam morphology). (*B*) Alpha angle is assessed on lateral view by: (1) drawing a circle approximating the femoral head, (2) drawing a line bisecting the femoral neck, and (3) drawing a line from FHC to point where bone extends beyond the femoral head circle. (4) Alpha angle is formed by lines 2 and 3 (alpha angle >55° indicates cam morphology).

MR IMAGING MAGNETIC RESONANCE ARTHROGRAPHY TECHNIQUE

Many studies have assessed the diagnostic accuracy of MRA and MR imaging. Results of three recent studies are shown in **Table 3**.[31–33] It is reasonable to question whether the moderate benefits of MRA outweigh the added risks, financial costs, and workflow burdens incurred by arthrography, especially given the potential of improved MR imaging with greater field strengths and improved hardware. This remains an active area of discussion within the literature.[34,35]

At our institution, we perform MRA on 3-T magnets using a surface coil and inherent spine coil segments (**Table 4**). The hip of interest is centered within the bore of the magnet to the extent possible. We first survey the entire pelvis with large field of view sequences. Next, we evaluate for marrow edema and musculotendinous injuries about the hip by acquiring fast spin echo sequences in true anatomic planes. We complete our protocol by acquiring sequences specifically tailored to assess for FAI (**Table 5**). Some institutions perform MRA with continuous leg traction, termed traction arthrography.[15] This serves to

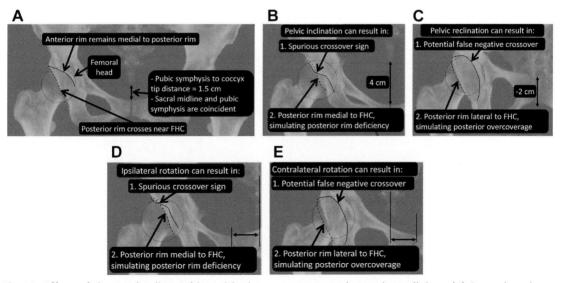

Fig. 10. Effects of abnormal radiographic positioning on crossover and posterior wall signs. (*A*) Coronal maximum intensity projection computed tomography with normal positioning and normal osseous landmarks. (*B*) Pelvic inclination of 30°. (*C*) Pelvic reclination of 30°. (*D*) Ipsilateral rotation of 15°. (*E*) Contralateral rotation of 15°.

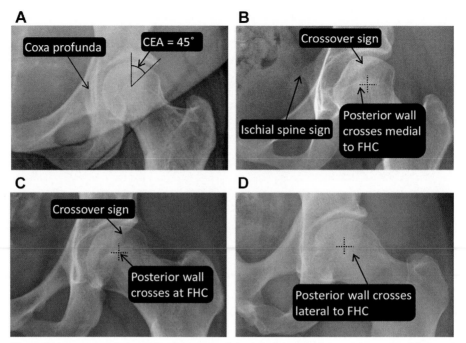

Fig. 11. Radiographic patterns of pincer impingement. (*A*) Global acetabular overcoverage. (*B*) Acetabular retroversion. (*C*) Focal anterior overcoverage. (*D*) Focal posterior overcoverage.

Table 2
Diagnostic criteria: pincer morphology on radiography

Global acetabular overcoverage	Acetabular retroversion
• Coxa profunda	• Crossover sign
• Protrusio acetabuli in severe cases	• Posterior wall crosses medial to FHC
• Increased center-edge angle (>40°)	• Ischial spine sign
Focal anterior rim overcoverage	Focal posterior rim overcoverage
• Crossover sign	• Posterior wall crosses lateral to FHC
• Posterior wall crosses near FHC	

Abbreviation: FHC, femoral head center.

Box 5
Cam morphology on radiography and MR imaging

- Asphericity of the femoral head
- Abnormal waisting at the FHNJ
- Femoral head-neck offset less than 10 mm
- Femoral head-neck offset to femoral head diameter ratio less than 0.17 (on cross-table axial radiographic projection)[26]
- Alpha angle greater than 55°

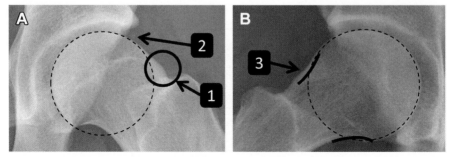

Fig. 12. Radiographic imaging appearance of cam-type morphology. (*A*) Frog-leg lateral radiograph demonstrates cam deformity at the anterior FHNJ (1) and labral mineralization (2). (*B*) Frog-leg lateral radiograph demonstrates asymmetry of the anterior FHNJ (3).

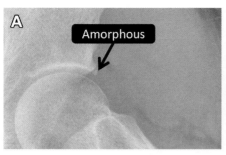
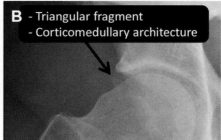

Fig. 13. Abnormal mineralization in setting of FAI. (*A*) Labral mineralization (*arrow*). (*B*) Os acetabulum (*arrow*).

break the seal effect of the labrum, allowing contrast material to interpose between and thereby separate the acetabular and femoral cartilage layers, potentially improving visualization of cartilage injury.

Cartilage assessment with MR imaging/MRA largely relies on detecting abnormal cartilage morphology, which occurs late in the course of injury. Earlier stages of cartilage injury occur at the histologic level and include increased water content, disruption of the collagen network, and loss of glycosaminoglycan.[20] This histologic injury leads to measurable changes in relaxation times of MR contrast parameters, such as T1 and T2. The goal of cMR imaging is to probe the histologic environment by quantifying these changes (**Table 6**).[20,36]

MR Imaging/Magnetic Resonance Arthrography Checklist, Anatomy, and Imaging Findings of Femoroacetabular Impingement

MR imaging/MRA findings of FAI are subtle, requiring the use of a checklist (**Box 6, Figs. 15–18**).[37,38]

Osseous

We first establish the osseous deformities present because these inform surgical decision-making

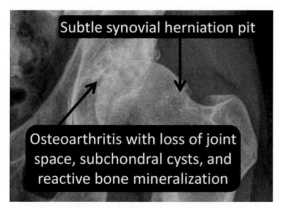

Fig. 14. Synovial herniation pit and moderate to severe osteoarthritis (*arrows*) on anteroposterior radiograph.

and direct the soft tissue search pattern. We classify any pincer deformities as global acetabular overcoverage or acetabular retroversion (**Fig. 19**, **Tables 7** and **8**). Advanced imaging techniques can further aid in visualization (**Fig. 20**). Next, we search for cam morphology on all planes and sequences and by using multiplanar reformatted images (see **Box 5**; **Fig. 21**). When detected, we provide a clock face localization. We typically do not provide alpha angles unless requested otherwise.

Cartilage

We next assess the hip articular cartilage, a potentially crucial contribution of MR imaging/MRA, because moderate-to-severe cartilage injuries may be a contraindication to joint preservation surgery.[30] Unfortunately, MR imaging/MRA has limited accuracy for chondral injury detection in the setting of FAI for multiple reasons (**Box 7**; see **Table 3**). This deficiency along with increasing use of joint preservation surgery has spurred research into compositional cMR imaging techniques, which have the potential to identify histologic cartilage injury before gross morphologic abnormalities develop (see **Table 6**). Early results are mixed, yet encouraging, and the clinical impact of cMR imaging remains to be established.[15,36,39–41] The remainder of this section focuses on the morphologic assessment of hip articular cartilage, which is currently in wide clinical use.

Hip articular cartilage is normally smooth in contour and uniformly intermediate in signal intensity (see **Fig. 18**). The femoral and acetabular cartilage layers each have a thickness of 1 to 3 mm.[19] These layers are often inseparable on MR imaging. Recall that isolated cam and isolated pincer FAI each have characteristic cartilage injury distributions (see **Fig. 3**). However, the morphology of cartilage injury is similar and includes chondrolabral separation, cartilage delamination, and surface defects.

We first assess for chondrolabral separation, indicated by abnormal signal at the chondrolabral junction. Defects may be partial-thickness or full-thickness. Acute and subacute injuries tend to

Table 3
Diagnostic accuracy of MRA and MR imaging

Study	Study Type	Acetabular Labrum Injury (%)		Acetabular Cartilage Injury (%)	
		MRA	MR Imaging	MRA	MR Imaging
Sutter, et al,[31] 2014	Direct comparison in 28 patients at 1.5 T	Sn: 85–89 Sp: 50–100	Sn: 77–89 Sp: 50	Sn: 71–92 Sp: 25–100	Sn: 58–83 Sp: 50–100
Smith, et al,[32] 2011	Meta-analysis	Sn: 87 Sp: 64	Sn: 66 Sp: 79	N/a	N/a
Smith, et al,[33] 2013	Meta-analysis	N/a	N/a	Sn: 62 Sp: 86	Sn: 59 Sp: 94

Results of three recent studies comparing the diagnostic accuracy of MRA and MR imaging for detection of soft tissue injuries in FAI.

Abbreviations: N/a, not applicable; Sn, sensitivity; Sp, Specificity.

Table 4
Suggested MRA protocol at 3 T

Sequences	TR/TE (ms)	FA	ETL	PB (Hz/pixel)	NEX	Matrix	FOV (cm)	Slice Thickness/Gap (mm)
Coronal STIR wide FOV	3100/40	90°	11	195	2	352 × 192	34 × 30	5/1
Coronal T1 FS	960/12	90°	6	244	2	256 × 256	16 × 16	3/0.5
Axial T1	600/10	90°	2	244	2	256 × 256	16 × 16	3/0.5
Coronal IW FS	3000/36	90°	7	195	2	256 × 256	16 × 16	3/0.5
Axial oblique IW FS	3600/36	90°	11	195	2	256 × 256	16 × 16	3/0.5
Sagittal IW	3600/36	90°	11	195	2	256 × 256	16 × 16	3/1
Radial IW FS	2900/24	90°	7	150	2	256 × 256	16 × 16	2.0[a]
3D axial GRE	5.9/2.7	10°	1	488	3	208 × 208	20 × 20	1.5

Abbreviations: 3D, three dimensional; ETL, echo train length; FA, flip angle; FOV, field of view; FS, fat-saturated; GRE, gradient-recalled echo; IW, intermediate-weighted; NEX, number of excitations; PB, pixel bandwidth; TE, echo time; TR, repetition time.

[a] For the radial sequence, 24 slices are acquired, spaced at 7.5° intervals.

Table 5
Sequences helpful in the evaluation of FAI

Axial oblique (Swiss axial)	• Obtained parallel to the femoral neck • Allows better visualization of the anterior and posterior labrum with decreased geometric distortion
Radial imaging	• Images are perpendicular to a double-oblique en face view of the acetabulum • Sequence is acquired directly from scout images (our preference) or reformatted from an isovoxel three-dimensional sequence • Minimizes geometric distortion and partial-volume average effects inherent when imaging spherical structures using routine anatomic planes
3D GRE	• Obtained with 1.5-mm isotropic voxels • Allows multiplanar assessment of osseous morphology
SS-FSE of the knee and hip	• Rapid acquisition of low-resolution images of the hip and knee with unchanged positioning to assess for femoral torsion

Abbreviations: 3D, three dimensional; GRE, gradient recalled echo; SS-FSE, single-shot fast spin echo.

Table 6		
Four common cartilage compositional MR imaging techniques		
Technique	Comments	Pathologic Findings
dGEMRIC	T1 map; detects loss of GAGs; requires intravenous or intra-articular contrast	T1 shortening
T2 mapping	Detects increased water content and collagen network disruption	T2 prolongation
T2* mapping	Detects increased water content, collagen network disruption, and calcium deposits in injured cartilage	T2* shortening
T1ρ imaging	Detects loss of GAG and collagen network disruption	T1ρ prolongation

Abbreviations: dGEMRIC, delayed gadolinium-enhanced MR imaging of cartilage; GAG, glycosaminoglycan.

imbibe contrast or approach fluid signal intensity (**Fig. 22**). Chronic injuries are usually characterized by intermediate signal that does not imbibe contrast. We have found margination of the defect

Box 6
MR imaging/MRA checklist approach to the assessment of FAI

1. Review recent pelvic radiograph
2. Acetabular depth (see **Fig. 15**)
3. Center-edge angle (see **Fig. 15**)
4. Equatorial and cranial acetabular version (see **Fig. 16, Table 7**)
5. Assessment of femoral head sphericity and FHNJ concavity (see **Fig. 17**)
6. Hip cartilage (see **Fig. 18**)
7. Acetabular labrum (see **Fig. 18**)

to be useful in distinguishing chondrolabral separation from a normal variant sublabral sulcus but not useful in determining chronicity. In some cases, distinguishing chondrolabral separation from a sublabral sulcus is not possible (**Fig. 23**). **Box 8** lists the criteria for sublabral sulcus.[42,43]

Cartilage delamination injuries, particularly carpet phenomenon, are difficult to identify. The most specific finding is fluid or contrast signal interposing between a cartilage flap and the subchondral bone plate (**Figs. 24** and **25**). However, the sensitivity of this finding is only 22% to 30%.[24] Linear T1 and T2 hypointensity within the acetabular cartilage has also been observed in delaminated cartilage, although the utility of this finding has been questioned.[24,36] Cartilage surface injuries manifest as surface irregularity, focal asymmetric cartilage thinning, or gross defects (see **Fig. 24**). Once characterized, cartilage injuries and chondrolabral separation are localized using a clock face.

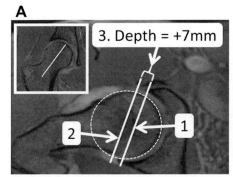 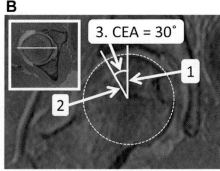

Fig. 15. Global acetabular overcoverage is evaluated on MR imaging using acetabular depth (AD) and center-edge angle (CEA). (*A*) AD is measured on oblique axial image parallel to the longitudinal axis of the femoral neck, at the level of the mid femoral neck by: (1) drawing a line connecting anterior and posterior osseous acetabular rims; and (2) drawing a parallel line through the femoral head center (FHC). (3) AD is the distance between (1) and (2). AD is positive when FHC is lateral to line (1), and negative when FHC is medial to line (1). (*B*) CEA is measured on coronal image through the FHC by: (1) drawing a line from FHC extending vertically; and (2) drawing a line from FHC to the lateral osseous rim. (3) CEA is the angle between lines (1) and (2).

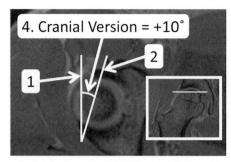
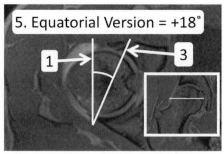

Fig. 16. Focal acetabular overcoverage is evaluated on MR imaging/MRA using cranial and equatorial angles, similar to computed tomography. Measurements are made on axial images by: (1) drawing a sagittal midline, which bisects the pubic symphysis and sacrum, correcting for patient rotation; (2) drawing a line connecting the anterior and posterior acetabular rims at the level of superior acetabulum where the femoral head is visualized; and (3) drawing a line connecting the anterior and posterior acetabular rims at the level of the mid-acetabulum. Cranial version angle is formed between lines (1) and (2), and equatorial version angle is formed between lines (1) and (3). Positive angles reflect acetabular anteversion, and negative angles reflect acetabular retroversion.

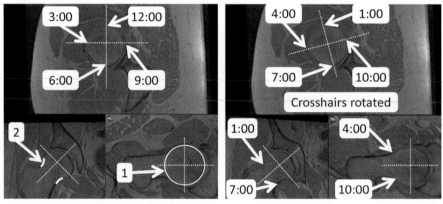

Fig. 17. Assessment for cam-type morphology using MR imaging/MRA (parallels radiographic approach). Reformat 3D sequences into radial images based off the longitudinal axis of the femoral neck. Axes are then rotated on the double-oblique sagittal view to circumferentially assess the FHNJ without geometric distortion. (1) Assess femoral head sphericity by approximating femoral head with a circle and searching for bone extending beyond this circle; and (2) assess symmetry of the FHNJ concavities on each slice.

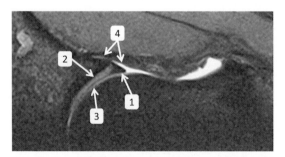

Fig. 18. Normal MR appearance of hip cartilage and acetabular labrum. Radial intermediate-weighted MRA at 1:00-clock position demonstrates: (1) triangular-shaped, uniformly hypointense labrum with smooth margins; (2) thicker homogeneously intermediate-signal intensity acetabular cartilage; (3) thinner homogeneously intermediate-signal intensity femoral cartilage; and (4) small normal pericapsular recess with contrast extending between the capsular margin of the labrum and adjacent capsule.

Labrum

Like cartilage injuries, moderate to severe labral injury is a contraindication to joint-preservation surgery.[30] The following section describes normal labrum, anatomic variants, and labral injuries. The acetabular labrum is normally triangular (see **Fig. 18**). The labrum may also be rounded, flattened, or teardrop in shape, which we consider variant anatomy provided there are no other morphologic labral abnormalities.[44] The articular and capsular margins of the labrum are smooth. The labrum should be uniformly hypointense on all sequences.

A normal-variant sublabral sulcus can occur at any location, although its existence and prevalence is controversial (see **Box 8, Fig. 23**).[44] A perilabral recess is normally located between the capsular edge of the labrum and the adjacent capsule (see **Fig. 18**). The transverse ligament is a histologically identical extension of the labrum

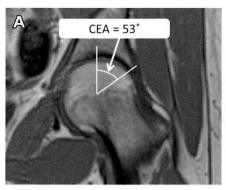

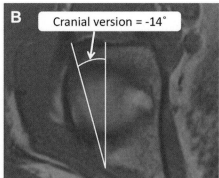

Fig. 19. Pincer FAI morphology on MR imaging. (*A*) Coronal image demonstrates global acetabular overcoverage, with a CEA of 53°. (*B*) Axial image shows acetabular retroversion, with cranial version of −14°.

Table 7
Normal and abnormal values for cranial and equatorial retroversion on MR imaging

Measurement Level	Normal Values	Abnormal Values
Cranial	13°–20°	<0°
Equatorial	5°–8°	<0°

Table 8
Pincer morphology on MR imaging

On MR imaging, we classify pincer deformities into global acetabular overcoverage or acetabular retroversion

Global acetabular overcoverage	Acetabular retroversion
• Negative acetabular depth (femoral head center medial to line connecting anterior and posterior acetabular rims) • Center-edge angle >39°	• Negative cranial or equatorial acetabular version ("retroversion")

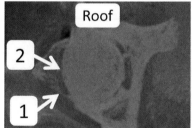

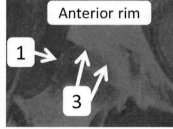

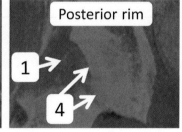

Fig. 20. Inverted gray-scale minimum intensity projection images illustrating normal acetabular morphology. Source data is a GRE sequence with TR/TE/FA of 5.9 ms/2.7 ms/10°. 1 = femoral head, 2 = acetabular roof, 3 = anterior rim, 4 = posterior rim.

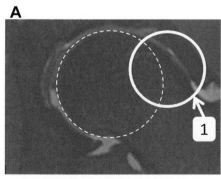

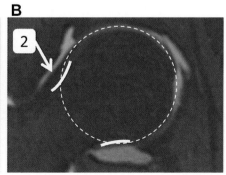

Fig. 21. MR imaging/MRA appearance of cam morphology. (*A*) Radial intermediate-weighted MRA at 1:30 demonstrates femoral head asphericity (*1 = solid circle*). *Dashed circle = femoral head*. (*B*) Radial intermediate-weighted MRA at 1:30 demonstrates asymmetric FHNJ (*2*).

Box 7
Reasons for modest diagnostic performance of MR imaging/MRA in the detection of hip articular cartilage injury

1. Hip articular cartilage is thin and spherical
2. MR imaging/MRA detects cartilage voids and is ill-suited to identify typical delamination cartilage injury of FAI
3. Seal effect of labrum, which tends to prohibit fluid entry into the central joint
4. Tightly congruent nature of the hip joint may keep damaged cartilage closely apposed to bone
5. Truncation artifacts can create artifactual hyperintensities (potential false positive) or generate spurious laminar appearance of cartilage (potential false negative)

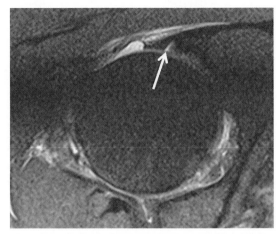

Fig. 23. Normal variant labral sulcus. Radial intermediate-weighted MRA at 11:00 demonstrates a partial-thickness defect (*arrow*) with smooth margins centered at the chondrolabral junction. Adjacent cartilage, labrum, and perilabral soft tissues are normal (intralabral signal is secondary to noise).

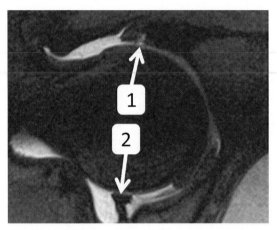

Fig. 22. Chondrolabral separation. Radial intermediate-weighted MRA centered posterosuperiorly at 11:00 demonstrates abnormal signal at the chondrolabral junction (1), indicating partial-thickness chondrolabral separation. Signal abnormality approaches fluid intensity, consistent with acute/subacute injury. The margins are irregular, excluding a normal variant sublabral sulcus; normal transverse ligament inferiorly (2).

Box 8
Criteria for sublabral sulcus

When a labral defect is encountered, we favor a sublabral sulcus when the following criteria are met:

1. The defect is partial-thickness.
2. The defect is centered at the chondrolabral junction.
3. The defect demonstrates smooth margins.
4. The adjacent cartilage and labrum otherwise appear normal.
5. There is absence of any other perilabral abnormalities to include osseous pathomorphologies. We view an otherwise benign-appearing labral defect with caution in the setting of cam or pincer morphology.

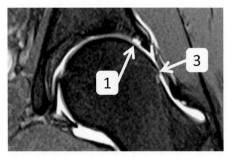
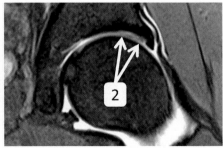

Fig. 24. Cartilage delamination. Contiguous coronal intermediate-weighted images centered superiorly at 12:00 demonstrate chondrolabral separation with associated full-thickness cartilage defect (1), adjacent cartilage delamination indicated by linear increased signal at the interface between subchondral bone and cartilage (2), and cam deformity (3).

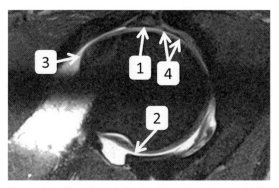

Fig. 25. Chronic labral hypertrophy. Radial intermediate-weighted MRA demonstrates relative labral hypertrophy and intrasubstance intermediate signal at 1:30, which does not reach an articular surface (1), consistent with degeneration. At surgery, the labrum was unstable (2 = normal labrum at 7:30 for comparison); (3) cam deformity; and (4) cartilage delamination at 1:30. At surgery, surface communication was not visualized (carpet phenomenon).

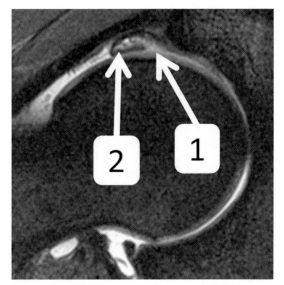

Fig. 26. Delaminating labral tear. Radial intermediate-weighted MRA demonstrates chondrolabral separation (1) and delaminating tear (2) extending into the substance of the labrum toward the free edge.

Box 9
Pearls, pitfalls, and variants

Pearls

- FAI is often bilateral, yet asynchronous with regard to symptoms: evaluate both hips when FAI is a consideration.
- On anteroposterior projections of the pelvis, pelvic tilt must be assessed.
- 42% of patients with cam FAI have an associated acetabular deformity (pincer).
- Look closely for cam deformity on the anteroposterior and lateral radiographs. The deformity is often only seen on one view.
- Ensure that the frontal radiograph is not laterally rotated and that the x-ray beam is centered on midline (as opposed to the hip). The patient should also be upright.

Pitfalls

- Systemic disorders with hip joint involvement may mimic FAI (eg, ankylosing spondylitis, diffuse idiopathic skeletal hyperostosis (DISH), congenital hip dysplasia).
- Rarely, hydroxyapatite deposition occurs in the acetabular labrum, which usually resolves on follow-up examination at 6 weeks.
- Greater trochanter enthesopathy in younger adolescent age group from gluteal tendon overuse.
- Suboptimal radiographic technique may overestimate, underestimate, or falsely diagnose FAI.

Variants

- Sublabral recesses or sulci can be positioned anywhere along the labrum, most commonly along the anterosuperior labrum and posteroinferior labrum.
- Supra-acetabular fossa in the acetabular roof (12:00) is present in about 10% of individuals. A type 1 fossa is a defect in subchondral bone and cartilage, filled with joint fluid. A type 2 fossa is a defect in the subchondral bone only, filled with cartilage. These should not be mistaken for osteochondral defects.
- Superior acetabular roof notch is a sharply delineated, more longitudinally oriented, fluid- or fat-filled pit in the medial aspect of the acetabular roof, distinct from the supraacetabular fossa.
- Stellate crease or stellate lesion is an area of the acetabular roof without cartilage coverage, located more medially than a supra-acetabular fossa.

inferiorly across the acetabular notch.[17] Clefts at the junction between the transverse ligament and labrum anteriorly and posteriorly are normal, provided they are shallow, centered at the chondrolabral junction, and smoothly marginated.

Abnormal labral signal may be present at the chondrolabral junction or within the substance of the labrum. Intrasubstance signal abnormality reflects tear if it extends to the articular surface and degeneration if it does not (see **Fig. 25**). Acute or subacute injuries typically imbibe contrast or approach fluid signal intensity. Chronic injuries are usually intermediate in signal intensity and do not imbibe contrast (see **Fig. 25**). Tears may be partial-thickness or full-thickness. A full-thickness tear can cause paralabral cyst formation. Delaminating labral tears propagate toward the free edge (**Fig. 26**).

Labral surface irregularity is an additional pathologic finding termed fraying. Marked abnormal labral morphology or hypertrophy, often without distinct intrasubstance signal abnormality, reflects degeneration and can also indicate labral instability (see **Fig. 25**).[45] Labral mineralization and ossification should be communicated in the report because labral repair is more difficult.[46] The labrum can be completely absent in long-standing FAI or osteoarthritis. Once detected and categorized, labral injuries are localized using a clock face.

SUMMARY

FAI morphology is prevalent and likely a primary contributor to idiopathic hip osteoarthritis. Early intervention in well-selected patients can provide symptomatic relief and delay progression to osteoarthritis. Radiologists contribute to patient care by identifying and properly characterizing subtle abnormalities on radiography and MR imaging and by generating comprehensive reports that advance clinical decision-making (see **Box 2; Box 9**).[47]

REFERENCES

1. Ito K, Minka MA II, Leunig M, et al. Femoroacetabular impingement and the cam-effect: a MRI-based quantitative anatomical study of the femoral head-neck offset. J Bone Joint Surg Br 2001;83-B:171–6.
2. Ganz R, Parvizi J, Beck M, et al. Femoroacetabular impingement: a cause for osteoarthritis of the hip. Clin Orthop Relat Res 2003;417:112–20.
3. Amanatullah DF, Antkowiak T, Pillay K, et al. Femoroacetabular impingement: current concepts in diagnosis and treatment. Orthopedics 2015;38: 185–99.
4. Banerjee P, Mclean CR. Femoroacetabular impingement: a review of diagnosis and management. Curr Rev Musculoskelet Med 2011;4:23–32.
5. Allen D, Beaulé PE, Ramadan O, et al. Prevalence of associated deformities and hip pain in patients with cam-type femoroacetabular impingement. J Bone Joint Surg Br 2009;91:589–94.
6. Laborie LB, Lehmann TG, Engesæter IØ, et al. Prevalence of radiographic findings thought to be associated with femoroacetabular impingement in a population-based cohort of 2081 healthy young adults. Radiology 2011;260:494–502.
7. Mascarenhas VV, Rego P, Dantas P, et al. Imaging prevalence of femoroacetabular impingement in symptomatic patients, athletes, and asymptomatic individuals: a systematic review. Eur J Radiol 2016; 85:73–95.
8. Beaulé PE, Speirs AD, Anwander H, et al. Surgical correction of cam deformity in association with femoroacetabular impingement and its impact on the degenerative process within the hip joint. J Bone Joint Surg Am 2017;99:1373–81.
9. Chinzei N, Hashimoto S, Fujishiro T, et al. Inflammation and degeneration in cartilage samples from patients with femoroacetabular impingement. J Bone Joint Surg Am 2016;98:135–41.
10. Nicholls AS, Kiran A, Pollard TCB, et al. The association between hip morphology parameters and nineteen-year risk of end-stage osteoarthritis of the hip: a nested case-control study. Arthritis Rheum 2011;63:3392–400.
11. Weinberg DS, Williamson DF, Millis MB, et al. Decreased and increased relative acetabular volume predict the development of osteoarthritis of the hip: an osteological review of 1090 hips. Bone Joint J 2017;99-B:432–9.
12. Beck M, Kalhor M, Leunig M, et al. Hip morphology influences the pattern of damage to the acetabular cartilage: femoroacetabular impingement as a cause of early osteoarthritis of the hip. J Bone Joint Surg Br 2005;87:1012–8.
13. Li AE, Jawetz ST, Greditzer HG, et al. MRI for the preoperative evaluation of femoroacetabular impingement. Insights Imaging 2016;7:187–98.
14. Diaz-Ledezma C, Casaccia M, Parvizi J. Reports of magnetic resonance images of the hip in patients with femoroacetabular impingement: is useful information provided to the orthopedic surgeon? Skeletal Radiol 2013;42:335–40.
15. Agten CA, Sutter R, Buck FM, et al. Hip imaging in athletes: sports imaging series. Radiology 2016; 280:351–69.
16. Volpon JB. Femoroacetabular impingement. Rev Bras Ortop 2016;51:621–9.
17. Seldes RM, Tan R, Hunt J, et al. Anatomy, histologic features, and vascularity of the adult acetabular labrum. Clin Orthop Relat Res 2001;382:232–40.

18. Ferguson SJ, Bryant JT, Ganz R, et al. An in vitro investigation of the acetabular labral seal in hip joint mechanics. J Biomech 2003;36:171–8.

19. Wyler A, Bousson V, Bergot C, et al. Comparison of MR-arthorgraphy and CT-arthrography in hyaline cartilage thickness measurement in radiographically normal cadaver hips with anatomy as gold standard. Osteoarthritis Cartilage 2009; 17:19–25.

20. Li X, Majumdar S. Quantitative MRI of articular cartilage and its clinical applications. J Magn Reson Imaging 2013;38:991–1008.

21. Roemer FW, Crema MD, Trattnig S, et al. Advances in imaging of osteoarthritis and cartilage. Radiology 2011;260:332–54.

22. Tannast M, Siebenrock KA, Anderson SE. Femoroacetabular impingement: radiographic diagnosis–what the radiologist should know. Am J Roentgenol 2007;188:1540–52.

23. Siebenrock KA, Ferner F, Noble PC, et al. The cam-type deformity of the proximal femur arises in childhood in response to vigorous sporting activity. Clin Orthop Relat Res 2011;469:3229–40.

24. Pfirrmann CWA, Duc SR, Zanetti M, et al. MR arthrography of acetabular cartilage delamination in femoroacetabular cam impingement. Radiology 2008;249:236–41.

25. Lerch S, Kasperczyk A, Bemdt T, et al. Ultrasound is as reliable as plain radiographs in the diagnosis of cam-type femoroacetabular impingement. Arch Orthop Trauma Surg 2016;136:1437–43.

26. Clohisy JC, Carlisle JC, Beaulé PE, et al. A systematic approach to the plain radiographic evaluation of the young adult hip. J Bone Joint Surg Am 2008;90(Suppl 4):47–66.

27. Jackson TJ, Estess AA, Adamson GJ. Supine and standing AP pelvis radiographs in the evaluation of pincer femoroacetabular impingement. Clin Orthop Relat Res 2016;474:1692–6.

28. Siebenrock KA, Kalbermatten DF, Ganz R. Effect of pelvic tilt on acetabular retroversion: a study of pelves from cadavers. Clin Orthop Relat Res 2003; 407:241–8.

29. Anderson LA, Kapron AL, Aoki SK, et al. Coxa profunda: is the deep acetabulum overcovered? Clin Orthop Relat Res 2012;470:3375–82.

30. Pfirrmann CWA, Mengiardi B, Dora C, et al. Cam and pincer femoroacetabular impingement: characteristic MR arthrographic findings in 50 patients. Radiology 2006;240:778–85.

31. Sutter R, Zubler V, Hoffmann A, et al. Hip MRI: how useful is intraarticular contrast material for evaluating surgically proven lesions of the labrum and articular cartilage? Am J Roentgenol 2014;202: 160–9.

32. Smith TO, Hilton G, Toms AP, et al. The diagnostic accuracy of acetabular labral tears using magnetic resonance imaging and magnetic resonance arthrography: a meta-analysis. Eur Radiol 2011; 21(4):863–74.

33. Smith TO, Simpson M, Ejindu V, et al. The diagnostic test accuracy of magnetic resonance imaging, magnetic resonance arthrography and computer tomography in the detection of chondral lesions of the hip. Eur J Orthop Surg Traumatol 2013;23(3):335–44.

34. Naraghi A, White LM. MRI of labral and chondral lesions of the hip. Am J Roentgenol 2015;205: 479–90.

35. Crespo-Rodriguez AM, De Lucas-Villarrubia JC, Pastrana-Ledesma M. The diagnostic performance of non-contrast 3-Tesla magnetic resonance imaging (3-T MRI) versus 1.5-Tesla magnetic resonance arthrography (1.5-T MRA) in femoro-acetabular impingement. Eur J Radiol 2017;88:109–16.

36. Ellermann J, Connor Z, Mikko JN, et al. Acetabular cartilage assessment in patient with femoroacetabular impingement by using T2* mapping with arthroscopic verification. Radiology 2014; 271:512–23.

37. Jesse MK, Petersen B, Strickland C, et al. Normal anatomy and imaging of the hip: emphasis on impingement assessment. Semin Musculoskelet Radiol 2013;17:229–47.

38. Bittersohl B, Hosalkar HS, Apprich S, et al. Comparison of pre-operative dGEMRIC imaging with intra-operative findings in femoroacetabular impingement: preliminary findings. Skeletal Radiol 2011;40:553–61.

39. Frank LR, Brossmann J, Buxton RB, et al. MR imaging truncation artifacts can create a false laminar appearance in cartilage. Am J Roentgenol 1997; 168:547–54.

40. Bulat E, Bixby SD, Siversson C, et al. Planar dGEMRIC maps may aid imaging assessment of cartilage damage in femoroacetabular impingement. Clin Orthop Relat Res 2016;474:467–78.

41. Samaan MA, Pedoia V, Zhang AL, et al. A novel MR-based method for detection of cartilage delamination in femoroacetabular impingement patients. J Orthop Res 2018;36(3):971–8.

42. Studler U, Kalberer F, Leunig M, et al. MR arthrography of the hip: differentiation between an anterior sublabral recess as a normal variant and a labral tear. Radiology 2008;249:947–54.

43. Saddik D, Troupis J, Tirman P, et al. Prevalence and location of acetabular sublabral sulci at hip arthroscopy with retrospective MRI review. Am J Roentgenol 2006;187:W507–11.

44. Kwee RM, Kavanagh EC, Miraude EA. Normal anatomical variants of the labrum of the hip at magnetic resonance imaging: a systemic review. Eur Radiol 2013;23:1694–710.

45. Blankenbaker DG, DeSmet AA, Keene JS, et al. Classification and localization of acetabular labral tears. Skeletal Radiolol 2007;36:391–7.

46. Hegazi TM, Belair JA, Eoghan JM, et al. Sports injuries about the hip: what the radiologist should know. Radiographics 2016;36:1717–45.

47. Dietrich TJ, Suter A, Pfirrmann CW, et al. Supraacetabular fossa (pseudodefect of acetabular cartilage): frequency at MR arthrography and comparison of findings at MR arthrography and arthroscopy. Radiology 2012;263:484–91.

Imaging of the Pelvis and Lower Extremity
Demystifying Uncommon Sources of Pelvic Pain

Daniel J. Mizrahi, MD[a], Alex E. Poor, MD[b],
William C. Meyers, MD[b], Johannes B. Roedl, MD, PhD[a],
Adam C. Zoga, MD[a],*

KEYWORDS

• Athletic pubalgia • Core muscle injury • Sports hernia • Pelvic pain • Musculoskeletal radiology

KEY POINTS

• Pelvic pain can result from gastrointestinal, gynecologic, urologic, neurologic, and musculoskeletal sources; it is crucial for the interpreter to recognize features of these sources of pelvic pain.
• Understanding musculoskeletal core anatomy and biomechanics is imperative for making an accurate diagnosis of musculoskeletal sources of pelvic pain.
• A multimodality approach is most useful for the accurate diagnosis of core muscle injuries; MR imaging is the primary imaging modality for identifying causes of pelvic pain.

INTRODUCTION

Although gastrointestinal, gynecologic, urologic, and neurologic sources of pelvic pain have been diagnosed and effectively treated for decades, some musculoskeletal lesions have been poorly understood until recent years. Over the past 10 years, the knowledge of musculoskeletal sources of pelvic pain and core injuries has evolved to optimize imaging for accurate diagnoses. Imaging has served as guidance for impactful conservative and interventional treatment plans. Between 2% and 5% of all sports injuries occur in the groin area.[1,2] Participation in sports that rely on quick acceleration, rapid changes in direction, kicking and frequent side-to-side motions (eg, soccer, ice hockey, American and Australian rules football, fencing, track and field events such as high jumping, and baseball) may subject athletes to injuries that lead to groin pain.

Between 2% and 8% of all athletic injuries involve the groin, and up to 13% of soccer injuries are groin related.[3–5] For this article, the authors use current terminology most prevalent in sports medicine clinics of North America, but this is not meant to diminish the value of other terminologies used effectively throughout the world. An understanding of the anatomy and biomechanics of the musculoskeletal core is the keystone to accurately diagnose and treat activity-related pelvic pain. With this knowledge, we can use imaging, particularly MR imaging, to confirm diagnoses, delineate extent of injury, and generate a roadmap for impactful treatment planning.

A primary step in the diagnostic process is obtaining a quality clinical history. Typically, we rely on the clinical history conveyed through our referring providers or on communication tools in the preimaging process. Reviewing clinical

Disclosures: The authors have nothing to disclose.
[a] Division of Musculoskeletal Radiology, Thomas Jefferson University, 132 South 10th Street, Suite 1096, Philadelphia, PA 19118, USA; [b] Vincera Institute, 1200 Constitution Avenue, Philadelphia, PA 19112, USA
* Corresponding author.
E-mail address: adam.zoga@jefferson.edu

Radiol Clin N Am 56 (2018) 983–995
https://doi.org/10.1016/j.rcl.2018.06.008
0033-8389/18/© 2018 Elsevier Inc. All rights reserved.

histories with the referring clinicians can reinforce a shared understanding of core injury and its unique terminology. Discussing injury patterns directly with the examining and treating clinicians builds a common understanding of the differential considerations and particular lesions most likely to fit a given clinical scenario. An imaging report must be clearly understood by the treating clinician if it is to be used effectively. If there is an incomplete understanding of the clinical syndrome, the radiologist is obligated to reach out to the referrer or the patient and gather as much information as possible regarding the reason for the patient's examination. Although direct interaction with the clinician is imperative, a great deal of valuable clinical information can be gained through thoughtfully constructed preimaging patient questionnaires. A core injury–specific musculoskeletal questionnaire is made available to patients both online at the time of scheduling and at the imaging center (**Fig. 1**). Information accrued through these means is added to the clinical input provided on the imaging examination order to comprise the ultimate clinical indication used in protocolling and interpreting the examination.

IMAGING TECHNIQUE

Once a quality clinical history has been established, the imaging modality and protocol should be chosen. The clinical context for most musculoskeletal indications for pelvic pain occur in an outpatient setting, and an MR imaging in 3 planes, generally noncontrast osseous pelvis protocol, is a valuable diagnostic examination across a wide spectrum of bony and soft tissue maladies. MR imaging should be the tertiary tool for musculoskeletal pain in the emergency department; typical indications in this setting include radiographically occult femoral neck or sacral ala fractures. Other helpful imaging modalities commonly used for the evaluation of pelvic pain outside of the musculoskeletal system include computed tomography (CT) (with oral and intravenous contrast for gastrointestinal conditions) and ultrasound (to evaluate abdominal wall hernias or as a first-line tool in evaluating gynecologic causes of pelvic pain). It is important to be aware of the other causes of pelvic pain extrinsic to the musculoskeletal system because these often can be isolated or concomitant causes observed on examinations tailored for the evaluation of clinically suspected musculoskeletal pelvic pain.

If there is a clinically suspected musculoskeletal core injury refractory to rest and physical therapy in an outpatient setting, a dedicated athletic pubalgia MR imaging protocol (**Table 1**) can provide the most valuable diagnostic information. This protocol differs from a typical MR imaging of the pelvis because the planes of imaging are optimized to evaluate the musculoskeletal core. This is a noncontrast MR imaging acquired in 4 planes with a phased array surface coil. Large field of view coronal and axial imaging covers from skin to skin in the AP and transverse planes and from the level of the umbilicus to the proximal third of the thighs. Higher resolution, smaller field of view imaging is then acquired in coronal oblique planes prescribed along the arcuate line of the pelvis (anterior crest of the iliac bones) and sagittal planes. This protocol can be performed at 1.5 T, and late model receiver coil technology allows for turning off the peripheral elements of the coil while acquiring the high-resolution sequences.

MUSCULOSKELETAL CORE ANATOMY

Understanding of the musculoskeletal core is an evolving science. Loosely, it includes all osseous, muscular, tendinous, ligamentous, and myofascial structures from the lower chest through the upper thighs.[6–9] The core concept is that when any of these structures is injured many others sustain a change in biomechanics. An injury to any part of the core alters the delicate biomechanical balance needed for optimal physical performance. With altered biomechanics, further injury occurs, sometimes involving different core structures.[10]

The center of the core is the pubic symphysis. The pubic symphysis is an amphiarthrodial joint, and although there is limited motion, injury to the perisymphyseal soft tissues can destabilize the symphyseal joint, allowing for abnormal joint motion and a vicious cycle of progressively abnormal biomechanics.[11,12] This joint with limited motion distributes forces from the center of the core to larger, lateralized structures, but it also withstands tractile forces from the numerous muscle attachments on and around it, which includes the rectus abdominis from above and the adductor longus from below the mesh as an aponeurosis with a broad attachment on the pubic tubercle anteroinferiorly just lateral to the symphysis itself. These left and right aponeuroses blend with a thick fibroaponeurotic plate that essentially covers the entire pubic symphysis region, which includes all of the perisymphyseal muscle attachments along with the ligamentous stabilizers at the anterior symphysis and even the periosteum of the pubic rami mesh with this fibroaponeurotic plate. Core muscles include the trunk flexors (rectus abdominis and obliques), the hip flexors (psoas, iliacus,

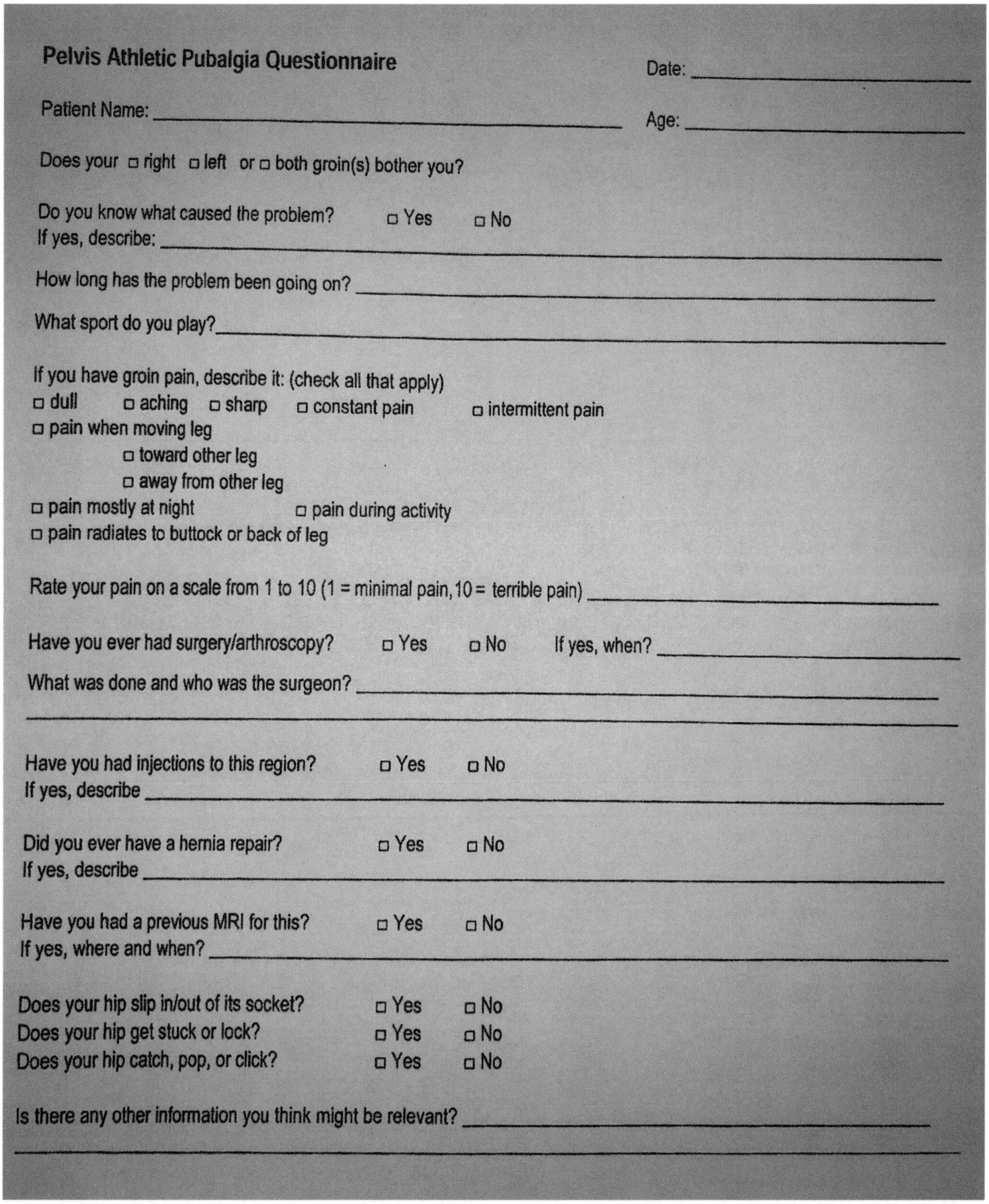

Pelvis Athletic Pubalgia Questionnaire

Date: _____

Patient Name: _____ Age: _____

Does your ☐ right ☐ left or ☐ both groin(s) bother you?

Do you know what caused the problem?   ☐ Yes   ☐ No
If yes, describe: _____

How long has the problem been going on? _____

What sport do you play? _____

If you have groin pain, describe it: (check all that apply)
☐ dull   ☐ aching ☐ sharp   ☐ constant pain   ☐ intermittent pain
☐ pain when moving leg
          ☐ toward other leg
          ☐ away from other leg
☐ pain mostly at night   ☐ pain during activity
☐ pain radiates to buttock or back of leg

Rate your pain on a scale from 1 to 10 (1 = minimal pain, 10 = terrible pain) _____

Have you ever had surgery/arthroscopy?   ☐ Yes   ☐ No   If yes, when? _____

What was done and who was the surgeon? _____
_____

Have you had injections to this region?   ☐ Yes   ☐ No
If yes, describe _____

Did you ever have a hernia repair?   ☐ Yes   ☐ No
If yes, describe _____

Have you had a previous MRI for this?   ☐ Yes   ☐ No
If yes, where and when? _____

Does your hip slip in/out of its socket?   ☐ Yes   ☐ No
Does your hip get stuck or lock?   ☐ Yes   ☐ No
Does your hip catch, pop, or click?   ☐ Yes   ☐ No

Is there any other information you think might be relevant? _____
_____

Fig. 1. Patient questionnaire provided to patients with clinically suspected core muscle injury before performing MR imaging.

and rectus femoris), the thigh adductors (pectineus, adductor longus, adductor brevis, adductor magnus and gracilis), the hip rotators, hip abductors, lumbar paraspinals, and even the trunk extensors. The most common core injuries, however, are centered at the fibroaponeurotic plate at the anterior symphyseal region, particularly involving the rectus abdominis and adductor longus. The hips also play a role in the musculoskeletal core, although understanding of the extent is still evolving. A preliminary cadaveric study showed a significant drop in intraarticular pressure of the hip joint when the ipsilateral lower psoas muscle was released.[13–15]

Table 1
Thomas Jefferson University 1.5 T MR imaging protocol for athletic pubalgia

Sequence	Plane	FOV (cm²)	Matrix	Section Thickness/ Gap (mm)	TR (msec)	TE (msec)	TI (msec)	BW (kHz)	ETL
STIR	Coronal	28–36	256 × 192	4/1	>2000	20–40	150	16	8
T1-weighted SE	Coronal	28	256 × 256	4/1	400–800	Min	NA	16	NA
T2-weighted fat-suppressed FSE	Axial	28	256 × 192	5/1	>2000	50–60	NA	16	8
PD-weighted fat-suppressed FSE	Sagittal	20–22	256 × 256	4/0.5	>2000	20–40	NA	16	8
PD-weighted fat-suppressed FSE	Axial oblique[a]	20	256 × 256	4/0.5	>2000	20–40	NA	16	8
PD FSE nonfat-suppressed	Axial oblique[a]	20	256 × 256	4/0.5	3000	15–30	NA	16	4–6

Indications for MR imaging with this protocol include suspicion of a rectus abdominis injury, adductor injury, osteitis pubis, or athletic pubalgia. All sequences should be centered on the symphysis pubis.

Abbreviations: BW, bandwidth; ETL, echo train length; FOV, field of view; FSE, fast spin echo; NA, not applicable; SE, spin echo; STIR, short inversion time inversion recovery; TE, echo time; TI, inversion time; TR, repetition time.

[a] The use of the axial oblique plane is recommended to maximize sensitivity for the detection of rectus abdominis–adductor longus myotendinous injuries.

The interconnectedness of the musculoskeletal core reinforces the need for early detection and treatment of core injuries for the prevention of more extensive, less manageable injuries. An injury sustained at any point from the lower costal margin to the hips can be considered a musculoskeletal core injury.[6] In recent years, the term "core injury" has evolved to be most used in the setting of a musculoskeletal injury anterior to or involving the pubic symphysis. Core injury or central core injury has, in some cases, replaced previously popular terms including "athletic pubalgia lesion" and "rectus abdominis/adductor aponeurosis injury." It has generally replaced the often inappropriately used "sports hernia" or "sportsman's hernia," because a true hernia is invariably lacking with these injuries.

MUSCULOSKELETAL CORE INJURIES

Most of the core injuries fall into 2 categories: (1) those that originate at the midline anterior to the pubic symphysis and (2) those that originate unilaterally at the level of the pubic tubercle. Although even midline core injuries tend to be symptomatic, both clinically and on imaging, distinguishing midline lesions from unilateral lesions is very useful in treatment planning. Meyers and colleagues[16] found a 4% incidence of contralateral core injury after unilateral pelvic floor repair, so identifying any bilaterality may justifiably warrant a bilateral treatment plan, even if symptoms are primarily unilateral. Tendinosis and interstitial tearing of the adductor longus can be a primary pain generator, so this phenomenon should be recognized and reported (**Fig. 2**).[17–19]

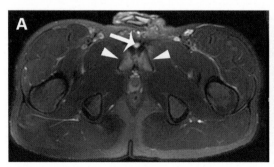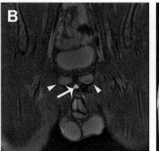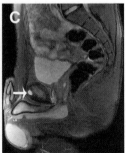

Fig. 2. Midline core lesion in a 20-year-old male soccer player with progressively worsening bilateral groin pain. Axial T2 fast spin echo (FSE) fat-suppressed (FS) (*A*), coronal oblique T2 FSE FS (*B*), and sagittal oblique T2 FSE FS (*C*) magnetic resonance (MR) images show a midline core muscle injury (*arrows*) extending to the left and right. There is associated bilateral pubic bone marrow edema (*arrowheads*).

Core injuries can be mild and subtle at imaging with only minimal detachment of the rectus abdominis/adductor aponeurosis from the pubic tubercle or the pubic symphysis, or they can be severe with complete detachment of the rectus abdominis from the osseous pubis and retraction of adductor tendons distal into the thigh. With these high-grade core injuries, often unilateral lesions, the adductors can avulse together as a unit, pulling a piece of pubic periosteum away from the pubic tubercle, or there can be an elongated region of periosteal disruption from the pubis superior to inferior, best seen in a sagittal plane, without tendinous retraction (**Fig. 3**). After identifying one of these core injuries at MR imaging, the report should be descriptive and anatomically detailed, offering as much information as possible to help guide construction of an appropriate treatment plan. Midline lesions should be detailed on both sides as extending to the lateral edge of the rectus abdominis or into the adductor longus. Unilateral lesions can be measured in both craniocaudal and transverse planes with any tendon retraction or hematoma described. Core structures should be assessed for symmetry, because posttraumatic atrophy is common, particularly involving the lower rectus abdominis. Such atrophy can effectively leave a more patulous superficial inguinal ring, with no structural support deep to the posteromedial aspect of the lower inguinal canal. Superior and secondary clefts are useful MR imaging observations, and osteitis pubis should be noted and graded, as should any visible ligamentous disruption or instability at the pubic symphysis. Ultimately, an MR imaging report detailing a core muscle injury should delineate estimated chronicity and severity of the injuries.[13,20–23]

ADDUCTOR LESIONS

Although the proximal adductor tendons are inherently involved in both midline and unilateral central core injuries, some core injuries are more centered in the lower extremity adductor compartment. This does not necessarily mean that the rectus abdominis is normal, but with these primary adductor lesions, the pain generator or injury most responsive to treatment is located distal to the pubic tubercles and pubic symphysis. Adductor tendons can suffer degenerative lesions more frequently seen in the rotator cuff tendons or the Achilles. The adductor longus hypertrophy leads to a hypoxic tendinopathy that worsens as pressure within the compartment increases. Hydroxyapatite deposition disease (calcific tendinosis) is not uncommon at the adductor longus, and it can be treated with similar techniques used elsewhere in the musculoskeletal system such as percutaneous tenotomy and lavage. In extreme cases of adductor tendinopathy, activity exacerbated by hypertrophy can even cause an exercise-induced compartment syndrome. More acutely, part of the adductor compartment can be traumatically strained, and accurate identification of the structure involved and location of injury can contribute to more impactful physical therapy planning. A distal adductor magnus strain should certainly be distinguished from a proximal adductor longus strain at MR imaging.[24,25]

One particularly troublesome adductor injury is a proximal myotendinous junction strain at the adductor longus with accompanying tearing of the muscle sheath leading to a more difficult treatment course. These strains are commonly encountered in the thighs of patients rehabilitating after a central core repair and have been termed "baseball pitcher–hockey goalie syndrome."[26] At

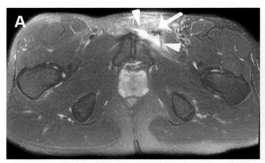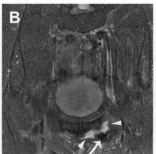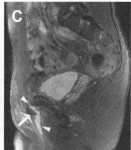

Fig. 3. Detachment of the midline and left rectus abdominis-adductor plate in a 35-year-old man with left greater than right groin pain for 3 to 4 weeks after squatting. Axial FSE T2 FS (*A*), coronal oblique FSE T2 FS (*B*), and sagittal oblique FSE T2 FS (*C*) MR images show detachment of the midline and left rectus abdominis-adductor plate including the distal rectus abdominis and proximal anterior adductor compartment (adductor longus, adductor brevis, and pectineus), which are completely avulsed as a unit (*arrows*). Fluid/hematoma fills the retraction gap (*arrowheads*).

MR imaging, look for a typical myotendinous strain pattern along with either a small fluid collection or visible disruption of the muscle sheath or fascia. Ultimately, these lesions will heal, but either percutaneous or open fascial release may be warranted to facilitate the healing (**Fig. 4**).[26]

Although many combinations of muscle and tendon injuries in the adductor compartment can be encountered, more diffuse and feathery edema in multiple muscles, often bilateral, indicate delayed onset muscle soreness or typical postworkout muscle tightness (**Fig. 5**).[27,28] A focal region of muscle edema away from a myotendinous junction might result from direct trauma and subsequent muscle contusion. As with adductor muscle injury, care should be taken to confirm normal flow signal in the femoral vasculature.

OTHER MUSCULOSKELETAL SOURCES OF PELVIC PAIN

As we move away from the pubic symphysis, specific musculoskeletal lesions become less common and often more elusive. These injuries are not typically "eye tests" with MR imaging but are almost always visible as T2-hyperintensity along or surrounding the injured structure on fluid sensitive, fat-suppressed images. Prescribing an MR imaging plane along the long axis of the soft tissue edema can sometimes help delineate injury extent. Rectus abdominal muscle strains can occur with trunk hyperextension and rotation. In the authors' experience, tennis players are prone to small tears of the rectus abdominis just below the level of the umbilicus on their dominant side during the serve. These are true muscle injuries and respond well to conservative treatment plans.

A core injury centered at the junction of the medial margin of the external oblique and the lateral margin of the rectus abdominis 8 to 10 cm cephalad to the pubic symphysis has been called hockey groin and can be clinically mistaken for

an abdominal wall hernia. More lateral, internal oblique and later the external oblique can avulse from the iliac crest with forceful rotation and extension. Our experience with this injury is limited to American football players, in particular quarterbacks evading a pass rush (**Fig. 6**).

Both apophysitis and avulsive tendinitis can occur at any of the attachments on the anterior superior iliac spine (ASIS) or the anterior inferior iliac spine (AIIS). Kicking athletes are particularly prone to an AIIS apophysitis with repeated stress across the rectus femoris on their plant leg (**Fig. 7**).[29,30] Subspinous impingement is a recently described syndrome where anterior soft tissues are impinged between the AIIS and the anterior femoral head-neck junction.[31] ASIS avulsion injuries are more commonly seen in women participating in a myriad of activities from running to rowing and even yoga and can involve origins of the sartorius, the tensor fascia lata, or the gluteus medius. Hip flexor lesions can manifest at MR imaging as iliopsoas bursitis, iliacus or psoas muscle strains, or psoas muscle atrophy.

More posteriorly, any paraspinal or hip rotator unit can be injured with overuse or a single trauma. Baseball outfielders have been reported to be prone to acute or chronic quadratus lumborum strain as they track a long fly ball while running away from the hitter (**Fig. 8**). Piriformis and quadratus lumborum strains can occur with activities that involve extension at the waist and change of direction, but piriformis syndrome is generally used to describe a lesion resulting from anomalous anatomy, as a part of the sciatic nerve essentially pierces between the bundles of the piriformis and becomes impinged during piriformis muscle contraction.[32] Hamstring complex injuries can loosely be considered core injuries, as can ischiofemoral impingement, where the quadratus femoris muscle is repeatedly compressed in a narrowed interval between the lesser trochanter of the femur and the ischial tuberosity or a hypertrophied

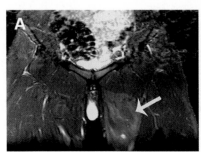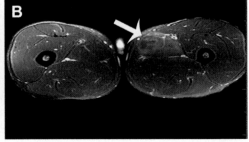

Fig. 4. "Baseball pitcher–hockey goalie syndrome" in a 25-year-old male baseball pitcher with left groin pain. Coronal FSE T2 FS (*A*) and axial FSE T2 FS (*B*) MR images show "baseball pitcher–hockey goalie syndrome" of the left adductor longus muscle with diffuse strain/edema (*arrows*) of the entire muscle.

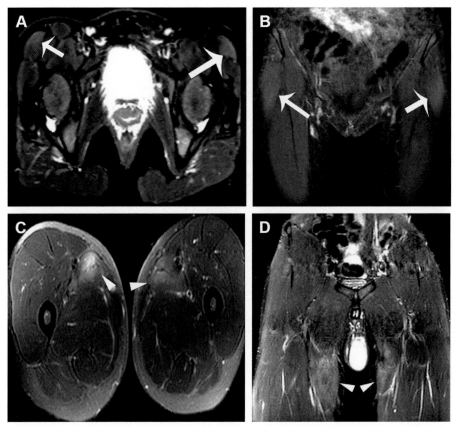

Fig. 5. Delayed onset muscle soreness in 2 different patients. Axial FSE T2 FS (*A*) and coronal FSE T2 FS (*B*) images from a 23-year-old woman with right lower abdominal pain and right groin pain after an injury lifting weights at the gym show mild, diffuse edema within both sartorius muscles (*arrows*). Axial FSE T2 FS (*C*) and coronal FSE T2 FS (*D*) images from a 24-year-old hockey player with bilateral inner thigh pain shows mild peritendinous edema and intramuscular edema within the proximal bilateral rectus femoris muscles, (*arrowheads*), typical for delayed onset muscle soreness.

hamstring complex origin, creating painful soft tissue edema.[33] Obturator externus and internus strains are often present in conjunction with central core injuries, especially when the adductor longus and pectineus are both involved.

Rower's rib and slipping rib syndrome are commonly used terms but particularly difficult diagnoses to delineate with imaging. An adapted musculoskeletal core MR imaging protocol uses large field of view imaging with a phased array

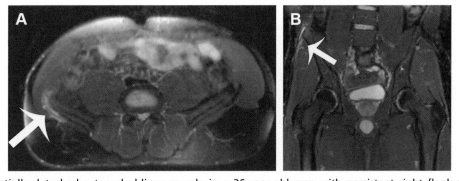

Fig. 6. Partially detached external oblique muscle in a 36-year-old man with persistent right flank pain after twisting injury. Axial FSE T2 FS (*A*) and coronal FSE T2 FS (*B*) images show partial detachment of the posterior margin of the external oblique from its attachment onto the iliac crest, with muscle edema and fluid (*arrows*) interposed between the detached external oblique muscle fibers and posterior superior iliac crest.

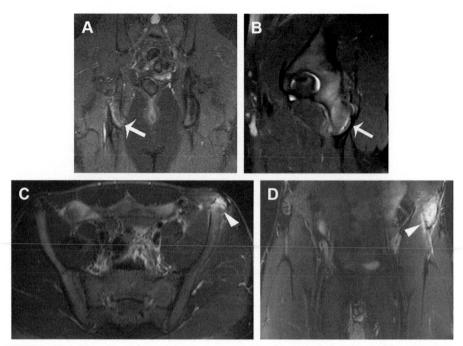

Fig. 7. Apophysitis in 2 different patients. Coronal FSE T2 FS (*A*) and sagittal FSE T2 FS (*B*) images from a 17-year-old woman with 4 months of right hip pain after hyperflexion injury show bone marrow edema (*arrows*) and mild bony remodeling of the apophysis of the right ischial tuberosity at the hamstring tendon origin. Axial FSE T2 FS (*C*) and coronal FSE T2 FS (*D*) images from a 17-year-old man with left hip and groin pain after basketball injury show intense bone marrow edema in the left ASIS apophysis (*arrowheads*) and fluid within the physis, consistent with acute apophysitis. Intense surrounding soft tissue edema on the left extends into the left rectus femoris muscle.

surface coil covering both sides of the body and centered on the level of symptoms. A skin marker is very useful in directing imaging; large field of view short inversion time inversion recovery (STIR) and T1-weighted images are most useful, because signal and fat suppression homogeneity are essential. Asymmetric soft tissue or osseous edema can be diagnostic, and care should be taken to identify skeletal asymmetry, including scoliosis. For rower's rib, the edema often reflects an overuse type avulsive mechanism at the serratus anterior or obliques intimate to the lower lateral ribs, either anteriorly or posteriorly. Another variant shows soft tissue avulsive edema at the inferior costal margin.[34]

Slipping rib syndrome most commonly refers to hypermobility of the anterior ends of the false rib costal cartilage leading to painful biomechanical friction. MR imaging findings are not clearly established, but again, large field of view STIR

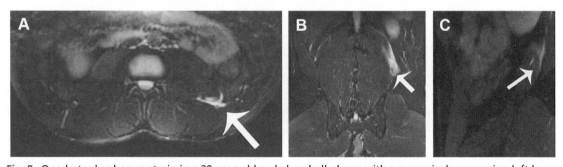

Fig. 8. Quadratus lumborum strain in a 29-year-old male baseball player with progressively worsening left lower flank pain. Axial FSE T2 FS (*A*), coronal FSE T2 F (*B*), and sagittal FSE T2 FS (*C*) images show fluid signal within the superolateral one-third of the muscle fibers involving the belly of the left quadratus lumborum muscle (*arrows*), compatible with a grade 2 strain.

sequences can sometimes identify the soft tissue or chondral edema.[35] Similar injuries are encountered with some frequency in the rib cages of powerful baseball hitters. The term used commonly here is "oblique strain," but edema is more often centered in the ribs themselves or the intercostal or costochondral cartilage.[36]

Sometimes the source of pelvic pain is anomalous osseous anatomy. Transitional anatomy at the lumbosacral junction is exceedingly common, but it is more often symptomatic when it is asymmetric. A partially sacralized L5 vertebra can exhibit a unilaterally enlarged transverse process and an anomalous, partially stable fusion with the sacral ala. When the partial fusion allows for partial instability during activity, a painful unilateral condition called Bertolotti syndrome can occur at this anomalous partial fusion, manifesting on MR imaging as bone marrow edema (**Fig. 9**). Although MR imaging is necessary to identify the bone marrow edema, the asymmetric anomaly (and sometimes sclerosis) can easily be identified on an anteroposterior radiograph.[37]

In young patients with posterior lumbosacral pain, particularly teen athletes, osseous stress response manifesting as bone marrow edema on MR imaging is encountered with some frequency at the pars interarticularis, particularly L5. This painful lesion is common in softball pitchers among others, but it is not clear if the osseous stress is a precursor of true spondylolysis. Sacroiliitis is most commonly inflammatory in this patient population, and facet arthritis can be painful, but is generally seen in an older cohort of patients.

Although shin splints are a well-known osseous stress syndrome, thigh splints are a similar lesion seen predominantly in young runners but centered along the medial femora. MR imaging shows

bilateral and often relatively symmetric findings of subcortical bone marrow edema at the femoral shafts, sometimes with accompanying periostitis (**Fig. 10**).[38] Osseous stress response can occur at several reproducible locations about the pelvis. In young athletes, osseous stress injury can occur at the site of the triradiate cartilage growth plate manifesting as linear bone marrow edema on axial fluid sensitive images.[39] The imager's threshold for femoral neck stress injury should be very low, particularly with female runners. Any bone marrow edema focal at the medial femoral neck should be suspicious for an early femoral neck stress fracture.

Intrinsic hip pathologies are beyond the scope of this review, but extrinsically, greater trochanteric pain syndrome (GTPS) is a common cause for imaging referral and is often treated by the musculoskeletal radiologist. Patients with GTPS generally fall into 2 groups: (1) middle-aged to older women with insertional gluteus medius tendinopathies and (2) young women with pain throughout the gluteus medius musculotendinous unit. The first group has positional pain local to the greater trochanter and often shows MR imaging findings of a trochanteric bursitis along with degenerative, rotator cuff–like lesions at the distal gluteus medius. The latter group can have abnormal Q angles on weight-bearing radiographs and diffuse gluteus medius muscle edema at MR imaging.[40–42]

NONMUSCULOSKELETAL SOURCES OF PELVIC PAIN

Pudendal neuralgia is an increasingly diagnosed source of pelvic and perineal pain. Although imaging findings are often elusive, magnetic resonance (MR) neurography protocols have shown promise

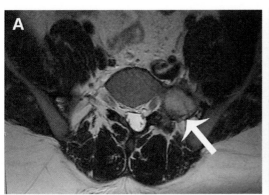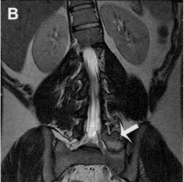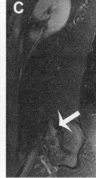

Fig. 9. Bertolotti syndrome in a 19-year-old man with left lower back pain. Axial FSE T2 (*A*), coronal FSE T2 FS (*B*), and sagittal FSE T2 FS (*C*) images show transitional lumbosacral anatomy (*arrows*) with partial sacralization of the left L5, with articulation between the left L5 transverse process and left sacral ala and associated bone marrow edema.

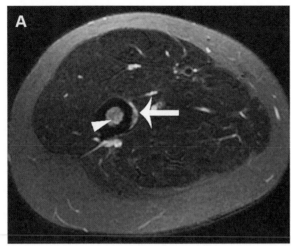
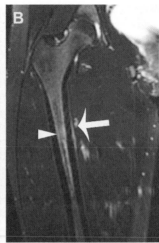

Fig. 10. Adductor insertion avulsion syndrome (thigh splints) in a 19-year-old female runner with right groin pain. Axial FSE T2 FS (*A*) and coronal FSE T2 FS (*B*) images show increased linear periosteal T2 signal along the medial cortex of the right proximal, mid femur (*arrows*), compatible with periostitis and osseous stress response. There is associated intramedullary edema (*arrowheads*).

in identifying some nerve lesions contributing to this painful, often bilateral syndrome. MR imaging sometimes shows expansive regions of abnormal neural edema or enlargement, but more focal sources of nerve impingement can be more difficult to identify. The most likely location for symptomatic pudendal nerve entrapment is within or just distal to Alcock's canal, medial to the ischial spine between the sacrotuberous and sacrospinous ligaments. Regardless of MR imaging protocol, with pudendal neuralgia or deep pelvic pain exacerbated by sitting, care should be taken to assess for causes or evidence of pudendal nerve entrapment in this location (**Fig. 11**).[43,44]

Ilioinguinal, iliohypogastric and genitofemoral nerve entrapment syndromes are also detailed in the sports medicine and general surgery literature as sources of pelvic pain, but reproducible imaging findings have been elusive. Systematic ultrasound assessment accompanied by dynamic maneuvers shows promise in helping to establish these difficult neurogenic lesions.

Other sources of nonmusculoskeletal pelvic pain can be gynecologic. Endometriosis is a difficult diagnosis with musculoskeletal MR imaging protocols, but multiple cakelike or masslike structures within the visceral pelvis can be seen. Endometrial deposits often proliferate in regions of prior intervention, around surgical scars or arthroscopy portals. If endometriosis is suspected, pre- and postcontrast MR imaging protocols should be considered (**Fig. 12**).

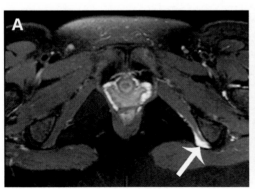
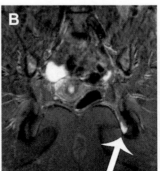
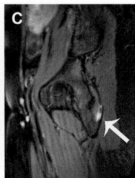

Fig. 11. Pudendal neuralgia in a 33-year-old woman with vulvodynia and pelvic floor dysfunction. Axial FSE T2 FS (*A*), coronal FSE T2 FS (*B*), and sagittal FSE T2 FS (*C*) images show abnormally increased fluid sensitive signal intensity about the enlarged left pudendal nerve (*arrows*) at the level of the ischial tuberosity, with tapering elongation toward the obturator internus.

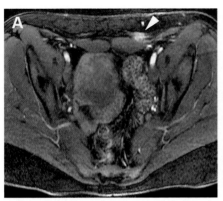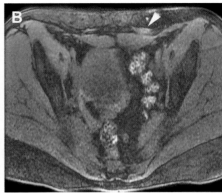

Fig. 12. Abdominal wall endometriosis in a 42-year-old woman with left lower quadrant abdominal pain. Axial FSE T2 FS (*A*) and enhanced axial T1 FS (*B*) images show an irregular T2 hyperintense, enhancing focus in the left anterior abdominal wall abutting the rectus abdominis muscle (*arrowheads*).

Uterine fibroids are a very common source of pelvic pain in women, particularly when causing mass effect on surrounding structures. Adenomyosis of the uterus can also be identified with noncontrast MR imaging protocols as an enlargement of the uterine junctional zone. However, fibroids and adenomyosis are so common that it is important for the imager to diligently search for other sources of musculoskeletal pain. More nefarious sources of pelvic pain can be enteric, including inflammatory bowel disease and adenocarcinoma. Free fluid in the dependent pelvis in men or excessive fluid in women may warrant further evaluation with an appropriate examination.

Hernias are relatively uncommon in young athletic patients, but they remain an important source of pelvic pain in the general population. Umbilical, Spigelian, and femoral hernias should all be observed at MR imaging, and if there is concern for a sliding hernia, assessment with dynamic ultrasound may be indicated. Inguinal hernias are the most common, and on the left, a painful varicocele can accompany an inguinal hernia and symptoms are often exacerbated by activity. Ultrasound

examination with Doppler flow analysis and dynamic maneuvers remains the study of choice for inguinal canals and varicoceles, but these lesions can often be identified with musculoskeletal MR protocols (**Fig. 13**).

Pitfalls

No single imaging modality can be considered optimal for diagnosing and delineating all sources of pelvic pain, particularly in active patients. The clinical scenario should be considered and as much clinical information as possible should be accrued before an imaging modality and an imaging protocol is chosen. An athletic pubalgia MR imaging protocol is the study of choice for identifying central core injuries and many musculoskeletal lesions about the pelvis, but with diligent review, it can also identify some nonmusculoskeletal sources of pelvic pain. In sedentary patients, a more succinct MR imaging osseous pelvis protocol is often a more reasonable option. Older and obese patients with groin pain are likely to have referred pain from the ipsilateral hip, and dedicated hip

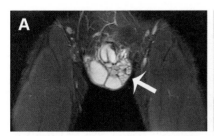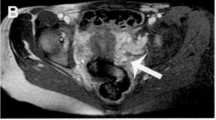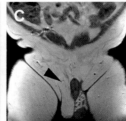

Fig. 13. Nonmusculoskeletal causes for groin/pelvic pain in 3 different patients. (*A*) Coronal FSE T2 FS image in a 31-year-old man shows dilated serpiginous tubules in the left hemiscrotum, compatible with a varicocele (*arrow*). (*B*) Axial FSE T2 FS image in a 60-year-old woman with pelvic pain shows numerous tortuous bilateral parauterine veins (*arrow*), compatible with pelvic congestion syndrome. (*C*) Coronal T1 image in a 74-year-old man with right hip pain shows a large right fat-containing inguinal hernia in the right hemiscrotum (*arrowhead*).

imaging should be considered. Ultrasound often offers the highest yield for lesions requiring a dynamic assessment such as hernias and varicoceles. When it comes to pelvic pain, imagers must leave their "silos" and consider the full clinical picture and also all organ systems that might play a role in causing symptoms. A musculoskeletal subspecialist should observe endometriosis, and a body imager should identify a core injury. Similarly, a central core lesion or sacroiliitis should be observed on a hip MR imaging, because there is frequently clinical overlap.

SUMMARY

Imaging has a central role in demystifying sources of pelvic pain. Armed with an understanding of musculoskeletal core anatomy and biomechanics as well as common gastrointestinal, urologic, and gynecologic confounders, imagers can provide essential value in the accurate diagnosis and treatment planning for patients with pain and dysfunction from pelvic sources. MR imaging is the primary imaging modality with its exquisite sensitivity for edema and inflammation, but focused sonographic, radiographic, and CT protocols are very useful for directed indications. Imagers should strive to problem solve and use the tools available to them to arrive at an accurate diagnosis and contribute to impactful treatment planning.

REFERENCES

1. Karlsson J, Sward L, Kalebo P, et al. Chronic groin injuries in athletes. Recommendations for treatment and rehabilitation. Sports Med 1994; 17:141–8.
2. Renstrom P, Peterson L. Groin injuries in athletes. Br J Sports Med 1980;14:30–6.
3. Ekstrand J, Gillquist J. The avoidability of soccer injuries. Int J Sports Med 1983;4:124–8.
4. Ekstrand J, Hilding J. The incidence and differential diagnosis of acute groin injuries in male soccer players. Scand J Med Sci Sports 1999;9:98–103.
5. Emery CA, Meeuwisse WH. Risk factors for groin injuries in hockey. Med Sci Sports Exerc 2001;33: 1423–33.
6. Farber AJ, Wilckens JH. Sports hernia: diagnosis and therapeutic approach. J Am Acad Orthop Surg 2007;15:507–14.
7. Hackney RG. The sports hernia: a cause of chronic groin pain. Br J Sports Med 1993;27:58–62.
8. Taylor DC, Meyers WC, Moylan JA, et al. Abdominal musculature abnormalities as a cause of groin pain in athletes. Inguinal hernias and pubalgia. Am J Sports Med 1991;19:239–42.
9. Malycha P, Lovell G. Inguinal surgery in athletes with chronic groin pain: the 'sportsman's' hernia. Aust N Z J Surg 1992;62:123–5.
10. Shortt CP, Zoga AC, Kavanagh EC, et al. Anatomy, pathology, and MRI findings in the sports hernia. Semin Musculoskelet Radiol 2008;12:54–61.
11. Williams A. Thigh. In: Stranding S, editor. Gray's anatomy: the anatomical basis of clinical practice. 39th edition. Edinburgh (Scotland): Elsevier Churchill Livingstone; 2005. p. 1465–7.
12. Gamble JG, Simmons SC, Freedman M. The symphysis pubis: anatomic and pathologic considerations. Clin Orthop Relat Res 1986;203:261–72.
13. Brennan D, O'Connell MJ, Ryan M, et al. Secondary cleft sign as a marker of injury in athletes with groin pain: MR image appearance and interpretation. Radiology 2005;235:162–7.
14. Omar IM, Zoga AC, Kavanagh EC. Athletic pubalgia and "sports hernia": optimal MR imaging technique and findings. Radiographics 2008;28: 1415–38.
15. Robinson P, Salehi F, Grainger A, et al. Cadaveric and MRI study of the musculotendinous contributions to the capsule of the symphysis pubis. AJR Am J Roentgenol 2007;188:W440–5.
16. Meyers WC, Foley DP, Garrett WE, et al. PAIN (Performing Athletes with Abdominal or Inguinal Neuromuscular Pain Study Group). Management of severe lower abdominal or inguinal pain in high-performance athletes. Am J Sports Med 2000;28: 2–8.
17. Zoga A, Mullens F, Meyers W. The spectrum of MR imaging in athletic pubalgia. Radiol Clin North Am 2010;48:1179–97.
18. Zoga AC, Kavanagh EC, Omar IM, et al. Athletic pubalgia and the "sports hernia": MR imaging findings. Radiology 2008;247:797–807.
19. Palisch A, Zoga AC, Meyers WC. Imaging of athletic pubalgia and core muscle injuries: clinical and therapeutic correlations. Clin Sports Med 2013;32: 427–47.
20. Meyers WC, McKechnie A, Philippon MJ, et al. Experience with "sports hernia" spanning two decades. Ann Surg 2008;248:656–65.
21. Khan W, Zoga AC, Meyers WC. Magnetic resonance imaging of athletic pubalgia and the sports hernia: current understanding and practice. Magn Reson Imaging Clin N Am 2013;21:97–110.
22. Kunduracioglu B, Yilmaz C, Yorubulut M, et al. Magnetic resonance findings of osteitis pubis. J Magn Reson Imaging 2007;25:535–9.
23. Murphy G, Foran P, Murphy D, et al. "Superior cleft sign" as a marker of rectus abdominis/adductor longus tear in patients with suspected sportsman's hernia. Skeletal Radiol 2013;42:819–25.
24. Mullens FE, Zoga AC, Meyers WC, et al. Review of MRI technique and imaging findings in athletic

pubalgia and the "sports hernia". Eur J Radiol 2012; 81:3780–92.

25. Robinson P, Barron DA, Parsons W, et al. Adductor-related groin pain in athletes: correlation of MR imaging with clinical findings. Skeletal Radiol 2004; 33:451–7.

26. Meyers WC, Lanfranco A, Castellanos A. Surgical management of chronic lower abdominal and groin pain in high-performance athletes. Curr Sports Med Rep 2002;1:301–5.

27. Evans GF, Haller RG, Wyrick PS, et al. Submaximal delayed-onset muscle soreness: correlations between MR imaging findings and clinical measures. Radiology 1998;208:815–20.

28. Page P. Pathophysiology of acute exercise-induced muscular injury: clinical implications. J Athl Train 1995;30:29–34.

29. Arnaiz J, Piedra T, de Lucas EM, et al. Imaging findings of lower limb apophysitis. AJR Am J Roentgenol 2011;196:W316–25.

30. McKinney BI, Nelson C, Carrion W. Apophyseal avulsion fractures of the hip and pelvis. Orthopedics 2009;32:42.

31. Sutter R, Pfirrmann CW. Atypical Hip Impingement. AJR Am J Roentgenol 2013;201:437–42.

32. Hopayian K, Song F, Riera R, et al. The clinical features of the piriformis syndrome: a systematic review. Eur Spine J 2010;19:2095–109.

33. Torriani M, Souto SC, Thomas BJ, et al. Ischiofemoral impingement syndrome: an entity with hip pain and abnormalities of the quadratus femoris muscle. AJR Am J Roentgenol 2009;193:186–90.

34. Dragoni S, Giombini A, Di Cesare A, et al. Stress fractures of the ribs in elite competitive rowers: a report of nine cases. Skeletal Radiol 2007;36:951–4.

35. Udermann BE, Cavanaugh DG, Gibson MH, et al. Slipping rib syndrome in a collegiate swimmer: a case report. J Athl Train 2005;40:120–2.

36. Gerrie BJ, Harris JD, Lintner DM, et al. Lower thoracic rib stress fractures in baseball pitchers. Phys Sportsmed 2016;44:93–6.

37. Brohn JL, van Royen BJ, Wuisman P. The Clinical Significance of Lumbosacral Transitional Anomalies. Acta Orthop Belg 2007;73:687–95.

38. Anderson MW, Kaplan PA, Dussault RG. Adductor insertion avulsion syndrome (thigh splints): spectrum of MR imaging features. AJR Am J Roentgenol 2001;177:673–5.

39. Ergen FB, Yildiz AE, Ayvaz M, et al. Bilateral triradiate cartilage injury: an overuse syndrome in an adolescent football player. Skeletal Radiol 2012;41:353–5.

40. Dwek J, Pfirrmann C, Stanley A, et al. MR imaging of the hip abductors: normal anatomy and commonly encountered pathology at the greater trochanter. Magn Reson Imaging Clin N Am 2005;13:691–704.

41. Chowdhury R, Naaseri S, Lee J, et al. Imaging and management of greater trochanteric pain syndrome. Postgrad Med J 2014;90:576–81.

42. Williams BS, Cohen SP. Greater trochanteric pain syndrome: a review of anatomy, diagnosis and treatment. Anesth Analg 2009;108:1662–70.

43. Robert R, Prat-Pradal D, Labat JJ, et al. Anatomic basis of chronic perianal pain: role of the pudendal nerve. Surg Radiol Anat 1998;20:93–8.

44. Wadhwa V, Hamid AS, Kumar Y, et al. Pudendal nerve and branch neuropathy: magnetic resonance neurography evaluation. Acta Radiol 2017; 58:726–33.

MR Imaging of Entrapment Neuropathies of the Lower Extremity

Elisabeth R. Garwood, MD[a],*, Alejandra Duarte, MD[b],
Jenny T. Bencardino, MD[b]

KEYWORDS

- Neuropathy • Entrapment • Lower extremity • MR neurography • Nerve • Denervation
- Peripheral nerve • Mononeuropathy

KEY POINTS

- Entrapment neuropathies are common and can impose a significant disease burden.
- Clinical diagnosis is challenging; advanced peripheral nerve imaging with MR neurography can guide diagnosis and treatment decisions.
- Advances in MR neurography have emphasized improved spatial and contrast resolution of the peripheral nerves to aid morphologic assessment.
- Emerging techniques to provide noninvasive functional assessment are promising.
- Radiologist familiarity with MR neurography protocols, peripheral nerve anatomy, and the appearance of the peripheral nerves in normal and pathologic states, is critical for timely diagnosis.

INTRODUCTION

Structural compression or entrapment, the most common mechanism of peripheral nerve injury, is frequently encountered in clinical practice. There are 14.2 million subspecialty referrals for peripheral neuropathy made annually in the United States.[1] Lower extremity peripheral neuropathies are a heterogeneous group of disorders with a broad range of clinical presentations and etiologies. Lower extremity peripheral neuropathies present a greater diagnostic challenge to clinicians as compared with upper extremity neuropathies and are more commonly underdiagnosed or misdiagnosed.[1] It is suspected that, for these reasons, rather than true lower prevalence, lower extremity peripheral neuropathies are diagnosed with less frequency than upper extremity neuropathies. When considered individually, entrapment neuropathies have a relatively low prevalence; for example, the most widespread entrapment mononeuropathy, carpal tunnel syndrome, affects only 3% to 6% of the population, however, when considered in aggregate, the societal burden is significant.[2] Twenty-six percent of patients between the ages of 65 and 74 years and 54% of patients over the age of 85 have at least 1 lower extremity motor or sensory deficit consistent with peripheral neuropathy.[3]

The current understanding of compression-related nerve damage is related to the mechanism of increased endoneural fluid pressure from the

Disclosure Statement: No disclosures (E.R. Garwood, J.T. Bencardino). Supported by grant number NIH R01-AR067789 from the National Institute of Arthritis and Musculoskeletal and Skin Diseases (NIAMS) of the National Institutes of Health (NIH) (A. Duarte).
[a] Department of Radiology, NYU Langone – Orthopedic Hospital, 301 East 17th Street 6th Floor, Room 600, New York, NY 10003, USA; [b] Department of Radiology, NYU Langone Medical Center, 660 First Avenue, New York, NY 10016, USA
* Corresponding author.
E-mail address: elisabeth.garwood@nyumc.org

Radiol Clin N Am 56 (2018) 997–1012
https://doi.org/10.1016/j.rcl.2018.06.012
0033-8389/18/© 2018 Elsevier Inc. All rights reserved.

blockage of normal fluid egress, which leads to intraneural microvascular congestion. Ultimately, nerve infarction and fibrosis can result, and these microstructural changes manifest as signal alterations on MR imaging.[4] There are 2 primary clinical classifications of nerve injury that correlate histology, clinical presentation, and prognosis and are used for neuropathy severity grading and guidance of treatment choice. The type of injury resulting from compression is classified as axonotmesis (Seddon classification) or Sunderland classification types II through IV (Table 1). The clinical presentation of nerve dysfunction related to entrapment depends on the types of fibers carried by that nerve (motor, sensory, or autonomic) and may manifest as alterations of sensory function (pain, paresthesia, dysesthesia, hypoesthesia), decreased motor function (muscle weakness, complete or total palsy or paralysis, muscle atrophy), or changes in autonomic function (anhidrosis and ulceration).[5]

Compression neuropathies are diagnosed through a combination of clinical assessment, physical examination, electrodiagnostic studies, and increasingly by MR neurography or musculoskeletal ultrasound. A course of treatment—conservative, interventional, or surgical—is selected based on the result of this evaluation. Conservative therapies include activity modification, biomechanical modification, physical therapy, and neuropathic pain medications. Percutaneous image-guided perineural injection with an anesthetic and a steroid in combination with conservative therapies is a common initial therapeutic strategy for lower extremity peripheral mononeuropathies.[6] For compression neuropathies nonresponsive to these measures, surgical management in the form of neurolysis, nerve wrapping, neuroma resection, or less commonly, neurectomy, can result in symptomatic relief.[7,8]

TECHNICAL CONSIDERATIONS

Peripheral nerves pose several imaging challenges related to the high spatial resolution required to assess these small anatomic structures, the relative poor contrast resolution of the peripheral nerves compared with the neighboring vasculature, and the technical challenge of imaging off-isocenter relative to the magnetic bore.[9] Current MR neurography protocols optimized for peripheral nerve visualization use a combination of 2-dimensional and 3-dimensional pulse sequences.[4] MR neurography, for most cases, is performed to optimize spatial resolution and contrast-to-noise ratio, including 3T field strength, high channel (>15 elements) phased array surface coils, small field of view, and isotropic voxel size when 3-dimensional sequences are used.[10]

DIAGNOSTIC CRITERIA

The interpretation of MR neurography currently hinges on the visual morphologic assessment of the peripheral nerves and regional anatomy. A normal nerve is T1-weighted isointense to muscle and slightly T2-weighted hyperintense. The caliber of a normal nerve is generally slightly smaller than the accompanying arterial vasculature with a gradual distal taper. Direct MR

Table 1
Sunderland and Seddon classifications of peripheral nerve injury severity grading with corresponding histology, MR appearance, clinical presentation, and clinical recovery expectations

Sunderland Classification	Seddon Classification	Histology	MR Appearance	Clinical Presentation	Recovery
II	Axonotmesis	Axon and myelin abnormal	Increased intrasubstance signal	Paresthesia Partial or total palsy	Usually full 1–6 mo
III		Axon, myelin, and endoneurium abnormal	Increased intrasubstance signal Increased caliber May have prominent fascicles	Paresthesia Dysesthesia Partial or total palsy	Partial 12–24 mo
IV		Only epineurium preserved (neuroma) Axon, myelin, endoneurium and perineurium abnormal	Heterogeneous intrasubstance signal Eccentric or fusiform neuroma formation	Hypoesthesia Dysesthesia Total palsy	None without repair

findings of peripheral nerve injury secondary to entrapment include changes in nerve caliber manifested by an increase in nerve size near the site of entrapment, irregular nerve contour, disruption of the uniform fascicular architecture, increased intraneural signal, abnormal anatomic course of the nerve, and, in the case of contrast administration, increased enhancement. Indirect signs include disruption of the normal perineural fat planes, mass effect, perineural edema, regional intramuscular signal alterations, or muscular atrophy indicative of denervation changes distal to the entrapment and within the appropriate innervation territory (**Table 2**).[10,11] MR neurography allows identification of the compressive lesion, level of entrapment, and severity of neural changes.

IMAGING PITFALLS

Magic angle can lead to the artifactual appearance of increased intrasubstance signal or increased signal to noise within a peripheral nerve along areas of normal anatomic curvature. The increase in contrast to noise produced by true pathologic lesions is greater than the increase in contrast to noise produced by magic angle artifact and can usually be distinguished by an experienced observer.[12] Knowledge of common areas of peripheral nerve magic angle artifact can aid in the distinction between artifact and true pathologic lesions. This phenomenon is commonly observed at the following sites: the sciatic nerve at the level of the greater sciatic notch, the femoral nerve as it exits the pelvis, the lateral femoral cutaneous nerve at the anterior superior iliac spine, and the medial plantar nerve branch of the tibial nerve at the level of the tarsal tunnel.[13]

FUTURE DIRECTIONS

The current standard of MR neurography is based on qualitative morphologic assessment of the peripheral nerves. The future of MR neurography lies in its ability to acquire and quantify functional information about the peripheral nerves. Adapting techniques established in imaging of the central nervous system including diffusion tensor imaging, which is widely used to assess the structural integrity of large axon bundles in the central nervous system, and diffusion tensor tractography, hold promise; however, these modalities currently remain limited to research applications owing to nonautomated postprocessing, data correction, and analysis techniques.[9] With PET/MR imaging techniques gaining traction, nuclear medicine applications, such as developing PET biomarkers specific to nerve injury or inflammation, may be an important area of future research for peripheral nerve imaging.[14]

DEEP GLUTEAL SYNDROME AND SUBGLUTEAL SPACE ENTRAPMENT OF SCIATIC NERVE
Anatomy

The sciatic nerve arises from the ventral divisions of the L4 through S3 nerve roots and exits the pelvis posteriorly through the greater sciatic foramen. The 2 divisions of the sciatic nerve—the tibial (medial) and the peroneal (lateral)—are enveloped in 1 nerve sheath and provide motor innervation to the posterior compartment musculature of the thigh and both sensory and motor innervation below the knee.[15]

The subgluteal space or posterior peritrochanteric space is a potential site of sciatic nerve entrapment where the sciatic nerve lies close to

---

Table 2
MR neurography findings in normal versus abnormal nerve morphology

	Normal Nerve	Abnormal Nerve
Signal intensity	T1-weighted isointense to muscle T2-weighted isointense to slightly hyperintense	T1-weighted isointense to hypointense T2-weighted hyperintense
Morphology	Uniform fascicular size	Nonuniform fascicular size, enlargement of some fascicles
	Nerve caliber slightly smaller than accompanying arterial vasculature	Nerve caliber larger than accompanying arterial vasculature
	Gradual distal tapering	Abrupt caliber change
Ancillary findings	Preserved perineural fat plane	Perineural edema (T2-weighted hyperintense) or fibrosis (low signal intensity)
	Normal muscle signal and bulk	Geographic intramuscular signal intensity changes or fatty atrophy

the posterior hip joint capsule and is bordered by the linea aspera laterally, sacrotuberous ligament medially, inferior border of the sciatic notch superiorly, and common hamstrings origin inferiorly. The subgluteal space contains the piriformis, superior, and inferior gemelli; the obturator internus; the quadratus femoris musculature; the superior and inferior gluteal nerves; and the sciatic nerve.

Pathologic Conditions

Subgluteal space entrapments present clinically with deep gluteal syndrome and encompass a variety of specific sciatic entrapment etiologies, including fibrovascular band entrapment, piriformis syndrome, ischiofemoral impingement, and entrapment related to proximal hamstrings tendon dysfunction or injury. The clinical presentation of patients with deep gluteal syndrome is nonspecific, most commonly characterized by posterior hip/thigh or buttock pain or dysesthesias exacerbated by sitting. Tenderness to palpation along the gluteal and posterior peritrochanteric region may be present.[16]

Imaging Findings

Perineural fibrous or fibrovascular bands can develop along the sciatic nerve course resulting in a reduction or loss of normal nerve mobility during hip or knee motion that precipitates a compression or traction-related sciatic neuropathy. Blunt trauma to the buttock is hypothesized to be the origin of these bands. The most common location for adhesive fibrovascular band formation, seen on MR imaging as a slightly T2-weighted hyperintense linear band, is lateral, extending from the posterior margin of the greater trochanter to the sciatic nerve. Adhesive bands are identified on MR imaging through close inspection of the perineural fat plane surrounding the sciatic nerve within the subgluteal space; however, although there is arthroscopic correlation, it has been noted that fibrovascular bands are not always evident on MR imaging. Piriformis muscle-related pathologies, although controversial, can include asymmetric hypertrophy of the piriformis and dynamic sciatic entrapment by the piriformis muscle, which may occur more commonly in the setting of variant neuromuscular anatomy. Piriformis muscle hypertrophy secondary to altered biomechanics/gait disturbance, excessive lumbar lordosis, and hip flexion deformities is also observed in asymptomatic individuals; the interpretation of asymmetric piriformis muscle hypertrophy in the clinical context is important and concomitant sciatic nerve signal abnormality or perineural edema improves diagnostic

sensitivity.[15,17] Ischiofemoral impingement is characterized on MR imaging by an anatomically narrowed ischiofemoral space with accompanying denervation changes of the quadratus femoris muscle, additionally, altered sciatic nerve signal intensity, nerve thickening, and perineural edema may be present (**Fig. 1**). Sciatic nerve entrapment related to proximal hamstrings tendon dysfunction, scarring, avulsion injury, and proximal hamstring repair has been observed owing to the close proximity of the sciatic nerve to the common hamstrings origin (**Fig. 2**).[18,19]

Treatment Options

If conservative management is not successful, treatment options include image-guided piriformis botulinum injection in the case of symptomatic piriformis hypertrophy and endoscopic decompression/perineural release in the setting of fibrovascular band entrapment or ischiofemoral impingement. Neurolysis and adhesion release is also indicated in cases of entrapment owing to postoperative scar in the setting of hamstring tendon repair at the ischial tuberosity.[19]

Mimics

Intraarticular or extraarticular hip pathology, and lumbar radiculopathy can present with similar symptoms as sciatic nerve entrapment.

PUDENDAL NEURALGIA
Anatomy

The pudendal nerve receives contributions from the S2 through S4 nerve roots and provides sensory, motor, and autonomic innervation to genitalia, rectum, and perineum. In the pelvis, the pudendal nerve can be found descending along the anterior/lateral border of the piriformis muscle; it then courses inferiorly to briefly exit the pelvis interposed between the sacrospinous and sacrotuberous ligaments at the greater sciatic foramen, ventral to the sciatic nerve. The pudendal nerve then reenters the pelvis through the lesser sciatic foramen winding around the sacrospinous ligament, then courses anteriorly and laterally through a fibroosseous tunnel, the pudendal or Alcock's canal where is it the most posteriorly positioned structure within the canal, accompanied by the internal pudendal vessels.[20]

Pathologic Conditions

Pudendal neuralgia owing to pudendal entrapment is being increasingly recognized as a source of chronic pelvic pain. Entrapment along the nerve course most commonly occurs at the pudendal

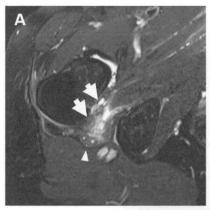
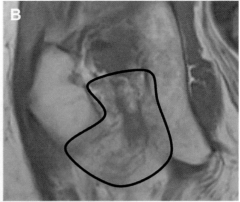
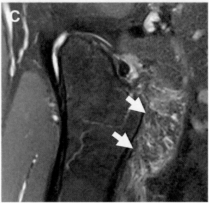

Fig. 1. Ischiofemoral impingement in 70-year-old woman presenting with right posterior hip and buttock pain. On physical examination, there is marked tenderness to palpation along the posterior peritrochanteric region and shooting pain is elicited with direct pressure over the greater sciatic notch. Axial T2-weighted (*A*), coronal proton density without fat suppression (*B*), and sagittal T2-weighted (*C*) fat-suppressed images show diffuse edema of the quadratus femoris muscle (*arrows*), fatty atrophy of the quadratus femoris (*outline*), mass effect on an enlarged sciatic nerve (*arrowhead*), and perineural edema interposed between the deep margin of the sciatic nerve and the quadratus femoris.

canal, but can also occur at the level of the ischial spine and along the nerve's interligamentous course between the sacrotuberous and sacrospinous ligaments (**Fig. 3**).[21] Clinically, patients present with pain along the pudendal distribution involving the genitalia, perineum, and/or anorectal regions exacerbated by sitting. Pudendal neuralgia has been described in the setting of competitive bicyclists, trauma/pelvic fractures, parturition-related injury, and iatrogenic injury during gynecologic or urologic surgery. Treatment options in addition to medical management and conservative measures include image guided pudendal nerve block, computed tomography-guided cryoablation, and minimally invasive neurolysis.[22,23]

Imaging Findings

Nerve enlargement or perineural fibrosis may be seen. Intrinsic nerve signal changes may be challenging to detect owing to the small size of the nerve and close proximity to vasculature.

Mimics

The differential diagnosis for pudendal neuralgia is broad and includes other causes of chronic pelvic pain. Gynecologic, urologic, and gastrointestinal etiologies must be considered, including endometriosis, inflammatory bowel disease, and chronic prostatitis.

OBTURATOR NEUROPATHY
Anatomy

The obturator nerve receives contributions from the L2 through L4 nerve roots. In the pelvis, the obturator nerve descends along the medial border of the psoas musculature and courses along the lateral pelvic sidewall and exits the pelvis through the obturator foramen.

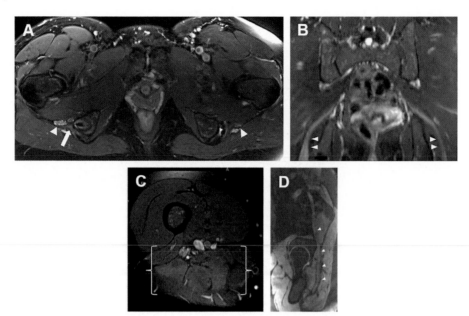

Fig. 2. Right sciatic nerve injury after right hip arthroscopy and hamstring tendon repair in 45-year-old woman. Subsequence sciatic neurolysis revealed subgluteal fibrovascular band compression of the right sciatic nerve. Axial T2-weighted spectral attenuated inversion recovery (SPAIR) (*A*) and reformatted coronal space short T1-weighted inversion recovery (*B*) sequences show asymmetric enlargement and a T2-weighted hyperintense signal abnormality of the distal subgluteal right sciatic nerve as compared with the normal contralateral side (*arrowheads*), consistent with neuritis. A fibrovascular band extends from the ischial tuberosity to the sciatic nerve, traversing the perineural fat (*arrow*). (*C*) An axial T2-weighted SPAIR sequence obtained at mid-thigh demonstrates patchy T2-weighted hyperintense signal abnormality within the posterior compartment musculature (*brackets*) reflective of denervation changes in a sciatic distribution. (*D*) Time-reversed fast imaging with steady state precession oblique sagittal reconstruction demonstrates thickening of the sciatic nerve rather than normal distal tapering (*arrowheads*).

The obturator nerve bifurcates into an anterior branch that continues superficial to the adductor brevis and a posterior branch that course deep to the adductor brevis before entering the thigh.

Pathologic Conditions

Isolated obturator neuropathy is uncommon. Entrapment neuropathies of the obturator nerve include obturator hernia (**Fig. 4**) and nerve entrapment by muscle herniation (baseball pitcher—hockey goalie syndrome). Space-occupying lesions such as paralabral cysts and ganglia at the hip may result in symptomatic obturator nerve compression. Injuries of the obturator nerve are most commonly seen in conjunction with femoral nerve injuries and include pelvic or hip fractures and iatrogenic injury related to hip arthroscopy.[20] Iatrogenic obturator nerve injury is a known but uncommon complication of female midurethral sling placement for stress urinary incontinence and is reported in less than 1% of cases.[24] Obturator neuropathy clinically presents with weakness of thigh adduction and hip internal rotation that can result in gait disturbance. If there is involvement of the anterior branch, cutaneous sensory changes may be present along the medial groin and thigh.

Imaging Findings

Space-occupying lesion of the obturator canal with displacement of the neurovascular bundle can be seen. Denervation changes within the adductor compartment musculature may be present.

Mimics

Obturator neuropathy can be confused with athletic pubalgia, osteitis pubis, inguinal hernia, and stress fracture.

LATERAL FEMORAL CUTANEOUS NERVE ENTRAPMENT/MERALGIA PARESTHETICA
Anatomy

The lateral femoral cutaneous nerve receives contributions from the L2 and L3 nerve roots and

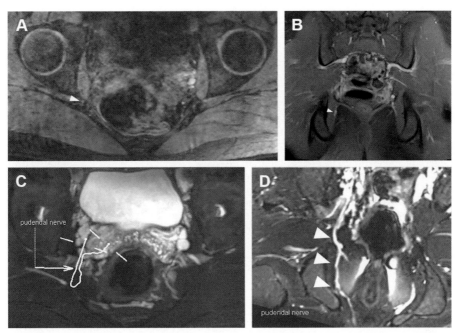

Fig. 3. Right pudendal neuralgia in 26-year-old man. Axial time-reversed fast imaging with steady state precession (*A*) and coronal T1-weighted postcontrast fat-suppressed (*B*) images show asymmetric enlargement, increased signal intensity, and enhancement of the right pudendal nerve (*arrowheads*) at the level of the ischial spine (*A*) and distal to Alcock's canal (*B*), reflective of neuritis. Subsequent image-guided therapeutic right pudendal perineural injection provided symptomatic relief. The course of the right pudendal (*line*) nerve in the axial plane (*C*) and 3-dimensional maximum intensity projection reconstruction (*D*) of the right pudendal neurovascular bundle in a healthy volunteer (*arrowheads*). Note the sharp turn of the nerve as it descends from the lumbosacral plexus into the lower pelvis bending forward at the level of Alcock's canal to end after a horizontal course along the floor of the pelvis.

provides sensory only innervation to the cutaneous anterolateral thigh. The nerve exits the pelvis slightly medial to the anterior superior iliac spine and deep to the inguinal ligament.

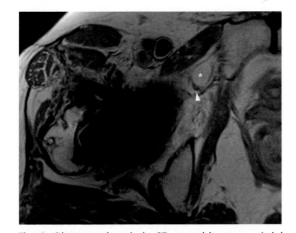

Fig. 4. Obturator hernia in 67-year-old woman. Axial T1-weighted sequence shows posterior displacement of the obturator neurovascular bundle (*arrowhead*) by a fat-containing right obturator hernia within the obturator canal (*asterisk*). Susceptibility artifact is due to right total hip arthroplasty.

Pathologic Conditions

Meralgia paresthetica is entrapment neuropathy of the lateral femoral cutaneous nerve as it exits the pelvis and occurs most frequently in obese patients. It is more common in those with diabetes. Entrapment neuropathy of the lateral femoral cutaneous nerve has been associated with tight clothing, seat belts, pregnancy, limb length discrepancy, and iatrogenic injury in the setting of pelvic fracture repair, inguinal herniorrhaphy, and abdominoplasty.[25,26] Diabetic patients are 7 times more likely to develop meralgia paresthetica compared with the general population.[27] The symptomatic presentation is specific, with pain, numbness, and paresthesias confined to the anterior/lateral cutaneous thigh. Perineural injection of anesthetic can be useful for both diagnostic and therapeutic purposes.[28,29]

Imaging Findings

Increased nerve caliber and altered nerve signal may be observed in the setting of lateral femoral cutaneous nerve entrapment (**Fig. 5**). Osseous hypertrophy at the anterior/inferior iliac spine or

A   B

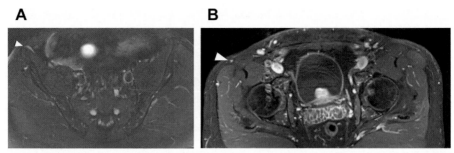

Fig. 5. Right meralgia paresthetica in 54-year-old man. (*A*) Axial T2-weighted spectral attenuated inversion recovery sequence shows thickening and increased T2-weighted signal of the right lateral femoral cutaneous nerve (*arrowhead*) as it exits the pelvis deep to the inguinal ligament at the level of the anterior superior iliac spine. (*B*) Axial T1-weighted postcontrast image with fat suppression shows asymmetric thickening and enhancement of the right lateral femoral cutaneous nerve (*arrowhead*) as it continues distally within the thigh.

thickening of the inguinal ligament are potential anatomic compressive lesions readily identified on MR imaging.

Mimics

Meralgia paresthetica may be confused clinically with L2/L3 radiculopathy and femoral mononeuropathy.

FEMORAL NERVE ENTRAPMENT
Anatomy

The femoral nerve, the largest branch of the lumbosacral plexus, receives contributions from the L2 through L4 nerve roots. In the pelvis, the femoral nerve courses through the psoas muscle then descends along the anterior margin of the psoas and iliacus musculature deep to the iliacus fascia, providing motor innervation to both. The femoral nerve exits the pelvis deep to the inguinal ligament and travels through the fibromuscular femoral triangle in the proximal thigh, where it bifurcates into anterior and posterior divisions. The anterior division provides motor innervation to the pectineus and sartorius muscles and gives of sensory branches that provide cutaneous sensory innervation to the anterior thigh. The posterior division provides motor innervation to the quadriceps musculature (rectus femoris, vastus lateralis, vastus intermedius, and vastus medialis). The terminal cutaneous sensory branch of the posterior division is the saphenous nerve that travels through the medial thigh within the adductor canal and supplies medial cutaneous sensory innervation from the level of the distal thigh through the medial malleolus, medial arch of the foot, and the great toe.

Pathologic Conditions

Femoral nerve entrapment most commonly occurs just distal to the pelvic exit, deep to the inguinal ligament.[30] Susceptibility to maximum compression occurs during hip flexion. Iatrogenic injury to the femoral nerve includes scarring from hernia repair or femoral vascular access and surgical procedures around the lower abdomen and pelvis.[31] Mass effect from psoas muscle hematoma and iliopsoas bursal distention have also been reported as compressive anatomic lesions.[32] Clinically, femoral neuropathy presents with knee weakness characterized by decreased knee extension (quadriceps weakness) and decreased hip flexion (iliopsoas muscle weakness). An absent knee jerk and sensory deficits in the anterior thigh, medial calf, and medial arch may also be present.[32]

Imaging Findings

In isolated femoral mononeuropathy, iatrogenic injury is more commonly implicated than entrapment. The most common site of anatomic entrapment is just distal to the pelvic exit deep to the inguinal ligament, where focal nerve enlargement and signal abnormality may be observed. Isolated denervation changes within the psoas musculature indicate a lesion along the intrapelvic course of the femoral nerve, whereas denervation changes that involve the quadriceps indicate a more distal lesion, occurring after the takeoff of the iliopsoas motor branch.[32,33]

Mimics

L4 radiculopathy, lumbar plexopathy, and upper motor neuron disease may mimic femoral nerve entrapment.

PERONEAL NEUROPATHY
Anatomy

The peroneal nerve receives contributions from the L4 through S2 nerve roots. In the thigh, the peroneal nerve travels as the peroneal component of the sciatic nerve positioned laterally within the sciatic nerve bundle and supplies motor innervation to the short head of the biceps femoris muscle. The common peroneal nerve takes off from the sciatic nerve at the apex of the popliteal fossa and then courses laterally, wraps around the fibular head/neck, and enters the anterior compartment musculature of the calf through the peroneal tunnel where it bifurcates into the superficial and deep peroneal nerves. The superficial branch innervates the ankle everters and continues as the superficial peroneal sensory nerve, supplying the lateral lower leg and foot. The deep division of the peroneal nerve runs along the anterior surface of the interosseous membrane and innervates the tibialis anterior, extensor digitorum longus, peroneus tertius, and extensor hallucis longus muscles, and gives off a sensory articular branch to the tibiotalar joint. The deep peroneal nerve bifurcates below the tibiotalar joint into a lateral and medial branch. The lateral branch provides motor innervation to the extensor digitorum brevis and extensor hallucis brevis; the medial branch provides purely sensory innervation to the first web space.

Pathologic Conditions

Compression neuropathy of the common peroneal nerve at the fibular head is the most common mononeuropathy of the lower extremity that clinically presents with foot drop or motor weakness of ankle dorsiflexion. Pain is an uncommon feature. At the level of the fibular head/neck, the common peroneal nerve is located superficially, protected only by a thin layer of subcutaneous fat and closely apposed to the underlying bone of the fibula, making it particularly susceptible to damage from external compression.[11] Traction- or contusion-related injuries to the common peroneal nerve can be seen in the setting of knee trauma, particularly with knee dislocation or multiligamentous knee injuries (**Fig. 6**).[34] Anatomic variations in the relationship between the common peroneal nerve and the distal biceps femoris tendon and lateral gastrocnemius may predispose to compression neuropathy of the common peroneal nerve above the level of the fibular neck.[35] Usually, the common peroneal nerve at the level just above the knee joint is surrounded by abundant fat as it courses superficial to the lateral head of the gastrocnemius musculature and at the level of the distal biceps femoris tendon. In about one-quarter of patients, at this level the common peroneal nerve is not cushioned by abundant fat but travels in a narrow tunnel interposed between the short head of the distal biceps femoris and lateral head of the gastrocnemius musculature. This configuration, with a particularly long

tunnel length, has been observed in a case of common peroneal nerve compression neuropathy.[35] Compression of the deep peroneal nerve within the proximal calf at the level of the peroneal tunnel is less common than compression at the level of the fibular head, and the dominant clinical feature of this compression syndrome is pain in the peroneal dermatome that can progress to foot drop.[36]

Imaging Findings

The primary role of MR imaging in the assessment of suspected common peroneal nerve entrapment at the fibula is the identification of space-occupying lesions or muscular denervation changes in the peroneal distribution. In this location, compressive lesions can include meniscal cysts, fibular head osteophyte or enthesophytes, large fabellae, ganglion cysts arising from the proximal tibiofibular articulation, intraneural ganglia (which likely reflect the dissection of synovial fluid from the superior joint capsule of the proximal tibiofibular joint along the articular branch of the nerve; **Fig. 7**), and fracture/hemorrhage along the proximal fibula.[36–39] Extrinsic compression such as from tight casting or prolonged leg crossing may result in common peroneal nerve abnormalities, such as increased caliber or increased intrasubstance signal or fascicular enlargement with or without muscle denervation changes. The common peroneal nerve should be closely inspected in all cases of severe knee trauma, such as dislocation and multiligamentous injury of the knee, because the surgeon may decide to perform common peroneal neurolysis or nerve wrapping at the time of ligament repair.[34] If the common peroneal nerve courses within a narrow tunnel between the short head of the distal biceps femoris tendon and the lateral gastrocnemius, careful inspection of common peroneal nerve morphology and the presence or absence of denervation changes within a common peroneal distribution is warranted.

Mimics

Peroneal neuropathy must be distinguished from L5 radiculopathy, sciatic neuropathy, motor neuron disease, and lumbar plexopathy.[40]

SUPERFICIAL PERONEAL NEUROPATHY
Anatomy

The superficial peroneal nerve takes off from the common peroneal nerve usually just after it courses around the fibular neck within the proximal calf. After its bifurcation from the common peroneal nerve, the superficial peroneal nerve

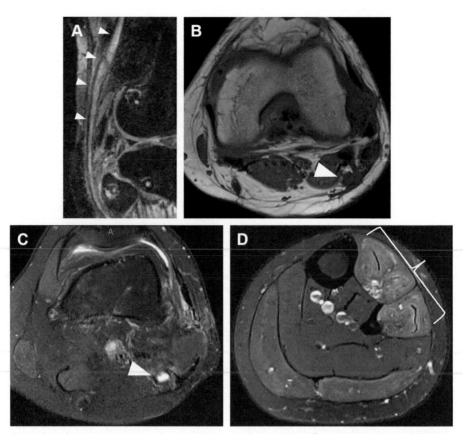

Fig. 6. Traction-related common peroneal nerve injury in the setting of posttraumatic multiligamentous knee injury and subsequent reconstruction in a 28-year-old woman. Oblique sagittal time-reversed fast imaging with steady state precession reformatted (A), axial proton density, (B) and T2-weighted fat-suppressed (C) sequences show long segment fusiform enlargement and a T2-weighted hyperintense signal abnormality of the common peroneal nerve above the level of the knee joint (arrowheads). (D) T2-weighted hyperintense denervation changes are seen involving the anterior compartment musculature of the calf including the tibialis anterior and extensor digitorum longus (bracket).

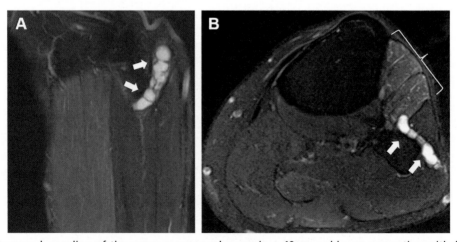

Fig. 7. Intraneural ganglion of the common peroneal nerve in a 49-year old man presenting with foot drop. Sagittal (A) and axial (B) T2-weighted fat-suppressed images at the level of the proximal fibula show a lobular T2-weighted hyperintense intraneural ganglion cyst dissecting along the course of the common peroneal nerve (arrows). T2-weighted hyperintense denervation changes are seen involving the anterior compartment musculature of the calf, including the tibialis anterior and extensor digitorum longus (bracket).

occupies a fascial plane between the peroneus longus and extensor digitorum longus musculature. The nerve transitions from a deep to a superficial course by exiting the crural fascia within the lateral calf in the lower one-third of the leg.[41] The superficial peroneal nerve provides motor innervation to the peroneus longus and brevis muscles along its proximal course and sensory innervation along the dorsum of the foot and toes.

Pathologic Conditions

Mechanical entrapment of the superficial peroneal nerve may occur as it exits the deep crural fascia. In a series of 480 patients presenting with chronic lower leg pain, 3.5% were found to have superficial peroneal nerve entrapment neuropathy.[41] This phenomenon is observed with greater frequency in athletes and dancers, attributed to repetitive plantar flexion and ankle inversion.[42] Scarring or fibrous bands, intraneural ganglion cyst, and muscle herniation through an enlarged crural fascial opening have been observed to compress the superficial peroneal nerve.[42–44] Patients with superficial peroneal neuropathy present with pain and sensory changes over the dorsum of the foot. A positive Tinel sign at the level of the crural fascial exit may be observed.

Imaging Findings

The fascial exit of the superficial peroneal nerve should be closely inspected for fascial defect, muscular herniation, and perineural fibrosis or scar.

Mimics

The differential diagnosis for superficial peroneal neuropathy includes exertional compartment syndrome, lumbar radiculopathy, and common peroneal neuropathy.

DEEP PERONEAL NEUROPATHY (ANTERIOR TARSAL TUNNEL SYNDROME)
Anatomy

The anterior tarsal tunnel is a fibroosseous tunnel along the dorsal midfoot bound superficially by the inferior extensor retinaculum, laterally by the fibula, medially by the medial malleolar process of the distal tibia, and posteriorly by the talonavicular joint. Contents include the extensor musculature of the foot (tibialis anterior, extensor halluces longus, and extensor digitorum longus), the dorsalis pedis artery and vein, and the deep peroneal nerve.[45]

Pathologic Conditions

The deep peroneal nerve may become entrapped at 3 anatomic locations, deep to the inferior extensor retinaculum along the superior border as the nerve dives under the retinaculum, deep to the extensor hallucis longus tendon at the level of the talonavicular joint, and deep to the extensor hallucis brevis muscle at the level of the first and second tarsal-metatarsal articulations.[46] Anatomic compressive lesions include dorsally directed osteophytosis at the talonavicular and/or navicular cuneiform articulations, dorsally directed ganglia, and intraneural ganglion formation have been described.[47] Clinically, patients with a lesion of the deep peroneal nerve experience sensory changes along the dorsal/medial foot, classically with pain radiating to the first web space dorsally. Extensor digitorum weakness may be seen.

Imaging Findings

Denervation changes within a deep peronal nerve distribution including the anterior tibial, extensor hallucis longus, extensor digitorum longus, and peroneus tertius musculature. Compressive lesions such as dorsally directed osteophytes at the talonavicular and navicular/cuneiform joints may be identified.

Mimics

Deep peroneal neuropathy must be distinguished from L5 radiculopathy, common peroneal neuropathy, and exertional anterior compartment syndrome.[45]

TIBIAL NEUROPATHY
Anatomy

The tibial nerve receives contributions from the L4 through S2 nerve roots. In the thigh, the tibial nerve, as the tibial component of the sciatic nerve positioned medially within the sciatic nerve sheath, supplies motor innervation to the hamstrings and one-half of the adductor magnus musculature. The sciatic nerve bifurcates into the common peroneal nerve and tibial nerve, which in turn gives off a medial sural cutaneous branch. The tibial nerve continues below the knee within the posterior compartment of the calf situated between the medial and lateral heads of the gastrocnemius, providing motor innervation to both the deep and superficial posterior compartment musculature. At the level of the ankle, the tibial nerve, now named the posterior tibial nerve, gives off the medial calcaneal nerve, which provides sensory innervation to the medial hindfoot then bifurcates at the level of the tarsal tunnel, the fibroosseous tarsal tunnel posterior to the medial malleolar process of the distal tibia and deep to the flexor retinaculum, into the medial plantar and lateral plantar nerves, which provide both motor and sensory innervation to the foot.

Compression neuropathies of the tibial nerve include tarsal tunnel syndrome, sural, medial plantar, lateral plantar, inferior calcaneal, and interdigital neuropathy.

POSTERIOR TIBIAL NERVE (TARSAL TUNNEL SYNDROME)
Pathologic Conditions

Compression of the posterior tibial nerve in the fibroosseous tarsal tunnel may occur secondary to abnormal hindfoot alignment, most commonly hindfoot valgus, space-occupying lesions within the tarsal tunnel, such as osteophytes that may project into the tunnel, scar formation from prior trauma, talocalcaneal coalition with associated osseous excrescence (**Fig. 8**), ganglia, and variant muscle anatomy (accessory flexor digitorum, accessory soleus).[5] In a series of 67 talocalcaneal coalitions, increased T2-weighted signal involving the medial plantar nerve branch of the posterior tibial nerve was observed in 31% of cases.[48] Symptoms of tarsal tunnel syndrome include neuropathic pain and paresthesias along the plantar foot.

Imaging Findings

Space-occupying lesions within the tarsal tunnel are readily identified on MR imaging with careful attention to hindfoot alignment, the presence of low signal intensity scar tissue within the tarsal tunnel, small ganglia arising from the subtalar joint or medial compartment tendon sheaths, accessory muscles, projectional osteophytes, and talocalcaneal coalition. The tibial nerve is closely inspected for caliber change, fascicular uniformity, and signal intensity, and these changes may be more difficult to detect owing to the small nerve size at this distal level. However, it is important to remember that 40% of patients with clinical tarsal tunnel syndrome will not have imaging abnormalities.[5]

Mimics

S1 radiculopathy, posterior tibial tendon dysfunction, and plantar fasciitis may mimic compression of the posterior tibial nerve.

INFERIOR CALCANEAL (BAXTER) NEUROPATHY
Anatomy

The inferior calcaneal nerve is the first branch of the lateral plantar nerve and provides motor innervation to the abductor digiti minimi muscle. After its takeoff, the nerve courses distally between the abductor hallucis and quadratus plantae musculature then curves laterally along the inferior margin of the calcaneus.

Pathologic Conditions

Entrapment typically occurs at 2 locations—as the nerve travels between the abductor hallucis and medial margin of the quadratus plantae and more distally, where the nerve closely approximates the medial calcaneal tuberosity anteriorly. Plantar calcaneal enthesopathy, plantar fasciitis, and hyperpronation alignment of the foot can contribute to entrapment at the level of the medial calcaneal tuberosity.[49]

Imaging Findings

Isolated denervation changes within the abductor digiti minimi muscle may be observed (**Fig. 9**). Mass effect on the inferior calcaneal nerve from calcaneal enthesopathy or plantar fasciitis can be identified by MR imaging. Intrinsic nerve signal abnormalities may be challenging to assess secondary to small size of the nerve.

Mimics

Inferior calcaneal (Baxter) neuropathy may be confused with plantar fasciitis, plantar fascia tear, calcaneal stress fracture, and inflammatory enthesopathy.[50]

INTERDIGITAL NEUROPATHY (MORTON NEUROMA)
Anatomy

The distal branches of the tibial nerve and the medial and lateral plantar nerves terminally divide into the interdigital nerves at the level of the metatarsal bases. The interdigital nerves travel through a fibroosseous tunnel formed by the metatarsal heads and intermetatarsal ligament.

Pathologic Conditions

Interdigital (Morton) neuroma is not a true neuroma or neoplastic process, but rather perineural fibrosis of the common plantar digital or interdigital nerve branches that occurs secondary to interdigital nerve entrapment between the metatarsal heads plantar to the intermetatarsal ligament.[51] The second and third intermetatarsal spaces are more commonly involved than the first and fourth web spaces owing to the smaller size of the second and third web space and larger size of the third interdigital nerve, which receives

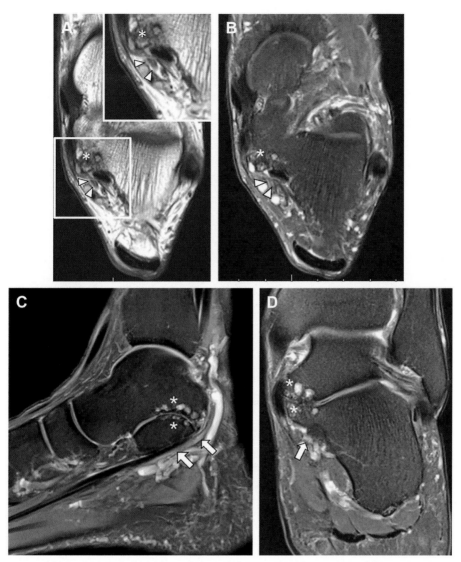

Fig. 8. A 50-year-old man presented with tarsal tunnel syndrome in the setting of fibroosseous posteromedial extraarticular talocalcaneal coalition. Axial T1-weighted (*A*), axial T2-weighted (*B*), sagittal T2-weighted (*C*), and coronal T2-weighted fat-suppressed (*D*) sequences show the osseous excrescence associated with the coalition projecting posteromedially into the tarsal tunnel (*asterisks*) with effacement of the anterior perineural fat plane surrounding the medial plantar nerve (*arrowheads*). The medial plantar nerve is thickened and T2-weighted hyperintense (*arrows*).

contributions from both the medial and lateral plantar nerves.[52] In a series of symptomatic interdigital neuromas, 58% were found in the third web space and 36% in the second web space.[52]

Imaging Findings

MR imaging demonstrates 90% sensitivity and 100% specificity for the identification of Morton neuroma.[53] Interdigital neuromas on MR imaging appear as dumbbell or tear drop–shaped T1-weighted and T2-weighted intermediate

signal intensity soft tissue centered within the fat of the interdigital web space (**Fig. 10**). Interdigital neuromas are common findings in the general population and 30% of Morton neuromas are incidental findings in asymptomatic subjects. Larger neuromas are more likely to be symptomatic, and 5 mm in transverse dimension has been suggested as a threshold.[52] Additionally, fluid within the first through third intermetatarsal bursa measuring less than 3 mm is common in asymptomatic individuals and may be physiologic.[53]

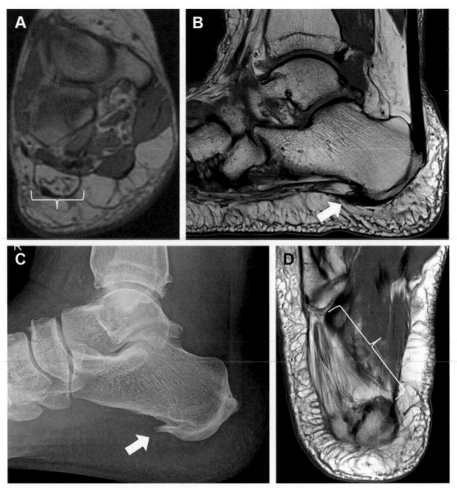

Fig. 9. A 43-year-old woman with late sequelae of Baxter neuropathy (entrapment of the inferior calcaneal nerve). Short axis proton density (*A*), sagittal proton density (*B*), lateral radiograph (*C*), and long axis proton density (*D*) sequences show moderate plantar calcaneal enthesopathy (*arrows*) and asymmetric marked fatty atrophy of the abductor digiti minimi musculature (*brackets*).

Mimics

Imaging mimics of interdigital neuropathy (Morton neuroma) include capsular scarring owing to plantar plate tear or other capsular injury, and intermetatarsal bursitis. Clinical mimics include stress fracture, Freiberg infraction, and ganglia.

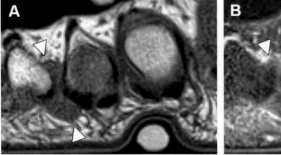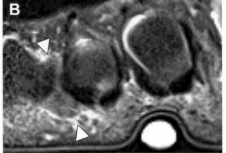

Fig. 10. A 47-year-old woman presented with plantar forefoot pain and paresthesias. Short axis T1-weighted (*A*) and T2-weighted with fat suppression (*B*) images show a bilobed T1-weighted and T2-weighted intermediate signal intensity nodule within the third web space reflective of interdigital (Morton) neuroma (*arrowheads*).

SUMMARY

Entrapment mononeuropathies of the lower extremity are common and present a significant societal disease burden. The clinical presentation, particularly of lower extremity neuropathies as compared with upper extremity neuropathies, can be mixed and, even with the aid of electrodiagnostic testing, diagnosis is challenging. MR neurography is a high-resolution, noninvasive, and operator-independent imaging modality that has proven useful in diagnosis, disease severity assessment, and informing treatment decisions in the management of lower extremity entrapment neuropathies. It is imperative for radiologists to be familiar with the complex peripheral nerve anatomy, common sites of anatomic compression, and common pathologic conditions resulting in various peripheral nerve entrapment neuropathies. Current assessment relies heavily on morphologic nerve changes; however, emerging innovative MR imaging sequences and PET/MR imaging hold the potential to supplement morphologic analysis with a noninvasive means of functional assessment.

REFERENCES

1. Lee AC, Drake DB, DeGeorge BR Jr. Medical student and primary care physician perception of the surgical management of upper- and lower-extremity peripheral nerve entrapment. Ann Plast Surg 2016;76:524–31.
2. Atroshi I, Gummesson C, Johnsson R, et al. Prevalence of carpal tunnel syndrome in a general population. JAMA 1999;282:153–8.
3. Mold JW, Vesely SK, Keyl BA, et al. The prevalence, predictors, and consequences of peripheral sensory neuropathy in older patients. J Am Board Fam Pract 2004;17:309–18.
4. Chhabra A, Madhuranthakam AJ, Andreisek G. Magnetic resonance neurography: current perspectives and literature review. Eur Radiol 2018;28:698–707.
5. Donovan A, Rosenberg ZS, Cavalcanti CF. MR imaging of entrapment neuropathies of the lower extremity. Part 2. The knee, leg, ankle, and foot. Radiographics 2010;30:1001–19.
6. Walter WR, Burke CJ, Adler RS. Ultrasound-guided therapeutic injections for neural pathology about the foot and ankle: a 4 year retrospective review. Skeletal Radiol 2017;46:795–803.
7. Kao DS, Cheng J. Peripheral neuropathy: surgical approaches simplified for the imagers. Semin Musculoskelet Radiol 2015;19:121–9.
8. Flanigan RM, DiGiovanni BF. Peripheral nerve entrapments of the lower leg, ankle, and foot. Foot Ankle Clin 2011;16:255–74.
9. Jeon T, Fung MM, Koch KM, et al. Peripheral nerve diffusion tensor imaging: overview, pitfalls, and future directions J. Magn Reson Imaging 2018;47(5):1171–89.
10. Carpenter EL, Bencardino JT. Focus on advanced magnetic resonance techniques in clinical practice: magnetic resonance neurography. Radiol Clin North Am 2015;53:513–29.
11. Kim SJ, Hong SH, Jun WS, et al. MR imaging mapping of skeletal muscle denervation in entrapment and compressive neuropathies. Radiographics 2011;31:319–32.
12. Kastel T, Heiland S, Baumer P, et al. Magic angle effect: a relevant artifact in MR neurography at 3T? AJNR Am J Neuroradiol 2011;32:821–7.
13. Subhawong TK, Wang KC, Thawait SK, et al. High resolution imaging of tunnels by magnetic resonance neurography. Skeletal Radiol 2012;41:15–31.
14. Shen B, Behera D, James ML, et al. Visualizing nerve injury in a neuropathic pain model with [(18)F]FTC-146 PET/MRI. Theranostics 2017;7:2794–805.
15. Martinoli C, Miguel-Perez M, Padua L, et al. Imaging of neuropathies about the hip. Eur J Radiol 2013;82:17–26.
16. Carro LP, Hernando MF, Cerezal L, et al. Deep gluteal space problems: piriformis syndrome, ischiofemoral impingement and sciatic nerve release. Muscles Ligaments Tendons J 2016;6:384–96.
17. Filler AG, Haynes J, Jordan SE, et al. Sciatica of non-disc origin and piriformis syndrome: diagnosis by magnetic resonance neurography and interventional magnetic resonance imaging with outcome study of resulting treatment. J Neurosurg Spine 2005;2:99–115.
18. Martin HD, Shears SA, Johnson JC, et al. The endoscopic treatment of sciatic nerve entrapment/deep gluteal syndrome. Arthroscopy 2011;27:172–81.
19. Wilson TJ, Spinner RJ, Mohan R, et al. Sciatic nerve injury after proximal hamstring avulsion and repair. Orthop J Sports Med 2017;5. 2325967117713685.
20. Soldatos T, Andreisek G, Thawait GK, et al. High-resolution 3-T MR neurography of the lumbosacral plexus. Radiographics 2013;33:967–87.
21. Wadhwa V, Hamid AS, Kumar Y, et al. Pudendal nerve and branch neuropathy: magnetic resonance neurography evaluation. Acta Radiol 2017;58:726–33.
22. Prologo JD, Lin RC, Williams R, et al. Percutaneous CT-guided cryoablation for the treatment of refractory pudendal neuralgia. Skeletal Radiol 2015;44:709–14.
23. Fritz J, Chhabra A, Wang KC, et al. Magnetic resonance neurography-guided nerve blocks for the diagnosis and treatment of chronic pelvic pain syndrome. Neuroimaging Clin N Am 2014;24:211–34.

24. Ramanathan A, Bryant S, Montoya TI, et al. Obturator neuropathy after retropubic tension-free vaginal tape placement. Obstet Gynecol 2015;125: 62–4.

25. Weng WC, Wei YC, Huang WY, et al. Risk factor analysis for meralgia paresthetica: a hospital-based study in Taiwan. J Clin Neurosci 2017;43: 192–5.

26. Lee SH, Shin KJ, Gil YC, et al. Anatomy of the lateral femoral cutaneous nerve relevant to clinical findings in meralgia paresthetica. Muscle Nerve 2017;55: 646–50.

27. Parisi TJ, Mandrekar J, Dyck PJ, et al. Meralgia paresthetica: relation to obesity, advanced age, and diabetes mellitus. Neurology 2011;77:1538–42.

28. Onat SS, Ata AM, Ozcakar L. Ultrasound-guided diagnosis and treatment of meralgia paresthetica. Pain Physician 2016;19:E667–9.

29. Cheatham SW, Kolber MJ, Salamh PA. Meralgia paresthetica: a review of the literature. Int J Sports Phys Ther 2013;8:883–93.

30. Chhabra A, Faridian-Aragh N. High-resolution 3-T MR neurography of femoral neuropathy. AJR Am J Roentgenol 2012;198:3–10.

31. Bohrer JC, Walters MD, Park A, et al. Pelvic nerve injury following gynecologic surgery: a prospective cohort study. Am J Obstet Gynecol 2009;201:531. e1-7.

32. Petchprapa CN, Rosenberg ZS, Sconfienza LM, et al. MR imaging of entrapment neuropathies of the lower extremity. Part 1. The pelvis and hip. Radiographics 2010;30:983–1000.

33. Busis NA. Femoral and obturator neuropathies. Neurol Clin 1999;17:633–53, vii.

34. Cho D, Saetia K, Lee S, et al. Peroneal nerve injury associated with sports-related knee injury. Neurosurg Focus 2011;31:E11.

35. Vieira RL, Rosenberg ZS, Kiprovski K. MRI of the distal biceps femoris muscle: normal anatomy, variants, and association with common peroneal entrapment neuropathy. AJR Am J Roentgenol 2007;189: 549–55.

36. Kim S, Choi JY, Huh YM, et al. Role of magnetic resonance imaging in entrapment and compressive neuropathy - what, where, and how to see the peripheral nerves on the musculoskeletal magnetic resonance image: part 1. Overview and lower extremity. Eur Radiol 2007;17:139–49.

37. Spinner RJ, Atkinson JL, Scheithauer BW, et al. Peroneal intraneural ganglia: the importance of the articular branch. Clinical series. J Neurosurg 2003; 99:319–29.

38. Young NP, Sorenson EJ, Spinner RJ, et al. Clinical and electrodiagnostic correlates of peroneal intraneural ganglia. Neurology 2009;72:447–52.

39. Loredo R, Hodler J, Pedowitz R, et al. MRI of the common peroneal nerve: normal anatomy and evaluation of masses associated with nerve entrapment. J Comput Assist Tomogr 1998;22:925–31.

40. Arnold WD, Elsheikh BH. Entrapment neuropathies. Neurol Clin 2013;31:405–24.

41. Paraskevas G, Tzika M, Natsis K. Entrapment of the superficial peroneal nerve: an anatomical insight. J Am Podiatr Med Assoc 2015;105:150–9.

42. Bregman PJ, Schuenke M. Current diagnosis and treatment of superficial fibular nerve injuries and entrapment. Clin Podiatr Med Surg 2016;33:243–54.

43. Kennedy JG, Baxter DE. Nerve disorders in dancers. Clin Sports Med 2008;27:329–34.

44. Stamatis ED, Manidakis NE, Patouras PP. Intraneural ganglion of the superficial peroneal nerve: a case report. J Foot Ankle Surg 2010;49:400.e1-4.

45. Ferkel E, Davis WH, Ellington JK. Entrapment neuropathies of the foot and ankle. Clin Sports Med 2015;34:791–801.

46. Beltran LS, Bencardino J, Ghazikhanian V, et al. Entrapment neuropathies III: lower limb. Semin Musculoskelet Radiol 2010;14:501–11.

47. Sillat T, Pivec C, Bernathova M, et al. Unusual cause of anterior tarsal tunnel syndrome: ultrasound findings. J Ultrasound Med 2017;36:837–9.

48. Alaia EF, Rosenberg ZS, Bencardino JT, et al. Tarsal tunnel disease and talocalcaneal coalition: MRI features. Skeletal Radiol 2016;45:1507–14.

49. Chundru U, Liebeskind A, Seidelmann F, et al. Plantar fasciitis and calcaneal spur formation are associated with abductor digiti minimi atrophy on MRI of the foot. Skeletal Radiol 2008;37:505–10.

50. Rosenbaum AJ, DiPreta JA, Misener D. Plantar heel pain. Med Clin North Am 2014;98:339–52.

51. Hochman MG, Zilberfarb JL. Nerves in a pinch: imaging of nerve compression syndromes. Radiol Clin North Am 2004;42:221–45.

52. Bencardino J, Rosenberg ZS, Beltran J, et al. Morton's neuroma: is it always symptomatic? AJR Am J Roentgenol 2000;175:649–53.

53. Zanetti M, Strehle JK, Zollinger H, et al. Morton neuroma and fluid in the intermetatarsal bursae on MR images of 70 asymptomatic volunteers. Radiology 1997;203:516–20.

Extreme Sports Injuries to the Pelvis and Lower Extremity

Preeti Arun Sukerkar, MD, PhD, Angela M. Fast, MD,
Geoffrey Riley, MD*

KEYWORDS

- Extreme sports • Injuries • Pelvis • Lower extremity

KEY POINTS

- Participation in extreme sports has increased over the past few decades.
- Many of these sports are associated with relatively high frequency of specific injury types.
- Imaging, particularly MR imaging and ultrasound, play key roles in evaluating these injuries and guiding clinical management.
- Specific imaging protocols should be used when evaluating for certain types of injuries, such as nerve pathologies and athletic pubalgia, because findings may be subtle.

INTRODUCTION

Extreme sports have been growing in popularity over the past few decades. These activities expose athletes to greater injury risks than traditional sports. They often take place in harsh environments at great speeds and/or heights and may require specialized equipment.[1] Given the risk of serious injuries or fatality, there is growing interest in specialized medical care for these extreme athletes. As with any injury, imaging plays a key role in the management of these patients. Here the authors describe pelvic and lower extremity injuries associated with various extreme sports.

GENERAL IMAGING STRATEGIES AND INJURIES

Extreme sports often take place in isolated environments with little access to advanced health care, requiring transfer to larger medical centers. In these conditions, assessment is limited to a physical examination and few modalities, such as plain radiography and ultrasound. However, advanced imaging like MR imaging or computed tomography (CT) is usually required given the relatively low sensitivity of plain radiography or ultrasound. In this section, the authors describe the imaging findings of general pelvic and lower extremity injuries that are frequently seen in sporting activities. When applicable, classification or grading schemes are described. Sport-specific injuries are discussed later in this review.

STRESS INJURIES

Stress injuries are overuse injuries that result from imbalance between osteoclastic and osteoblastic activity and may occur after recent changes in training regimens. Radiography has relatively low sensitivity (15%–35%) for detecting acute stress fractures on initial imaging. At follow-up, this increases up to 30% to 70% because of the more extensive bone reaction.[2] Findings in cortical bone include endosteal/periosteal callus formation, circumferential periosteal reaction with

Disclosures: The authors have no conflicts to disclose.
Department of Radiology, Stanford University, 300 Pasteur Drive, Stanford, CA 94305, USA
* Corresponding author.
E-mail address: griley@stanford.edu

Radiol Clin N Am 56 (2018) 1013–1033
https://doi.org/10.1016/j.rcl.2018.06.013

fracture line through one cortex, or frank fracture.[2] In cancellous bone, findings include flakelike patches of new bone formation, cloudlike mineralized bone, or focal linear sclerosis perpendicular to the trabeculae.[2]

Triple-phase technetium-99m biphosphate bone scintigraphy was previously used for its higher sensitivity compared with plain radiography.[2] However, MR imaging has essentially replaced bone scans with higher specificity and sensitivity.[2] MR imaging also provides more information about injury location and severity with better correlation to clinical severity.[3]

MR imaging demonstrates excellent sensitivity of 100% and specificity of 85% for detecting stress fractures. Findings include periosteal or bone marrow edema (high signal on T2-weighted and short tau inversion recovery [STIR] sequences). MR imaging also demonstrates these changes very early before the progression to a frank cortical fracture according to the Fredericson classification system (**Figs. 1–4**, **Table 1**).[4,5] Although this system was developed for tibial injuries, the findings are similar for stress injuries elsewhere.

The Fredericson classification helps determine clinical management. MR imaging findings correlate with both injury severity and time to return to activity, therefore, helping guide rehabilitation plans, as more severe injuries require longer rest times.[5] Additionally, MR imaging differentiates stress reaction from stress fracture, which shows a frank fracture line and/or cortical disruption, and can be used to monitor injuries over time during rehabilitation. Although stress reactions generally respond well to rest and occasional casting, stress fractures sometimes require surgical treatment if they do not heal or if they progress with more conservative measures.

MUSCLE, LIGAMENT, AND TENDON INJURY

The most common type of muscle injury in adults from sporting activity is muscle strain. These injuries generally involve the myotendinous junction and can extend to the epimysium.[6] Strains are classified into 3 clinical grades (**Table 2**). The imaging hallmark is edema and possibly hemorrhage at the site of tearing near the myotendinous junction. In some cases, there is edema at the muscle periphery along the epimysium. Severe strains show hematomas and torn/interrupted muscle fibers. Muscle belly tears are less common but can occur. Muscle injuries can also be due to overuse and are classified as fatigue-induced disorders or delayed-onset muscle soreness. Other muscle injuries include direct injuries such as lacerations and contusions. There are multiple classification schemes for imaging findings in muscles injuries (**Tables 3 and 4**).[6]

Ligamentous injuries in the lower extremity involve the knee, ankle, and foot. These injuries are directly visualized on MR imaging and ultrasound. Severity can range from minor sprains to severe sprains/partial tears to complete rupture. Tendon injuries are also directly visualized on ultrasound and MR imaging. Ultrasound offers the advantage of dynamic imaging. Chronic injuries appear as tendon thickening on ultrasound and MR imaging with intermediate signal on MR imaging. Tenosynovitis can also be easily visualized as increased fluid surrounding the tendon. Imaging

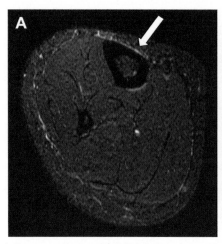
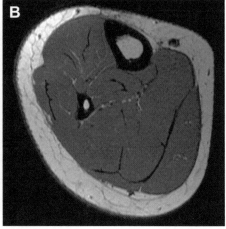

Fig. 1. Fredericson grade 1 medial tibial stress injury. Axial T2 fat-suppressed (*A*) and T1 (*B*) images demonstrate mild periosteal edema (*arrow*) on T2 imaging without underlying edema or T1 correlate.

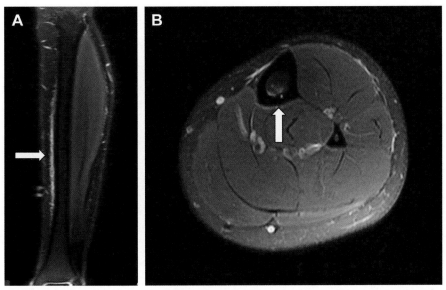

Fig. 2. Fredericson grade 2 medial tibial stress injury. Coronal T2 fat-suppressed (FS) image (*A*) demonstrates periosteal edema (*arrow*) and axial T2 FS (*B*) images demonstrates mild bone marrow edema (*arrow*), which did not have a T1 correlate.

evaluation of these injuries plays a key role in determining clinical management. For example, complete pectoralis major tendon tears and myotendinous junction tears generally require surgery, whereas partial tears and muscle belly tears may be treated conservatively. Discerning between complete and partial tears is best performed via imaging.

NERVE INJURIES

Although neuropathies can be chronic or acute, sports-related nerve injuries are more often chronic because of stretching or compression from positioning, muscle hypertrophy, or adjacent soft tissue injury.[7] These injuries are best diagnosed clinically and/or by electromyography

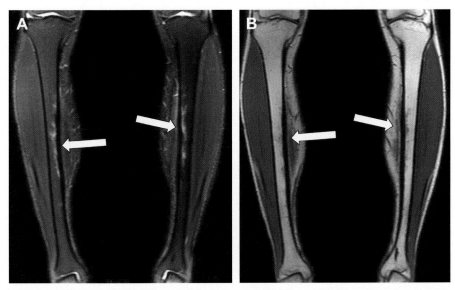

Fig. 3. Fredericson grade 3 medial tibial stress injury. Coronal T2 (*A*) and T1 (*B*) images demonstrate ill-defined bone marrow edema within the medial aspect of the bilateral tibial diaphysis with associated periosteal edema and T1 hypointensity (*arrows*). No discrete fracture is identified.

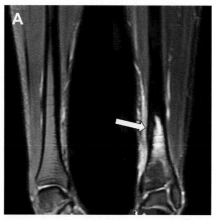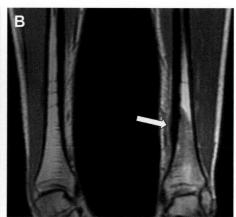

Fig. 4. Fredericson grade 4a medial tibial stress injury. Coronal T2 (*A*) and T1 (*B*) images demonstrate bone marrow edema on both T1 and T2 images with multiple focal areas of intracortical signal abnormality (*arrows*). No discrete fracture is identified.[8]

(EMG). However, imaging can be useful to diagnose subclinical injuries, grade and assess the extent of injuries, evaluate damage to surrounding structures, and determine clinical management. Magnetic resonance neurography (MRN) and ultrasound are the two most commonly used imaging methods for assessing peripheral nerves.[8]

The main sequences used in MRN include non–fat-suppressed T1-weighted images to evaluate nerve caliber/course and for perineural fibrosis, and fluid-sensitive fat-suppressed T2-weighted images to assess the fascicular morphology and signal. Three-dimensional (3D) imaging is useful for multiplanar reformats and maximum intensity projections. For example, at the authors' institution neurography studies include 3D dual-echo

steady-state sequences (**Table 5**). Contrast can be administered to evaluate for mass lesions. Finally, diffusion-weighted imaging or diffusion-tensor imaging can be used to suppress vascular signal and improve the signal-to-noise ratio of nerves.

Indirect and direct signs of nerve injury are assessed by imaging. Indirect imaging findings are related to denervation. There are 3 main patterns of denervation, although these can occur simultaneously (**Table 6**). In the acute/early subacute phase (<1 month), there will initially be no magnetic resonance (MR) abnormality, followed by edema starting within approximately 1 week (increased signal in the affected muscle on fat suppressed T2-weighted and STIR images). There may also be paradoxic muscle hypertrophy.[9] The late subacute phase (1–6 months) demonstrates edema early on and progressive muscle atrophy, which is reversible and appears on all sequences as decreased muscle bulk. The chronic phase (>6 months) shows atrophy and extensive fatty infiltration, which appears as replacement of much of muscle fibers with fat.[9] This injury is

---

Table 1
Fredericson grading scheme for tibial stress injuries

Grade	MRI Findings
0	No abnormality
1	Periosteal edema
2	Grade 1 with additional bone marrow edema on T2-weighted images
3	Grade 2 with bone marrow edema also visible on T1-weighted images
4a	Grade 3 with multiple additional intracortical foci of signal abnormality
4b	Grade 3 with linear fracture

Data from Kijowski R, Choi J, Shinki K, et al. Validation of MRI classification system for tibial stress injuries. AJR Am J Roentgenol 2012;198:878–84.

Table 2
Clinical grading of muscle injury

Grade	Clinical Findings
1	Pain only
2	Pain and weakness
3	Pain, weakness, and loss of function

Data from Guermazi A, Roemer FW, Robinson P, et al. Imaging of muscle injuries in sports medicine: sports imaging series. Radiology 2017;282(3):646–63.

Table 3
Overview of imaging classification of muscle injury

Grading System	Modality	Imaging Findings for Grade
British Athletics Muscle Injury Classification	MR or US	Grade 0: No abnormality OR patchy high signal Grade 1: Small muscle tear with high signal intensity <10% extension/involvement of muscle and measuring <5 cm Grade 2: Moderate muscle tear with high signal intensity involving 10%–50% of muscle, measuring >5 and <15 cm, and <5 cm fiber disruption Grade 3: Extensive muscle tear with high signal intensity involving >50% of muscle, measuring >15 cm, and >5 cm fiber disruption without discontinuity Grade 4: Complete tear/discontinuity of the muscle or tendon
Chan et al,[82] 2018	MR or US	Grade 1: Strain; ≤5% fiber disruption and edema Grade 2: Partial tear; >5% fiber disruption, edema, and hemorrhage Grade 3: Complete tear; complete disruption of muscle fibers with retraction and hemorrhage
Modified Peetrons	MR only	Grade 0: No abnormality Grade 1: Edema only; no evidence of tear or architectural distortion Grade 2: Partial muscle tear indicated by architectural disruption Grade 3: Complete/total muscle or tendon rupture
Peetrons	US only	Grade 1: No abnormality OR focal/diffuse hemorrhage with <5% fiber disruption Grade 2: Partial rupture with >5% fiber disruption with or without fascial injury Grade 3: Complete muscle rupture with retraction of fibers

Abbreviations: MR, magnetic resonance; US, ultrasound.
Adapted from Guermazi A, Roemer FW, Robinson P, et al. Imaging of muscle injuries in sports medicine: sports imaging series. Radiology 2017;282(3):646–63. © Radiological Society of North America.

irreversible, indicating long-term denervation, and is best seen on non–fat-suppressed T1-weight imaging.[7,10,11] Similar denervation findings are seen on CT and ultrasound.

Direct imaging via MRN and ultrasound is useful to evaluate the nerve injury severity. Nerve injury classification was initially divided into neurapraxia, axonotmesis, and neurotmesis

---

Table 4
Munich consensus statement on clinical and imaging grading of muscle injury

Grade	Clinical Findings and/or Severity	Imaging Findings
Grade 1A	Fatigue-induced muscle disorder	No abnormality
Grade 1B	Delayed-onset muscle soreness	No abnormality OR edema only
Grade 2A	Spine-related neuromuscular disorder	No abnormality OR edema only
Grade 2B	Muscle-related neuromuscular disorder	No abnormality OR edema only
Grade 3A	Minor partial muscle tear	Fiber disruption and hemorrhage
Grade 3B	Moderate partial muscle tear	Significant fiber disruption with some retraction, fascial injury, and hemorrhage
Grade 4	Subtotal or total muscle tear and/or tendinous avulsion	Subtotal or complete discontinuity of the muscle or tendon with fascial injury and hemorrhage; with or without wavy tendon morphology and retraction
Contusion	Direct injury	Diffuse or focal hemorrhage/hematoma

Data from Guermazi A, Roemer FW, Robinson P, et al. Imaging of muscle injuries in sports medicine: sports imaging series. Radiology 2017;282(3):646–63.

Table 5
Generalized neurogram protocol (3T scanner is optimal)

Sequence	Details and Caveats
Axial T1 Axial T2 fat saturated Axial STIR	It is possible do multiple stations for axial sequences for a smaller FOV; the workhorse of the neurogram protocol is the axial series. If use of contrast is desired, include axial fat-saturated precontrast and axial T1 fat-saturated with contrast.
Sagittal STIR Coronal STIR	Large FOV sequences are optional and generally used for further evaluation. It is not standard to acquire postcontrast imaging in these planes.
Axial DESS	This sequence is an optional sequence that is only used with 3T scanners.

Abbreviations: DESS, double echo steady state; FOV, field of view.

(grades I–III) by Seddon and colleagues[12] and later expanded to grades I to V by Sunderland.[7,12–14] The characteristics of these grades and their expected imaging correlates are summarized in **Table 7**.[7,14,15] This information provides guidelines for radiology reports commenting on the neuropathy severity and should be supplemented with any denervation findings to suggest the relative chronicity of the injury. Extrinsic lesions, such as hematomas or masses, should be reported.

Table 6
Denervation phases on MR imaging

Phase	MR Finding
Acute phase	No MR abnormality
Early subacute (phase 1)	Edema within the muscle with or without paradoxic hypertrophy
Late subacute (phase 2)	Edema within the muscle with progressive muscle atrophy
Chronic phase (phase 3)	Muscle atrophy and extensive fatty infiltration without edema

Abbreviation: MR, magnetic resonance.
Adapted from Kamath S, Venkatanarasimha N, Walsh MA, et al. MRI appearance of muscle denervation. Skeletal Radiol 2008;37:397–404; with permission.

Extreme Sports–Specific Injuries

Climbing

This section focuses on injuries related to indoor and outdoor rock climbing and bouldering, deep water soloing, ice climbing, and canyoneering. Literature describing the incidence of upper versus lower extremity injuries in climbing sports is inconsistent. Most studies show most climbing injuries are from overuse and occur in the upper limbs, particularly finger injuries.[16–18] Some studies found lower extremity injuries were more frequent than or of similar incidence to upper extremity injuries.[19–21] It is likely that chronic injuries are more frequent in upper extremities, whereas acute injuries are more common in lower extremities.[19,20] Lower extremity injuries often result from falls, usually involving the foot/ankle followed by the knee.[21] In one study of 515,337 visits to an indoor wall over 5 years, 30 injuries were recorded.[21] Twelve were in the lower extremity and 6 were in the upper extremity, with the remainder of the injuries occurring in the trunk or head and neck. Most lower extremity injuries were fractures, sprains, or dislocations. Another study of 40,282 emergency department visits for rock-climbing injuries between 1990 and 2007 showed that the lower extremities were the most frequently injured body part (46.3% of all injuries, with ankle injuries alone accounting for 19.2% of those).[22] The most common injuries in this study were fractures, sprains, or strains; most were related to falls.[22]

Another study of 699 injuries between 2002 and 2006 demonstrated a similar incidence of upper and lower extremity injuries.[23] Ligament injury, contusions, and tendon injuries were most common. Ligament and tendon injuries were more frequent in the fingers, whereas contusions were more common in the feet. Fractures were also relatively common, with almost 50% occurring in the feet. Similarly, a study of climbing accidents in Yosemite showed that the most common injuries were to the skin followed by the lower extremities, predominantly ankle fractures.[24]

Typical rock climbing foot and ankle injuries include contusions, fractures of the ankle bones, and lateral ankle ligament sprains.[19] This foot/ankle predominance is likely related to smaller-sized, tighter climbing shoes relative to normal footwear increasing the chance of foot injury during falls or collision with the wall.[19,25] Rare case reports of acute peroneal tendon dislocation have also occurred because of failure of the superior peroneal retinaculum during foot plantar flexion with maximum inversion and high tension onto the big toe.[26]

Table 7
Nerve injury imaging characteristics (Seddon-Sunderland classification)

Grade	Classification	Cause/Pathology	EMG Findings	Imaging Findings on MR
I	Neurapraxia	Nerve compression injury; local myelin injury with axon intact and functional	Normal to decreased recruitment	No abnormality OR increased T2 signal within the nerve; no muscular abnormality
II	Axonotmesis	Nerve crush injury; axon and myelin disruption with intact neuronal connective tissue	Absent nerve conduction distal to lesion and decreased amplitude and recruitment immediately	Increased T2 signal and diffusely enlarged nerve; no muscular abnormality
III	Axonotmesis	Nerve crush injury; axon, myelin, and endoneurium disruption		Increased T2 signal, fascicular enlargement or effacement secondary to edema, and muscular denervation
IV	Axonotmesis	Nerve crush injury; axon, myelin, endoneurium, and perineurium disruption		Focal nerve enlargement with heterogeneous T2 signal, muscular denervation, underlying diffuse abnormality with or without fascicular disruption
V	Neurotmesis	Nerve transection injury; axon, myelin, endoneurium, perineurium, and epineurium injury	Same as axonotmesis	Complete nerve disruption with or without hemorrhage and fibrosis in the nerve gap, epineural thickening, and muscular denervation

Data from Mitchell CH, Brushart TM, Ahlawat S, et al. MRI of sports-related peripheral nerve injuries. AJR Am J Roentgenol 2014;203:1075–84.

One recent study described a bouldering-specific lower leg injury-causing technique called the heel hook, in which the heel is used to apply pressure onto the hold, while pulling on the foot by flexing the hamstrings. The knee is also rotated outwardly, applying a high force onto the back and lateral structures of the knee and leg. In a study of 17 patients who complained of injury after performing a heel hook, all had sudden dorsal pain in the pelvis, thigh, or knee.[27] Given the outward rotation of the knee, most knee injuries were along the lateral and posterior stabilizers, including the lateral collateral ligament, iliotibial band, dorsal joint capsule, popliteus, and biceps femoris (**Fig. 5**). Most pelvic injuries resulted in complete or partial tendon avulsions. MR imaging was deemed more effective than ultrasound for evaluating these injuries given its ability to evaluate cruciate ligament injury and pelvic injury.[27]

There are few studies of injuries specifically related to ice climbing. In one retrospective study of 88 ice climbers, most acute injuries were open wounds and hematomas. Overuse injuries generally involved the upper extremity, although some reported calf strain injuries.[23,28] In another study during the Ice Climbing Festival held during the 2014 Olympics, the most common injuries were penetrating and superficial soft tissue injuries at the anteromedial aspect of the thigh and knee.[29]

Climbing-related chronic injuries in the pelvis and lower extremities are less well-studied than those of the upper extremities. However, the tight fit of the climbing shoe and the foot in malposition within the shoe can lead to chronic problems.[21] In a study of chronic foot and ankle injury in 144 climbers, the most common injury was nail disease (65.3% of patients), followed by recurrent ankle sprains (27.8%), retrocalcaneal bursitis (19.4%), Achilles tendinitis (12.5%), metatarsalgia (12.5%), and plantar fasciitis (5.6%).[30] Foot deformity has also been seen with a relatively high incidence of hallux valgus and increasing frequency of hallux rigidus (**Fig. 6**).[19,25]

Skiing and snowboarding

Lower extremity injuries are more common than upper extremity injuries in skiing. Previously, fractures were common due twisting forces transferred from the ski to the lower leg, but below-the-knee fractures have decreased in incidence with

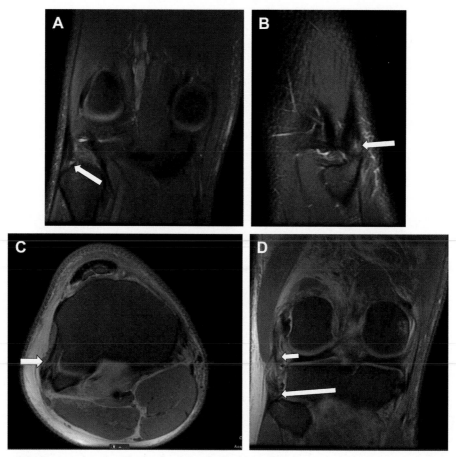

Fig. 5. Knee injuries associated with the heel hook climbing technique. Coronal (*A*) and sagittal (*B*) T2 fat-suppressed (FS) images demonstrate increased signal in the distal biceps femoris tendon at the insertion on the proximal fibula, compatible with partial avulsion of the biceps femoris (*arrows*). Axial (*C*) and coronal (*D*) T2 FS images demonstrate complete disruption of the lateral collateral ligament with proximal retraction (*C, D; short arrows*) and partial avulsion of the biceps femoris tendon at the insertion on the proximal fibula (*D; long arrow*).

modern ski boots and release bindings.[1,6,31] However, ligamentous injuries have risen in incidence.[6] Skiing injuries most frequently involve soft tissue and ligamentous injuries of the knee (one-third of all skiing injuries) (**Fig. 7**).[32] The most common knee injuries are medial collateral ligament (MCL) sprain and complete anterior cruciate ligament (ACL) rupture.[1,6,33] MCL injury from valgus force and/or external rotation comprises 15% to 20% of skiing injuries.[34] ACL injury in skiers occurs from mechanisms such as the anterior drawer mechanism from off-balance landing, flexion-internal rotation/phantom foot in which the skier's weight is positioned over the back of the skis and the tail of the ski catches on snow causing sudden internal rotation, and the valgus-external rotation/forward twisting fall.[16,35] Lateral collateral ligament injuries are usually associated with other ligament injuries and are uncommon in isolation, accounting

for only 4% of knee injuries in skiing.[34] Injury to the posterior cruciate ligament constitutes less than 1% of all skiing-related knee injuries and most commonly results from collisions.[34] Isolated meniscal tears are rare and more commonly occur with ACL tears.

Although below-the-knee fracture incidence has decreased, some studies show that lower leg fractures remain the next most common injury after soft tissue and ligamentous injury.[36] A recent study of skiers and snowboarders in Finland found that spiral tibial shaft fractures are the most common skiing-associated lower extremity fractures, although there is a relatively high incidence of tibial plateau injuries in adult skiers.[37] The incidence of skiing-associated tibial plateau fractures has in fact increased over the years.[6] These fractures result from varus or valgus stress in combination with axial loading.[38]

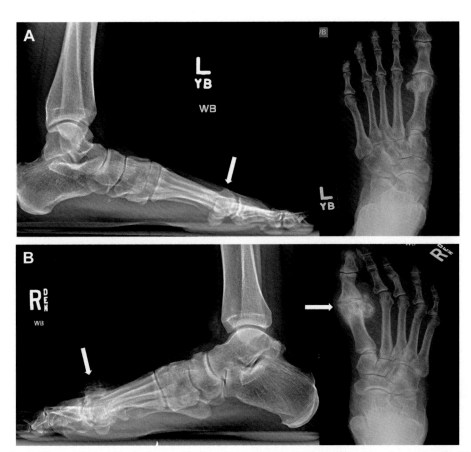

Fig. 6. Early and late radiographic findings of hallux rigidus. (*A*) Lateral and frontal radiographs of a 35-year-old woman demonstrate early hallux rigidus with dorsal projecting osteophytosis (*arrow*) and mild joint space narrowing. (*B*) Lateral and frontal radiographs in a 55-year-old man demonstrate late-stage hallux rigidus with bone-on-bone formation and extensive osteophyte formation most pronounced dorsolateral (*arrows*).

Skiing is associated with peroneal tendon dislocation when the strength of the peroneal retinaculum is exceeded during resistance to dorsiflexion or inversion stress. Peroneal tendon dislocation comprises 0.5% of all skiing injuries, whereas superior retinaculum sprain makes up about 2.5% of skiing injuries.[39] These injuries are often misdiagnosed in the acute phase as ankle

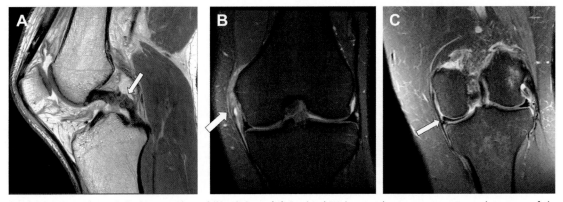

Fig. 7. Common knee injuries seen in a skiing injury. (*A*) Sagittal T1 image demonstrates a complete tear of the posterior cruciate ligament (*arrow*). (*B*) Coronal T2 fat-suppressed (FS) image demonstrates a near-complete tear of the medial collateral ligament with high T2 signal seen both superficially and deep to the ligament (*arrow*). (*C*) Coronal PD FS image shows an oblique tear through the body of the medial meniscus (*arrow*).

sprains and can lead to chronic disability.[40] Imaging with ultrasound or MR imaging can confirm the diagnosis (**Fig. 8**).

The injury rate is 2 times higher in snowboarders than skiers with different injury patterns.[1,16,41] Lower extremity injuries are overall less common with snowboarding than skiing, although ankle injuries occur slightly more frequently in snowboarding because of the softer boots.[32,33,42] Most injuries are caused by collisions and falls.[16,33] In one study of 7793 snowboarding injuries with 961 involving the lower extremity, laceration/contusion due to collision was the most common injury. Most injuries involved the leading extremity. The most common fracture site was the ankle.[43] Other studies have shown that ankle injuries make up about 15% to 20% of snowboarding injuries with half involving fractures.[44,45]

The snowboarder's fracture involving the lateral process of the talus is relatively unique to the sport (**Figs. 9** and **10**).[16] The likely mechanism is compression and forced inversion and

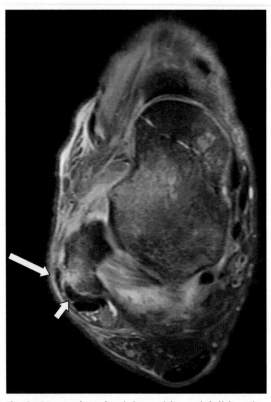

Fig. 8. Peroneal tendon injury with partial dislocation in a ski injury. Axial PD fat-suppressed image demonstrates a longitudinal split tear of the peroneal brevis (*short arrow*). The peroneal retinaculum is disrupted, and there is lateral dislocation of the lateral component of the split tear (*long arrow*).

dorsiflexion when landing from a jump.[16,33,46] This injury can lead to disability and osteoarthritis if anatomic alignment is not maintained. The fracture is often missed on radiograph (40%–50% of cases) and misdiagnosed as an ankle sprain.[47] CT or MR imaging are recommended for snowboarders presenting with ankle injury after falling from a jump. These injuries can be graded and treated according to the Hawkins Criteria scale (**Table 8**).[47,48]

Pelvic/hip injuries account for about 20% of snowboarding injuries and include hip chondrolabral injuries. Although hip dislocations are overall rare in snowboarding, they are 5 times more common in snowboarders than in skiers, likely because of differences in stance and aerial maneuvers between snowboarders and skiers.[49] Posterior dislocations are more common in snowboarders, whereas anterior dislocations occur more frequently in skiers. The rate of dislocation with concurrent femoral head fracture is higher in snowboarders than skiers.[49] Pelvic fractures are not common, comprising only 2% of snowboarding injuries.[35]

Knee injuries are less common in snowboarding than in skiing, comprising only 6% of injuries, likely due to the nonreleasable binding system preventing valgus stress.[45] When ACL tears occur, they are usually due to improper landings from a large jump. This injury may result from eccentric quadriceps contraction while landing on flat terrain with a flexed knee.[44] ACL injury may also occur during falls when only one foot is attached to the board, for example, when loading and unloading from the chairlifts.[16]

Chronic skiing and snowboarding injuries of the lower extremity also occur, although these are less well studied. For example, malleolar bursitis can result because of friction from stiff boots, appearing as focal T2-hyperintense and T1-hypointense fluid collections next to a bony prominence with occasional adjacent bone marrow or soft tissue edema. Ankle pseudotumor can occur with compression of the soft tissues between the lateral malleolus and the boot.[35,45,50] These injuries appear as subcutaneous poorly defined supramalleolar masses, generally with high T2 and low T1 signal and enhancement with contrast. They may be associated with more proximal fibular stress reaction or peroneal hypertrophy.[35,50] Skiers have also developed peripheral neuropathies, including femoral neuropathy from repetitive hip flexion and extension and deep peroneal neuropathy from poorly fitting footwear.[7] Although these are generally diagnosed clinically, MR neurography may play a role in determining management.

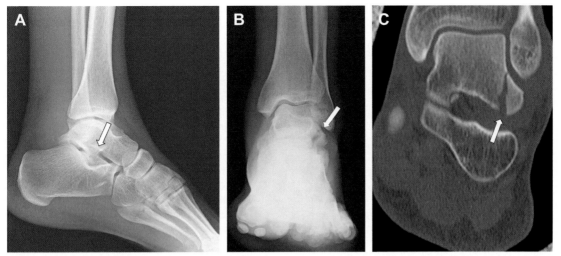

Fig. 9. Snowboarder's fracture of the ankle. Lateral (*A*) and frontal (*B*) views of the left ankle show a comminuted intra-articular fracture through the lateral process of the talus (*arrows*). The fracture extends to posterior subtalar joint and sinus tarsi, with 2 to 3 mm of displacement. The findings are often subtle and can be mistaken for an ankle sprain on radiograph. (*C*) Coronal CT clearly shows a fracture through the lateral talar process (*arrow*). CT or MR imaging is recommended for snowboarders presenting with ankle injury.

Ultrarunning

Ultramarathons include any race distance longer than traditional 42.2-km marathons. Ultrarunners face rugged terrain, elevation changes, and inclement weather. Overall, they have similar injury rates compared with other distance runners.[51] Not surprisingly, younger and less experienced ultrarunners tend to be most at risk for injury.[51]

Most injuries in ultrarunners are chronic from overuse, most often involving the knee with an incidence of 24%.[51] Patellofemoral pain syndrome/fat pad impingement is the most common

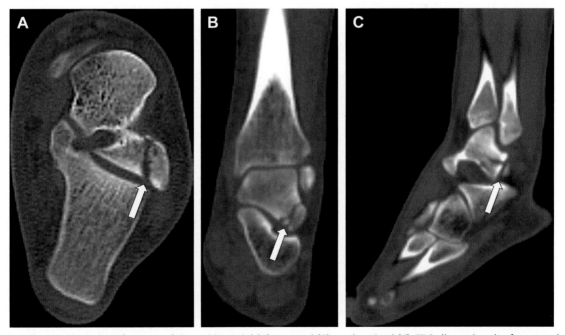

Fig. 10. Snowboarder's fracture of the ankle. Axial (*A*), coronal (*B*), and sagittal (*C*) CT 2-dimensional reformatted images (from same patient in **Fig. 9**) more clearly demonstrate the comminuted intra-articular fracture of the lateral process of the talus extending to the lateral portion of the posterior subtalar joint and sinus tarsi (*arrows*).

Table 8		
Hawkins classification of talar neck fractures on radiography or computed tomography			
Type	Imaging Findings	Treatment
---	---	---
I	Nondisplaced vertical fracture of the talar neck	8 wk in a cast followed by 4 wk in CAM cast
II	Displaced fracture with subtalar joint subluxation or dislocation; normal tibiotalar joint alignment	Closed reduction attempted first with anatomic reduction delaying surgical treatment
III	Displaced fracture with subluxation or dislocation of both the ankle and subtalar joint	Open reduction using a combined anteromedial and anterolateral surgical approach
IV	Type III findings with talonavicular joint displacement	Same as type III

Abbreviation: CAM, controlled ankle motion.

Data from Melenevsky Y, Mackey RA, Abrahams RB, et al. Talar fractures and dislocations: a radiologist's guide to timely diagnosis and classification. Radiographics 2015;35:765–79; and Hawkins LG. Fracture of the lateral process of the talus. J Bone Joint Surg Am 1965;47:1170–5.

injury, presenting as anterior knee pain behind the kneecap (**Fig. 11**).[52,53] The mechanism is unclear but may be related to patellofemoral joint stress and cartilage wear.[54] Iliotibial band issues occur with an incidence of 15.8%, usually presenting with lateral knee pain (**Fig. 12**). Ultrasound can dynamically visualize the iliotibial band, whereas MR imaging classically shows ill-defined increased T2 signal/edema in the fat between the iliotibial band and lateral femoral condyle with occasional bursae.[55,56] Chronic findings include iliotibial band thickening and sometimes edema superficial to it.[57] Muscle strains occur frequently, predominantly of the hamstrings and calf with an incidences of 13.1% and 11.8%, respectively. Ankle sprains, Achilles tendinitis, and plantar fasciitis are relatively common, with an incidence of 10.6% to 10.8%.[51]

Medial tibial stress injuries and other stress fractures occur frequently in this population. An example of a sacral stress fracture in a long-distance runner is shown in **Fig. 13**. However, while a recent study showed that ultrarunners have fewer stress fractures compared with other distance runners, they tend have a higher proportion of stress fractures in the foot compared with the lower leg, thigh, or pelvis.[51,58]

Nerve injuries can also occur, although the incidence in ultrarunners is not well-studied. Morton neuromas are the most common injuries due to compression and stretch of the interdigital nerves during push-off. Tarsal tunnel syndrome may occur because of tibial nerve compression at the ankle in runners with predisposing anatomy or malalignment. Jogger's foot can result from entrapment of the medial plantar nerve.

Groin pain in ultrarunners also merits discussion, as the differential is broad, including causes such as hip acetabular tears, adductor longus

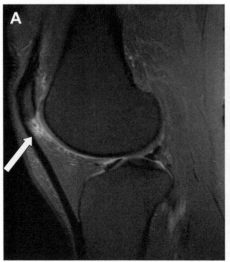
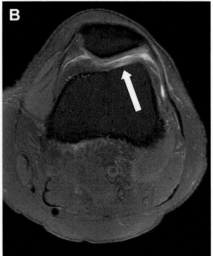

Fig. 11. Patellofemoral fat pad impingement syndrome. Sagittal T2 fat-suppressed (FS) (*A*) and axial proton-density FS (*B*) images demonstrate edema within the superolateral aspect of Hoffa fat pad (*arrows*), suggestive of patellofemoral fat pad impingement syndrome.

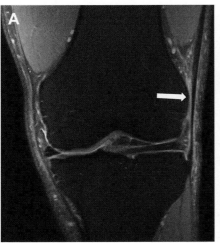
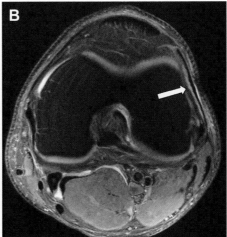

Fig. 12. Iliotibial band syndrome in ultrarunning athlete. Coronal (A) and axial (B) PD FS images demonstrate moderately increased signal both superficial and deep to the iliotibial band (arrows), compatible with iliotibial band friction syndrome. This overuse injury is common in ultrarunners and presents with lateral knee pain.

tendinosis, osteitis pubis, inguinal hernias, snapping hip, pubic stress fractures, and athletic pubalgia. Given the wide range of causes and the difficulty in discerning the cause with physical examination alone, imaging plays a key role in identifying the cause of the groin pain and determining management.[59]

Athletic pubalgia is a significant cause of injury in high-level athletes, although the specific incidence in ultrarunners has not been well studied. The term refers to various pathologies around the pubic symphysis with mechanisms of injury, usually involving chronic repetitive torque.[59] These injuries can generally only be diagnosed with MR imaging, although specific protocols must be used because of the subtle findings.[59] At the authors' institution, they perform axial and sagittal T1-weighted and fat-suppressed T2-weighted imaging with a small field of view

centered at the pubic symphysis and small field-of-view oblique proton density and fat-suppressed T2-weighted imaging along the arcuate line to evaluate the rectus abdominis and adductor attachments (Table 9). Larger field-of-view imaging is included to rule out more remote pathologies. MR imaging findings include injury along the lateral border of the rectus abdominis just above the pubic attachment or of the adductor longus origin. Eventually, there is extension of the lesion through the aponeurosis into both the rectus abdominis and adductor longus. Further extension under the pubic periosteum causes disruption of the aponeurosis from its pubic attachment. In severe cases, these lesions can extend to include the adductor origins and the contralateral side. Tendons may be completely avulsed.[59] An example of athletic pubalgia in an ultrarunner is shown in Fig. 14.

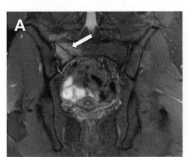
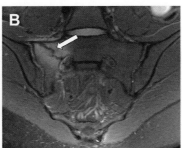
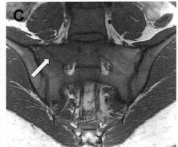

Fig. 13. Sacral MR imaging demonstrating stress fracture in a 21-year-old woman training for a half marathon. (A) Coronal T2 fat-suppressed (FS) image demonstrates increased signal within the right sacral ala with a linear hypointense fracture line (arrow). (B) Coronal T2 FS oblique image through the sacrum demonstrates increased signal within the right sacral ala with a linear hypointense fracture line (arrow). (C) Coronal T1 oblique image through the sacrum demonstrates a linear hypointense fracture line surrounded by hypointense edema within the sacral ala (arrow).

Table 9
Specialized sequences for athletic pubalgia protocol

Sequence	Description	Scan Plane and Example
Axial T1 SMFOV Axial T2 fat-saturated SMFOV	Center FOV on pubic symphysis	
Sagittal T1 SMFOV Sagittal T2 fat-saturated SMFOV	Center on the pubic symphysis over the entire femoral head through the opposite femoral head	
Coronal oblique PD SMFOV Coronal oblique T2 fat-saturated SMFOV	FOV from the arcuate line from sagittal T1 through the pubic symphysis	

Abbreviations: FOV, field of view; PD, proton density; SMFOV, small field of view.

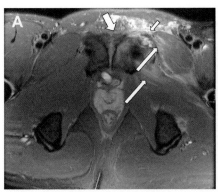
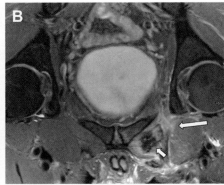

Fig. 14. Sports hernia in ultrarunning athlete. Axial T2 fat-suppressed (FS) (A) and coronal oblique T2 FS (B) small field-of-view images demonstrate severe left-sided partial tearing of the distal left rectus abdominus (A; thick arrow), partial avulsion of the origin of the left adductor longus (A, B; short arrows), and mild tears of the left pectineus and obturator externus (A, B; long arrows).

Osteitis pubis is a more common cause of groin pain in long-distance runners resulting from instability of the pubic symphysis from chronic shear and distraction injuries and unbalanced tensile strength from muscle attachments (Fig. 15).[59] MR imaging generally shows para-symphyseal bone marrow edema, occasionally with symphyseal fluid and peri-pubic soft tissue edema. Periostitis, erosive changes, subchondral cyst formation, and osteophytes may also be present when chronic.[59] Pubic stress fractures, most commonly in the inferior pubic ramus, can also cause groin pain. However, femoral neck stress fractures are more common and can sometimes cause groin pain as well.[6,59]

Most acute race-day injuries involve blisters, abrasions, hematomas, or chafing.[60–62] Tendonitis is the next most common race-day injury.[62] An acute injury unique to ultrarunners is anterior tibial tendinopathy from repeated or strained dorsiflexion while running on steep hills. Patients present with anterior ankle pain with swelling and occasionally erythema in the region of the anterior tibial tendon. The other extensor tendons passing under the extensor retinaculum may also be involved. The frequency of this injury is as high as 19%.[63] Ultrasound and MR imaging can confirm this injury.[64]

Bungee jumping
Bungee involves jumping from tall objects, such as bridges, buildings, or hot air balloons, while attached to an elastic cord via an ankle or body harness. Injuries during bungee jumping can be divided into those due to equipment malfunction, such as harness failure, and those that occur despite properly functioning equipment. The most common injuries that occur with proper functioning equipment involve retinal hemorrhage-induced impaired vision from the abrupt change in intravascular pressure during the upward recoil. Whiplash is also relatively common. More serious injuries include quadriplegia and carotid dissections.

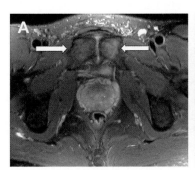
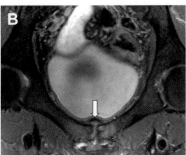
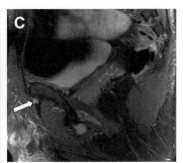

Fig. 15. Osteitis pubis in ultrarunning athlete. Axial T2 fat-suppressed (FS) (A) and coronal oblique T2 FS (B) small field-of-view images demonstrate bone marrow edema in the pubic bones (A; arrows) with capsular hypertrophy and fluid within the symphyseal cleft (B; arrow). (C) Sagittal T2 FS small field-of-view image demonstrates partial avulsion of the proximal adductor longus tendon (arrow).

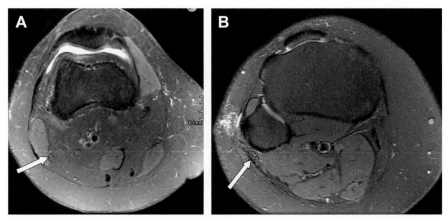

Fig. 16. Peroneal nerve injury. (*A*) Axial proton-density (PD) fat-suppressed (FS) image demonstrates normal common peroneal nerve (*arrow*) at the level of the distal femur. (*B*) Axial PD FS image at the level of the fibula shows fascicular thickening with hyperintense signal within several fascicles in the common peroneal nerve (*arrow*), compatible with peroneal nerve injury/neuropathy.

Bungee-related injuries specifically involving the lower extremities are less well studied. Besides strains, sprains, and fractures, most injuries involve peroneal nerve trauma. Classic signs of peroneal nerve palsy include cutaneous loss of sensation along the lateral leg, foot, and ankle, along with weakened eversion and dorsiflexion of the foot.[65] The common peroneal nerve can be injured anywhere from its origin in the popliteal fossa to its termination distal to the fibular tunnel.[66]

Mechanisms of peroneal nerve injury include external compression, direct trauma, traction, masses (including hematomas), entrapment, vascular, and other diseases. In bungee jumping, the most common mechanism is likely traction stretching of the nerve. Stretch injuries tend to involve longer segments and heal poorly.[65] Although the diagnosis is often made clinically or by EMG, MRN can help with management decisions by assessing the severity of the lesion and injury to surrounding structures and determining which patients need more urgent surgical referral (**Fig. 16**).

Ultrasound can also be used to assess for peroneal nerve injury, with nerve impairment presenting as enlarged nerve caliber with decreased fascicular pattern, increased hypoechogenicity, and blurring of the outer lining due to edema.[67] Severe damage can be seen as incomplete or complete nerve tear, with visualization of interrupted fascicles or a nerve stump.[67] Ultrasound can also evaluate for surrounding hematoma and soft tissue scarring.[67] Similarly to MR neurography, ultrasound can also significantly impact clinical management.

Mountain biking

Mountain biking is a common cause of fractures, causing up to 7.4% of sports-related fractures, mostly in the upper extremity.[68–72] Soft tissue injuries predominate in the lower extremities. Morel-Lavallée lesions are commonly seen in the greater trochanter region and lateral knee during falls from shearing/frictional forces and abrupt separation of the skin and subcutaneous fat from the underlying fascia.[16,68] These lesions are best evaluated by MR imaging and ultrasound, which show hemolymphatic fluid collections between the subcutaneous tissue and underlying fascia (**Fig. 17**).

Overuse injuries in the lower extremities are common with 20% to 27% of mountain bikers presenting with chronic knee pain. Patellofemoral pain syndrome and iliotibial band friction syndrome are common culprits. Pes anserine bursitis and medial plica syndrome can also be a source of anterior knee pain in bikers. Chronic foot injuries, such as metatarsalgia and Morton neuroma, are also prevalent in cross-country biking, likely related to the clipless stiff-soled shoes.[68] Biking is unique compared with other extreme sports because of the prolonged period of time sitting on a hard saddle, which can cause pudendal nerve impingement (**Fig. 18**), genital area numbness, and erectile dysfunction.[68] Female riders can develop unilateral vulvar hypertrophy.[71]

Water sports

Extreme water sports also place participants at risk of injury to the pelvis and lower extremity. Surfing, which continues to increase in popularity, presents with unique injuries. In a recent study of surfing injuries over a 12-year period, lower extremity injuries were found to be the most common acute injury. Lacerations were the most common injury overall, followed by strains and sprains. Fractures made up 11.9% of injuries and were

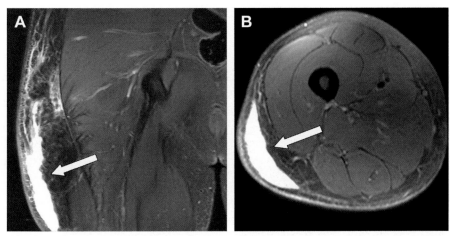

Fig. 17. Morel-Lavallee lesion. Coronal (*A*) and axial (*B*) T2 fat-suppressed images of the upper thigh demonstrated a T2 hyperintense collection (*arrows*) between the skin and subcutaneous fat from the underlying fascia, consistent with a Morel-Lavallee lesion. These lesions result from shearing and frictional force injuries and are commonly seen adjacent to the greater trochanter, as above, or lateral knee when related to sports injuries.

slightly more frequent in upper extremities than in lower extremities.[72] In another recent Australian study, there was a high incidence of acute ankle injuries, which was thought to be due to a change in surfing style and performance of more aerial techniques.[73] Surfer's myelopathy is another potential injury that presents with lower limb pain, numbness, paresthesia, and paraparesis. It is thought to be due to hyperextension of the lower thoracic and upper lumber spine. MR imaging may show central T2-hyperintense signal in the spinal cord and conus as well as spinal cord and conus swelling, although MR imaging findings do not necessarily correlate with symptom severity (**Fig. 19**).[16,35]

Skimboarding is another water sport prone to lower extremity injuries. Lower extremity fractures are most common, particularly at the ankle, followed by soft tissue injuries and lacerations.[16] An entity coined *skimboarder's toe* was also recently described, resulting from hyperdorsiflexion of the metatarsophalangeal joints while mounting a skimboard. MR imaging findings include soft tissue edema (particularly dorsally), bone marrow edema, and disrupted extensor expansion at the metatarsophalangeal joint.[74]

Another water sport in which lower extremity injuries are common is windsurfing. Foot strap injuries are specific to windsurfing and occur after falls or bad landings. Rotational force on the leg when the foot is wedged in the foot strap leads to twisting at the knee with a fixed foreleg, causing fractures of the femoral shaft, fibular head, and tibial plateau, as well as knee injury. Foot and ankle injuries, including of the Lisfranc ligament, also occur when the foot is acutely pronated while in the strap (**Fig. 20**). Kitesurfing is also associated with lower extremity injuries, most frequently of the ankle, although knee injuries are also common.[16,75]

Airborne sports
Skydiving is the most popular and well-studied of airborne extreme sports. Modern equipment has

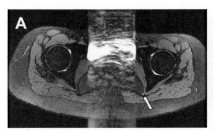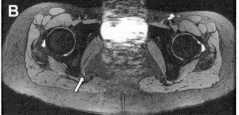

Fig. 18. Pudendal neuropathy in 22-year-old woman with bilateral labial pain and numbness. (*A, B*) Axial double echo steady state sequences demonstrate focally increased signal of the enlarged bilateral pudendal nerves (*arrows*) as they course along the obturator internus muscles, compatible with pudendal neuropathy.

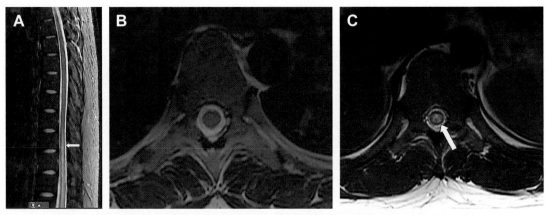

Fig. 19. Surfer's myelopathy in 24-year-old male surfer. (*A*) Sagittal STIR image of the spine demonstrates abnormal signal of the cord from T9 and extending inferiorly, with mild expansion of the involved cord (*arrow*). (*B*) Axial T2 images demonstrate normal signal at the T6 level. (*C*) In contrast, there is abnormal T2 signal and mild cord expansion at the T10 level (*arrow*). Given the patient's clinical history of back pain, bilateral lower extremity weakness, and antalgic gait, findings are consistent with surfer's myelopathy.

led to decreased injury and fatality associated with this sport, which has a relatively low injury and mortality rate compared with other extreme sports.[16] In one study of 8976 skydivers, it was found that 66% of injuries were minor; of the more severe injuries, 50% were due to extremity trauma mostly involving the lower limbs.[76] Another study in Sweden also showed a relative high frequency of lower extremity injuries.[77]

BASE (building, antenna, span, earth) jumping involves parachuting from tall fixed structures.[16] It is one of the most dangerous adventure sports in the world, with a 5- to 8-fold higher injury rate than skydiving.[1,78] Given that the sport is relatively

new, there are only a few studies of injuries associated with BASE jumping, and most focus on fatalities. Of the studies that have been performed, object strikes and bad landings are the cause of most injuries, most frequently involving the lower extremities.[79] In one study of 9914 jumps between 35 BASE jumpers, the estimated injury rate was about 0.4%, of which 72% involved the lower extremities.[78] Another study of BASE jumping injuries in Norway demonstrated a similar nonfatal injury rate with most involving ankle sprains or fractures.[80]

The use of wingsuits in skydiving and BASE jumping is more recent, with modern wingsuits

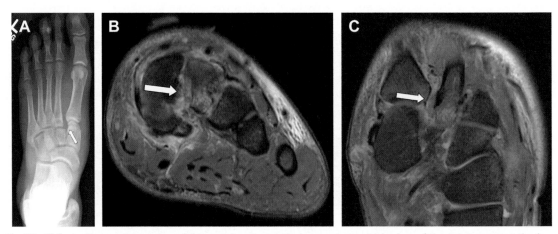

Fig. 20. Lisfranc ligamentous injury. (*A*) Frontal radiograph demonstrates widening of the joint space at the base of the first and second metatarsals, suspicious for underlying Lisfranc ligamentous injury. Axial T2 fat-suppressed (FS) (*B*) and coronal proton-density FS (*C*) images demonstrate high-grade tearing of the Lisfranc ligament (*arrows*) with associated mild widening between the first and second metatarsal bases. Bone marrow edema is present in the second metatarsal, and there is extensive overlying soft tissue edema.

developed in the 1990s. These suits help athletes control their flights and allow them to steer close to terrain, such as near the cliff faces. This sport is even less well studied than BASE jumping, although in one recent study of wingsuit BASE jumping fatalities it was found that most deaths are related to cliff or ground impact due to flight miscalculation.[81]

SUMMARY

Extreme sports continue to increase in popularity. As a result, injuries sustained from participation in such sports are more frequent. As many of these activities take place in remote regions, the specific sport, mechanism of injury, and physical examination are the first-line methods of assessing these patients. In addition, imaging plays a central role, with plain film and ultrasound as the most accessible modalities. MR imaging has also become more and more valuable in evaluating the extent and severity of many of these injuries, especially those involving soft tissues and nerves. As described earlier, these imaging studies make significant impacts on clinical management of extreme sports injuries.

REFERENCES

1. Laver L, Pengas IP, Mei-Dan O. Injuries in extreme sports. J Orthop Surg Res 2017;12:59.
2. Berger FH, de Jonge MC, Maas M. Stress fractures in the lower extremity. The importance of increasing awareness amongst radiologists. Eur J Radiol 2007;62:16–26.
3. Beck BR, Bergman AG, Miner M, et al. Tibial stress injury: relationship of radiographic, nuclear medicine bone scanning, MR imaging, and CT severity grades to clinical severity and time to healing. Radiology 2012;263:811–8.
4. Nattiv A, Kennedy G, Barrack MT, et al. Correlation of MRI grading of bone stress injuries with clinical risk factors and return to play: a 5-year prospective study in collegiate track and field athletes. Am J Sports Med 2013;41:1930–41.
5. Kijowski R, Choi J, Shinki K, et al. Validation of MRI classification system for tibial stress injuries. AJR Am J Roentgenol 2012;198:878–84.
6. Guermazi A, Roemer FW, Robinson P, et al. Imaging of muscle injuries in sports medicine: sports imaging series. Radiology 2017;282:646–63.
7. Mitchell CH, Brushart TM, Ahlawat S, et al. MRI of sports-related peripheral nerve injuries. AJR Am J Roentgenol 2014;203:1075–84.
8. Ohana M, Moser T, Moussaouï A, et al. Current and future imaging of the peripheral nervous system. Diagn Interv Imaging 2014;95:17–26.
9. Kamath S, Venkatanarasimha N, Walsh MA, et al. MRI appearance of muscle denervation. Skeletal Radiol 2008;37:397–404.
10. Van den Bergh FR, Vanhoenacker FM, De Smet E, et al. Peroneal nerve: normal anatomy and pathologic findings on routine MRI of the knee. Insights Imaging 2013;4:287–99.
11. Kim SJ, Hong SH, Jun WS, et al. MR imaging mapping of skeletal muscle denervation in entrapment and compressive neuropathies. Radiographics 2011;31:319–32.
12. Seddon HJ, Medawar PB, Smith H. Rate of regeneration of peripheral nerves in man. J Physiol 1943;102:191–215.
13. Sunderland S. A classification of peripheral nerve injuries producing loss of function. Brain 1951;74:491–516.
14. Chhabra A, Andreisek G, Soldatos T, et al. MR neurography: past, present, and future. AJR Am J Roentgenol 2011;197:583–91.
15. Chhabra A, Ahlawat S, Belzberg A, et al. Peripheral nerve injury grading simplified on MR neurography: as referenced to Seddon and Sunderland classifications. Indian J Radiol Imaging 2014;24:217–24.
16. Feletti F. Extreme sports medicine [Chapters 11–21]. New York: Springer Berlin Heidelberg; 2016. p. 123–274.
17. Jones G, Asghar A, Llewellyn DJ. The epidemiology of rock-climbing injuries. Br J Sports Med 2008;42:773–8.
18. Backe S, Ericson L, Janson S, et al. Rock climbing injury rates and associated risk factors in a general climbing population. Scand J Med Sci Sports 2009;19:850–6.
19. Schöffl V, Küpper T. Feet injuries in rock climbers. World J Orthop 2013;4:218–28.
20. Schöffl V, Morrison A, Schöffl I, et al. The epidemiology of injury in mountaineering, rock and ice climbing. Med Sport Sci 2012;58:17–43.
21. Schöffl V. Adventure and extreme sports injuries: epidemiology, treatment, rehabilitation and prevention. In: Mei-Dan O, Carmont MR, editors. Rock and ice climbing. London: Springer; 2013. p. 7–35.
22. Nelson NG, McKenzie LB. Rock climbing injuries treated in emergency departments in the U.S., 1990-2007. Am J Prev Med 2009;37:195–200.
23. Neuhof A, Hennig FF, Schöffl I, et al. Injury risk evaluation in sport climbing. Int J Sports Med 2011;32:794–800.
24. Bowie WS, Hunt TK, Allen HA. Rock-climbing injuries in Yosemite National Park. West J Med 1988;149:172–7.
25. Killian RB, Nishimoto GS, Page JC. Foot and ankle injuries related to rock climbing. The role of footwear. J Am Podiatr Med Assoc 1998;88:365–74.
26. Schöffl V, Popp D, Küpper T, et al. Injury trends in rock climbers: evaluation of a case series of 911

injuries between 2009 and 2012. Wilderness Environ Med 2015;26:62–7.

27. Schöffl V, Lutter C, Popp D. The "heel hook"- a climbing-specific technique to injure the leg. Wilderness Environ Med 2016;27:294–301.

28. Schöffl V, Morrison A, Schwarz U, et al. Evaluation of injury and fatality risk in rock and ice climbing. Sports Med 2010;40:657–79.

29. Mashkovskiy E, Beverly JM, Stöcker U, et al. Ice climbing festival in Sochi 2014 Winter Olympics: medical management and injury analysis. Wilderness Environ Med 2016;27:117–24.

30. Buda R, Di Caprio F, Bedetti L, et al. Foot overuse diseases in rock climbing: an epidemiologic study. J Am Podiatr Med Assoc 2013;103:113–20.

31. Stenroos A, Handolin L. Incidence of recreational alpine skiing and snowboarding injuries: six years experience in the largest ski resort in Finland. Scand J Surg 2015;104:127–31.

32. DeFroda SF, Gil JA, Owens BD. Epidemiology of lower extremity injuries presenting to the emergency room in the United States: snow skiing vs. snowboarding. Injury 2016;47:2283–7.

33. Langran M. Adventure and extreme sports injuries: epidemiology, treatment, rehabilitation and prevention. In: Mei-Dan O, Carmont MR, editors. Alpine skiing and snowboarding injuries. London: Springer; 2013. p. 37–67.

34. Paletta GA, Warren RF. Knee injuries and alpine skiing. treatment and rehabilitation. Sports Med 1994;17:411–23.

35. Guermazi A, Roemer FW, Crema MD. Imaging in sports-specific musculoskeletal injuries [Chapters 16–17]. London: Springer; 2016. p. 381–448.

36. Stenroos AJ, Handolin LE. Alpine skiing injuries in Finland - a two-year retrospective study based on a questionnaire among ski racers. BMC Sports Sci Med Rehabil 2014;6:9.

37. Stenroos A, Pakarinen H, Jalkanen J, et al. Tibial fractures in alpine skiing and snowboarding in Finland: a retrospective study on fracture types and injury mechanisms in 363 patients. Scand J Surg 2016;105:191–6.

38. Gill TJ, Moezzi DM, Oates KM, et al. Arthroscopic reduction and internal fixation of tibial plateau fractures in skiing. Clin Orthop Relat Res 2001;383: 243–9.

39. Arrowsmith SR, Fleming LL, Allman FL. Traumatic dislocations of the peroneal tendons. Am J Sports Med 1983;11:142–6.

40. Brage ME, Hansen ST. Traumatic subluxation/dislocation of the peroneal tendons. Foot Ankle 1992; 13:423–31.

41. Kim S, Endres NK, Johnson RJ, et al. Snowboarding injuries: trends over time and comparisons with alpine skiing injuries. Am J Sports Med 2012;40: 770–6.

42. Coury T, Napoli AM, Wilson M, et al. Injury patterns in recreational alpine skiing and snowboarding at a mountainside clinic. Wilderness Environ Med 2013; 24:417–21.

43. Ishimaru D, Ogawa H, Sumi H, et al. Lower extremity injuries in snowboarding. J Trauma 2011;70:E48–52.

44. Sachtleben TR. Snowboarding injuries. Curr Sports Med Rep 2011;10:340–4.

45. Madden CC, Putukian M, Young CC, et al. Netter's sports medicine [Chapters 77–79]. 2nd edition. Philadelphia: Elsevier; 2018. p. 598–611.

46. McCrory P, Bladin C. Fractures of the lateral process of the talus: a clinical review. "Snowboarder's ankle". Clin J Sport Med 1996;6:124–8.

47. Melenevsky Y, Mackey RA, Abrahams RB, et al. Talar fractures and dislocations: a radiologist's guide to timely diagnosis and classification. Radiographics 2015;35:765–79.

48. Hawkins LG. Fracture of the lateral process of the talus. J Bone Joint Surg Am 1965;47:1170–5.

49. Matsumoto K, Sumi H, Sumi Y, et al. An analysis of hip dislocations among snowboarders and skiers: a 10-year prospective study from 1992 to 2002. J Trauma 2003;55:946–8.

50. Anderson SE, Weber M, Steinbach LS, et al. Shoe rim and shoe buckle pseudotumor of the ankle in elite and professional figure skaters and snowboarders: MR imaging findings. Skeletal Radiol 2004;33:325–9.

51. Hoffman MD, Krishnan E. Health and exercise-related medical issues among 1,212 ultramarathon runners: baseline findings from the Ultrarunners Longitudinal TRAcking (ULTRA) study. PLoS One 2014;9:e83867.

52. Khodaee M, Ansari M. Common ultramarathon injuries and illnesses: race day management. Curr Sports Med Rep 2012;11:290–7.

53. Krabak BJ, Waite B, Lipman G. Injury and illnesses prevention for ultramarathoners. Curr Sports Med Rep 2013;12:183–9.

54. Collado H, Fredericson M. Patellofemoral pain syndrome. Clin Sports Med 2010;29:379–98.

55. Murphy BJ, Hechtman KS, Uribe JW, et al. Iliotibial band friction syndrome: MR imaging findings. Radiology 1992;185:569–71.

56. Ekman EF, Pope T, Martin DF, et al. Magnetic resonance imaging of iliotibial band syndrome. Am J Sports Med 1994;22:851–4.

57. Muhle C, Ahn JM, Yeh L, et al. Iliotibial band friction syndrome: MR imaging findings in 16 patients and MR arthrographic study of six cadaveric knees. Radiology 1999;212:103–10.

58. Hoffman MD. Injuries and health considerations in ultramarathon runners. Phys Med Rehabil Clin N Am 2016;27:203–16.

59. Omar IM, Zoga AC, Kavanagh EC, et al. Athletic pubalgia and "sports hernia": optimal MR imaging

technique and findings. Radiographics 2008;28: 1415–38.

60. Scheer BV, Murray A. Al Andalus ultra trail: an observation of medical interventions during a 219-km, 5-day ultramarathon stage race. Clin J Sport Med 2011;21:444–6.

61. Graham SM, McKinley M, Chris CC, et al. Injury occurrence and mood states during a desert ultramarathon. Clin J Sport Med 2012;22:462–6.

62. Krabak BJ, Waite B, Schiff MA. Study of injury and illness rates in multiday ultramarathon runners. Med Sci Sports Exerc 2011;43:2314–20.

63. Fallon KE. Musculoskeletal injuries in the ultramarathon: the 1990 Westfield Sydney to Melbourne run. Br J Sports Med 1996;30:319–23.

64. Krabak BJ, Waite B, Lipman G. Evaluation and treatment of injury and illness in the ultramarathon athlete. Phys Med Rehabil Clin N Am 2014;25: 845–63.

65. Vanderford L, Meyers M. Injuries and bungee jumping. Sports Med 1995;20:369–74.

66. Torre PR, Williams GG, Blackwell T, et al. Bungee jumper's foot drop peroneal nerve palsy caused by bungee cord jumping. Ann Emerg Med 1993;22: 1766–7.

67. Gruber H, Peer S, Meirer R, et al. Peroneal nerve palsy associated with knee luxation: evaluation by sonography-initial experiences. AJR Am J Roentgenol 2005;185:1119–25.

68. Ansari M, Nourian R, Khodaee M. Mountain biking injuries. Curr Sports Med Rep 2017;16:404–12.

69. Nelson NG, McKenzie LB. Mountain biking-related injuries treated in emergency departments in the United States, 1994-2007. Am J Sports Med 2011; 39:404–9.

70. Ashwell Z, McKay MP, Brubacher JR, et al. The epidemiology of mountain bike park injuries at the Whistler Bike Park, British Columbia (BC). Wilderness Environ Med 2012;23:140–5.

71. Carmont MR. Mountain biking injuries: a review. Br Med Bull 2008;85:101–12.

72. Klick C, Jones CM, Adler D. Surfing USA: an epidemiological study of surfing injuries presenting to US EDs 2002 to 2013. Am J Emerg Med 2016;34: 1491–6.

73. Furness J, Hing W, Walsh J, et al. Acute injuries in recreational and competitive surfers: incidence, severity, location, type, and mechanism. Am J Sports Med 2015;43:1246–54.

74. Donnelly LF, Betts JB, Fricke BL. Skimboarder's toe: findings on high-field MRI. AJR Am J Roentgenol 2005;184:1481–5.

75. van Bergen CJ, Commandeur JP, Weber RI, et al. Windsurfing vs kitesurfing: injuries at the north sea over a 2-year period. World J Orthop 2016;7: 814–20.

76. Barrows TH, Mills TJ, Kassing SD. The epidemiology of skydiving injuries: world freefall convention, 2000-2001. J Emerg Med 2005;28:63–8.

77. Westman A, Björnstig U. Injuries in Swedish skydiving. Br J Sports Med 2007;41:356–64.

78. Monasterio E, Mei-Dan O. Risk and severity of injury in a population of BASE jumpers. N Z Med J 2008; 121:70–5.

79. Mei-Dan O, Carmont MR, Monasterio E. The epidemiology of severe and catastrophic injuries in BASE jumping. Clin J Sport Med 2012;22:262–7.

80. Soreide K, Ellingsen CL, Knutson V. How dangerous is BASE jumping? An analysis of adverse events in 20,850 jumps from the Kjerag Massif, Norway. J Trauma 2007;62:1113–7.

81. Mei-Dan O, Monasterio E, Carmont M, et al. Fatalities in wingsuit BASE jumping. Wilderness Environ Med 2013;24:321–7.

82. Chan O, Del Buono A, Best TM, et al. Acute muscle strain injuries: a proposed new classification system. Knee Surg Sports Traumatol Arthrosc 2012;20(11): 2356–62.

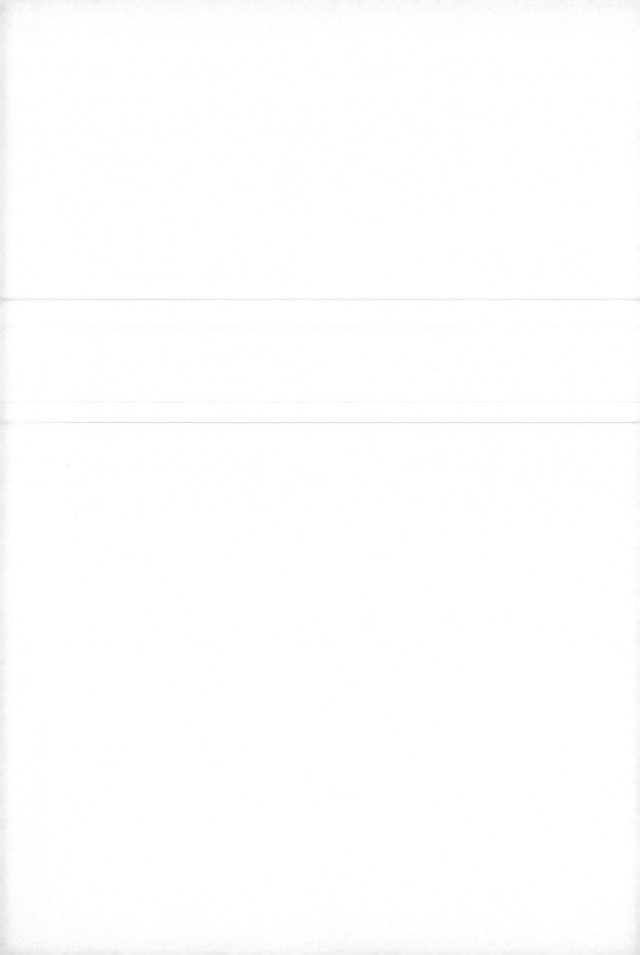

Ultrasound Intervention of the Lower Extremity/Pelvis

Brian Y. Chan, MD*, Kenneth S. Lee, MD

KEYWORDS

• Ultrasound • Injection • Corticosteroid • PRP • Pelvis • Hip • Knee • Ankle

KEY POINTS

- Musculoskeletal conditions are common, affect patients across all demographics, and are increasing in prevalence.
- Ultrasound is increasingly used to provide image-guided therapeutic interventions for management of musculoskeletal conditions, including in the pelvis and lower extremity.
- Intraarticular, intramuscular, perineural, bursal, and tendon sheath corticosteroid injections can be effective in providing prolonged symptomatic relief for a wide variety of musculoskeletal conditions.
- Platelet-rich plasma contains growth factors that may stimulate tendon healing following intratendinous instillation.
- Understanding the relevant anatomy and technical considerations of commonly performed ultrasound-guided interventions is key to ensuring patient safety and procedural accuracy.

INTRODUCTION

Musculoskeletal (MSK) conditions are common and affect patients across all demographics. Up to 30% of American adults experience joint pain, swelling, or restricted range of motion at any given moment.[1] Given the projected growth of the elderly population in the United States, the prevalence of MSK disorders is anticipated to increase.[2]

Ultrasound (US) is increasingly used in MSK radiology not only as a cost-effective diagnostic tool[3] but also for image guidance during therapeutic interventions.[4] Numerous studies have demonstrated superiority of US over landmark-guided injections, including in the hip,[5] knee,[6] and ankle.[7,8] In addition, US enables real-time visualization of soft tissue structures during interventions. Finnoff and colleagues[9] demonstrated significantly increased accuracy of US compared with fluoroscopic-guided piriformis injections in cadavers (95% vs 30%, respectively). A separate study by Rutten and colleagues[10] showed that US-guided glenohumeral joint injections were better tolerated by patients with shorter procedure times compared with fluoroscopy.

As MSK US becomes more widespread, familiarity and comfort with US-guided interventions will become increasingly important. The objective of this article is to highlight the growing number of US-guided interventions in the pelvis and lower extremity. In this article, the authors cover general concepts regarding therapeutic US-guided injection of corticosteroid and platelet-rich plasma (PRP) for the treatment of MSK conditions. The authors then review relevant anatomy and technique for US-guided pelvic and lower extremity interventions commonly performed at their institution.

Disclosure Statement: None (B.Y. Chan). Research support from National Basketball Association, General Electric, Mitek; Consultant – Echometrix; Royalties – Elsevier (K.S. Lee).
Department of Radiology, University of Wisconsin School of Medicine and Public Health, E3/366, 600 Highland Avenue, Madison, WI 53792, USA
* Corresponding author.
E-mail address: bchan@uwhealth.org

Radiol Clin N Am 56 (2018) 1035–1046
https://doi.org/10.1016/j.rcl.2018.06.011

Interventions

Technical considerations

Equipment selection is tailored to the specific intervention. A high-frequency (eg, 6–15 MHz) linear array transducer is typically used for superficial structures, whereas a low-frequency (eg, 5–12 MHz) curved array transducer may be required for deeper targets or patients with a larger body habitus. A small footprint linear "hockey stick" probe can facilitate guidance during superficial interventions where limited space is a consideration, such as in small joints of the foot and ankle.

Before intervention, a preprocedural anatomic survey of the target is performed to determine a safe and unobstructed route for intervention. Appropriate patient positioning is crucial to picking the ideal approach. Grayscale and Doppler US are used to identify and avoid sensitive structures such as vessels and nerves. Once the approach is determined, a mark is drawn on the skin to indicate the needle entry site. As with any procedure, standard sterile precautions are taken. Superficial and deep local anesthesia is performed with buffered 1% lidocaine.

Advancing the needle in-plane with the transducer is preferred so the entire length of the needle can be visualized. A large volume of US gel may be necessary to create a standoff pad in areas with undulating contours that make maintaining skin contact difficult. Visibility is maximized when adopting a needle trajectory as parallel to the transducer as possible. Jiggling the needle or instilling a small volume of lidocaine (a.k.a. hydrodissection) can aid localization of the needle tip. The most important consideration is to avoid advancing the needle haphazardly without identifying the needle tip.

Corticosteroid injection

Typical injection mixtures and volumes used at the authors' institution are shown in **Table 1**. For lower extremity injections, they most commonly use triamcinolone acetonide, 40 mg/mL (Kenalog -40, Bristol-Myers Squibb) mixed with varying amounts of short-acting anesthetic. For more superficial injections (ie, the foot), a soluble, nonparticulate steroid such as dexamethasone, 10 mg/mL, is often substituted to decrease the risk of cutaneous atrophy and depigmentation.

Table 1
Example pelvis and lower extremity injection volumes

	Ropivacaine HCl 0.5% (Naropin)[a] 5 mg/mL	Lidocaine HCl 1% Preservative-Free 10 mg/mL	Triamcinolone Acetonide (Kenalog-40)[b] 40 mg/mL	Dexamethasone Sodium Phosphate 10 mg/mL	Volume Injected
Hip					
Hip Joint	2 mL	2 mL	1 mL	—	5 mL
Iliopsoas Bursa	2 mL	2 mL	1 mL	—	5 mL
Lateral Femoral Cutaneous Nerve	—	3 mL	—	1 mL	4 mL
Greater Trochanteric Bursa	1 mL	1 mL	1 mL	—	3 mL
Ischial Gluteal Bursa	1 mL	1 mL	1 mL	—	3 mL
Ischiofemoral Space	1 mL	1 mL	1 mL	—	3 mL
Knee					
Knee Joint	4 mL	4 mL	1 mL	—	9 mL
Baker Cyst	1 mL	1 mL	1 mL	—	3 mL
Ankle					
Tibiotalar Joint	1 mL	1 mL	1 mL	—	3 mL
Peroneal Tendon Sheath	—	6 mL	—	1 mL	7 mL
Retrocalcaneal Bursa	—	1 mL	1 mL	—	2 mL
Plantar Fascia	—	2 mL	1 mL	—	3 mL

[a] Naropin, AstraZeneca.
[b] Kenalog-40, Bristol-Myers Squibb.

At the authors' institution, injection efficacy is assessed by tracking pre- and postinjection pain scores on a 10-point scale with a 2-week pain survey. Patients are counseled that 3 to 5 days may pass before onset of pain relief from the corticosteroid, and up to 1 week may be necessary to achieve maximal relief. Patients are also educated about the more common side effects of corticosteroids, including steroid flare, transient facial flushing, hyperglycemia, and chest fluttering.

Platelet-rich plasma

PRP contains growth factors that recruit inflammatory agents and stimulate tendon healing. PRP is produced by centrifugation of autologous venous blood drawn before the procedure. Following PRP preparation, a 22-gauge needle is advanced into portions of the tendon that seem hypoechoic or hyperemic. Afterward, the needle tip is advanced to the adjacent osseous attachment, and a portion of the PRP is instilled directly over the periosteum at the enthesis. The needle is subsequently withdrawn into the diseased tendon, and the remainder of the PRP is instilled into the region of tendinopathy.

The patient is advised not to take antiinflammatory medications before and after the procedure, which would inhibit inflammatory mediators involved in tendon healing. The affected extremity should be placed in an immobilization device immediately after the procedure, and the patient is cautioned to avoid strenuous activity for at least 8 weeks. It is important to note that PRP injections are considered experimental and are not reimbursed by most insurance companies.

Pelvis

Corticosteroid injection

Anterior hip

Hip joint Patients with intraarticular hip pathology may lack localizing signs or symptoms to the hip joint, and evaluation may be confounded by concomitant spine and knee pathology. Intraarticular hip corticosteroid injections are useful for providing symptomatic relief in patients responding poorly to conservative measures and can predict good surgical outcomes following hip arthroplasty.[11]

The patient is positioned supine with the hip in neutral rotation. The transducer is placed in an oblique axis parallel to the anterior femoral head-neck junction. Findings indicating presence of a joint effusion include convex bulging of the joint capsule, greater than 7 mm between the femoral neck and joint capsule, or asymmetry with the contralateral hip by greater than 1 mm.[12] If no joint fluid is present, the joint capsule layers appear as a single hyperechoic line. The needle is advanced in-plane from caudal to cranial into the anterior hip joint recess at the femoral head-neck junction. Instillation of injectate should result in uplifting of the joint capsule from the femoral neck (**Fig. 1**).

Iliopsoas bursa The iliopsoas bursa lies deep to the iliopsoas tendon and superficial to the acetabulum and anteromedial hip joint. Iliopsoas bursitis can be seen with pathologic conditions of the iliopsoas tendon, which is predisposed to friction during hip flexion as it crosses over the acetabular rim and hip joint. US-guided injection of the iliopsoas bursa can provide symptomatic relief and confirm the site of pain before further intervention such as iliopsoas tendon release.[13] Notably, the iliopsoas bursa can communicate normally with the hip joint in 14% of normal individuals, and fluid within the bursa may reflect intraarticular rather than iliopsoas pathology.[14]

The patient is positioned supine with the hip in neutral rotation. The transducer is placed parallel to the inguinal ligament over the hip joint. The probe is moved superiorly until the echogenic round iliopsoas tendon is identified over the iliopectineal eminence. The needle is advanced in-plane from lateral to medial until the tip contacts the iliac bone deep to the lateral margin of the iliopsoas tendon. The needle tip should remain superior to the hip joint to avoid an inadvertent intraarticular injection. Instillation of injectate should result in uplifting of the iliopsoas tendon from the underlying iliac bone (**Fig. 2**), and fluid should ideally flow medial to the iliopsoas tendon.

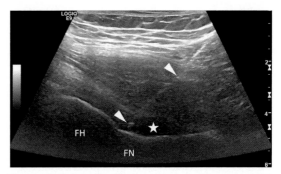

Fig. 1. Hip joint injection in a 41-year-old woman with right hip pain and primary osteoarthritis. Oblique longitudinal sonographic grayscale image of the anterior proximal femur during an intraarticular hip joint injection demonstrates the needle (*arrowheads*) advanced in-plane from caudal to cranial. The needle tip is positioned adjacent to the cortex at the junction of the femoral head (*FH*) and neck (*FN*). The joint capsule of the anterior recess is distended by anechoic injectate (*star*).

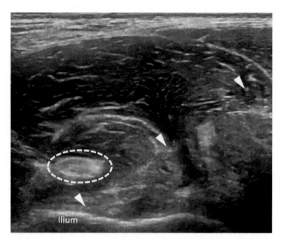

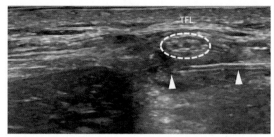

Fig. 2. Iliopsoas bursal injection in a 19-year-old male basketball player with an 8-month history of anterior right hip snapping. Transverse sonographic grayscale image during an iliopsoas bursa injection demonstrates a needle (*arrowheads*) advanced in-plane from lateral to medial. The needle tip contacts the anterior cortex of the ilium above the level of the hip joint. The round echogenic iliopsoas tendon (*circled*) is uplifted from the iliac bone by injectate.

Fig. 3. Lateral femoral cutaneous nerve injection in a 36-year-old man with left-sided "meralgia paresthetica" following a work-related injury. Transverse sonographic grayscale image below the level of the inguinal ligament during an LFCN injection demonstrates a needle (*arrowheads*) advanced in-plane from lateral to medial. The needle tip is positioned subjacent to the LFCN (*circled*), which lies deep to the tensor fascia lata (TFL). Anechoic injectate distends the fascial plane containing the LFCN and uplifts the overlying nerve.

ideally spread circumferentially around the nerve. Using larger volumes of anesthetic may be useful for hydrodissection in cases of perineural scarring.

Lateral femoral cutaneous nerve The lateral femoral cutaneous nerve (LFCN) is a superficial nerve that provides sensory innervation to the anterior and lateral thigh. It originates from the lumbar plexus, exits the pelvis beneath the inguinal ligament, and courses inferiorly in the fat plane interposed between the tensor fascia lata and sartorius muscles. However, due to variation in course of the LFCN, the use of image guidance during intervention is advocated to ensure a precise injection.[15,16] LFCN neuropathy, also known as "meralgia paresthetica," is often caused by compression as it crosses underneath the inguinal ligament. Numerous spontaneous and iatrogenic causes of LFCN neuropathy have been reported, including overly constrictive clothing, obesity, pregnancy, trauma, and bone graft harvesting.[17] LFCN neuropathy is also commonly seen following interventions using an anterior approach to the hip.[18]

The patient is positioned supine. The transducer is placed in the transverse plane over the anterior superior iliac spine (ASIS). The probe should be moved inferomedially from the ASIS toward the proximal thigh until the LFCN is visualized, approximately 1 cm medial to the ASIS, inferior to the inguinal ligament, and within the subcutaneous fat deep to the tensor fascia lata and superficial to the sartorius. The needle is advanced from lateral to medial until the tip is positioned immediately subjacent to the hyperechogenic epineurium of the LFCN (**Fig. 3**). Instillation of injectate should

Lateral hip
Greater trochanteric bursa There are 4 major facets of the greater trochanter: anterior, lateral, posterior, and superoposterior. The gluteus minimus inserts on the anterior facet, and the gluteus medius inserts on the lateral and superoposterior facets. The gluteus maximus courses over the gluteus medius and inserts directly on the femur and iliotibial tract. The greater trochanteric proper bursa (GT bursa) overlies the posterior and lateral facets of the greater trochanter and is interposed between the gluteus medius tendon and gluteus maximus muscle.

GT pain syndrome is a spectrum of disorders that present as pain and tenderness over the lateral aspect of the greater trochanter, reproducible with resisted abduction or external rotation.[19] Causes are multifactorial and include tendinopathy, tendon tears, and bursitis. Although inflammation and bursitis play a limited role in GT pain syndrome,[20–22] patients may experience prolonged symptomatic relief after a bursal injection.[23] At least one study showed that therapeutic injections of the GT bursa may provide greater symptomatic relief than subgluteus medius bursal injections.[24]

The patient is placed in lateral decubitus position with the affected side up. The transducer is placed in the transverse plane over the greater trochanter for visualization of the gluteus medius insertion on the lateral facet of the greater trochanter. The gluteus maximus muscle is seen superficial to the gluteus medius tendon. Preprocedural imaging infrequently reveals fluid within the GT bursa; however, if no fluid is present, a curvilinear echogenic line interposed between the gluteus medius tendon and gluteus maximus muscle is targeted. The needle is advanced in-plane from posterior to anterior until the tip is positioned within the GT bursa (**Fig. 4**). Instillation of injectate should result in GT bursal distension and uplifting of the overlying gluteus maximus muscle.

Posterior hip

Ischial bursa The hamstring muscle complex originates at the ischial tuberosity and is composed of the semimembranosus, semitendinosus, and the biceps femoris. An adventitial space known as the ischial bursa lies immediately superficial to the hamstring origin. Ischial bursitis presents as gluteal region pain and most commonly occurs secondary to chronic irritation from prolonged sitting, especially when vibration is involved (eg, tractor driving).[25] When conservative measures such as avoidance of sitting, antiinflammatory medications, and physical therapy fail, corticosteroid injection may provide symptomatic relief of sterile bursitis.[26]

The patient is positioned prone. The transducer is placed in the transverse plane over the ischial tuberosity. Preprocedural imaging may reveal fluid within the ischial bursa, bursal wall thickening, or hyperemia superficial to the hypoechoic hamstring

origin.[27] The sciatic nerve courses in close proximity to the hamstring origin and should also be identified to avoid unintentional contact or anesthetization. If the sciatic nerve obstructs entry to the ischial bursa, placing the patient in lateral decubitus position with the affected hip up and in flexion may move the sciatic nerve laterally away from the hamstring origin.[28] The needle is advanced in-plane from lateral to medial until the tip is immediately superficial to the hamstring origin. Instillation of injectate should result in pooling of fluid over the hamstring origin within the ischial bursa (**Fig. 5**).

Ischiofemoral space Ischiofemoral impingement (IFI) is defined by narrowing of the ischiofemoral space (IFS) with associated abnormal morphology and/or signal intensity of the quadratus femoris.[29] The IFS, or the space between the lateral cortex of the ischial tuberosity and the medial cortex of the lesser trochanter, measures approximately 20 mm in normal subjects.[29] Narrowing of the IFS may be positional, congenital, or acquired.[30] Hip pain associated with IFI is usually nonspecific and often bilateral. One study of patients with IFI demonstrated superior pain relief following US-guided corticosteroid injection of the quadratus femoris muscle compared with conservative measures.[31] Patients who fail nonoperative measures may ultimately require iliopsoas tendon release and resection of the lesser trochanter.[32]

The patient is positioned prone. The transducer is placed in the transverse plane over the IFS. Both the ischial tuberosity and lesser trochanter should be visualized, and the gluteus maximus

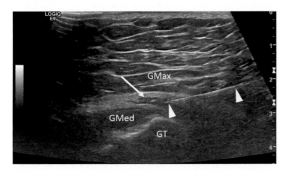

Fig. 4. Greater trochanteric bursal injection in a 64-year-old woman with lateral left hip pain and tenderness to palpation over the left greater trochanter. Transverse sonographic grayscale image during a GT bursa injection demonstrates a needle (*arrowheads*) advanced in-plane from posterior to anterior. The needle tip is positioned within the GT bursa at the level of the bony apex between the anterior and lateral facets. A small volume of anechoic fluid distends the left GT bursa (*arrow*). The gluteus maximus muscle (*GMax*) and gluteus medius tendon (*GMed*) insertion lie superficial and deep to the GT bursa, respectively.

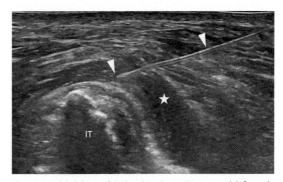

Fig. 5. Ischial bursal injection in a 59-year-old female tennis player with a 2-year history of pain over the left ischial bursa. Transverse sonographic grayscale image of the ischial tuberosity (*IT*) during an ischial bursa injection demonstrates a needle (*arrowheads*) advanced in-plane from lateral to medial. The needle tip is positioned immediately superficial to the hamstring origin. Anechoic injectate (*star*) distends the overlying ischial bursa.

lies superficial to these bony landmarks. The quadratus femoris is located within the IFS deep to the gluteus maximus. Care should be taken to identify the sciatic nerve, which courses in the fat plane between the gluteus maximus and quadratus femoris muscles. The nerve is typically seen just lateral to the hamstring tendon origin. The needle is advanced in-plane from lateral to medial and positioned with tip within the quadratus femoris muscle (**Fig. 6**).

Platelet-rich plasma

Hamstring origin Acute hamstring injuries occur during activities requiring abrupt contraction of the hamstring tendon, such as sprinting, football, or soccer. Hamstring injuries treated with PRP injections range from acute muscle strains to chronic tendinopathy from repetitive microtrauma. Literature on the effectiveness of PRP for symptomatic management is mixed and largely of low quality. One randomized controlled trial did not show shorter time to return to play following PRP injection as compared with platelet-poor plasma injection or conservative therapy.[33]

The patient is positioned prone. The transducer is placed in the transverse plane over the ischial tuberosity for visualization of the hamstring origin. The hamstring tendon origin should be assessed for tendinosis, tears, calcification, or hyperemia. The needle is advanced in-plane from lateral to medial, and the most tendinopathic and hyperemic portions of the tendon are targeted (**Fig. 7**).

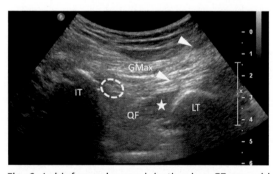

Fig. 6. Ischiofemoral space injection in a 57-year-old woman with chronic left groin pain and IFS narrowing on MRI. Transverse sonographic grayscale image during an IFS injection demonstrates a needle (*arrowheads*) advanced in-plane from lateral to medial. The ischial tuberosity (*IT*) and lesser trochanter of the femur (*LT*) define the medial and lateral margins of the IFS, respectively. The needle tip is advanced through the overlying gluteus maximus (*GMax*) and positioned within the quadratus femoris (*QF*) in the IFS. Anechoic injectate (*star*) is instilled directly into the quadratus femoris muscle. Note the sciatic nerve (*circle*) is remote from the injection site.

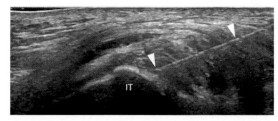

Fig. 7. Hamstring tendon PRP injection in a 31-year-old female runner with partial tear and tendinopathy of the right semimembranosus tendon origin. Transverse sonographic grayscale image at the level of the ischial tuberosity (*IT*) during hamstring tendon PRP instillation demonstrates a needle (*arrowheads*) advanced in-plane from lateral to medial. The needle tip is positioned within the thickened and heterogeneous hamstring origin.

The PRP should be instilled at the enthesis and into the diseased tendon origin as it is being withdrawn. Postprocedural imaging is typically performed to assess for resolution of hyperemia.

Knee

Corticosteroid

Knee joint The most common indication for intraarticular corticosteroid injections in the knee is primary osteoarthritis, with nearly half of all adults developing symptomatic knee osteoarthritis by age 85 years.[34] A systematic review in 2015 suggested a moderate improvement in pain and small improvement in physical function with intraarticular corticosteroids, although the results remain inconclusive due to the low quality of evidence.[35] The duration of symptomatic relief is variable, and a recent study by McAlindon and colleagues[36] found significantly greater cartilage volume loss and no significant difference in knee pain after 2 years of intraarticular injections with triamcinolone as compared with saline.

The patient is positioned supine with the knee in 20° of flexion. The transducer is placed in the transverse plane over the suprapatellar recess. If no joint effusion is seen, varying the degree of knee flexion and/or manually compressing other areas of the knee joint may displace fluid into the suprapatellar recess. The needle is advanced in-plane from lateral to medial until the tip is positioned within the suprapatellar recess, deep to the quadriceps fat pad (**Fig. 8**). Distension of the suprapatellar recess should be seen in real-time, and pooling of fluid around the tip or excessive patient pain may result from injection into the fat pad.

Popliteal (Baker) cyst Popliteal (Baker) cysts are commonly encountered popliteal fossa cysts that communicate with the posterior knee joint via a

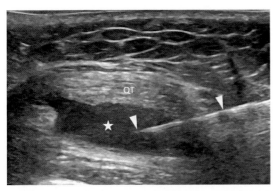

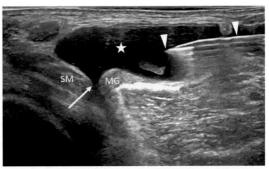

Fig. 8. Knee injection in a 52-year-old woman with right medial meniscus tear and knee pain. Transverse sonographic grayscale image during an intraarticular knee joint injection demonstrates a needle (*arrowheads*) advanced in-plane from lateral to medial. The needle tip is positioned subjacent to the distal quadriceps tendon (*QT*) within the fluid-distended suprapatellar recess (*star*).

Fig. 9. Baker cyst aspiration and injection in a 60-year-old man with right medial meniscus tear and posterior knee fullness. Transverse sonographic grayscale image of the posterior knee during Baker cyst aspiration and injection demonstrates a needle (*arrowheads*) advanced in-plane from lateral to medial. The needle tip is positioned within the center of the fluid-distended Baker cyst (*star*) at the level of cyst neck (*arrow*). The narrow neck is marginated by the medial head of the gastrocnemius (*MG*) and the semimembranosus (*SM*) tendons.

neck interposed between the medial head of the gastrocnemius and the semimembranosus tendons. Baker cysts may herald intraarticular pathology, including primary osteoarthritis or internal derangement.[37] These cysts can compress neurovascular structures in the popliteal fossa, leading to peripheral neuropathy, ischemia, or thrombosis.[38] Cyst rupture can cause acute-onset severe calf pain and swelling. Pain, stiffness, and limitations in physical function from Baker cysts have been found to respond well to US-guided aspiration followed by corticosteroid injection.[39] Recurrence rates after aspiration have been reported as 12.7%, which is favorable compared with arthroscopic resection.[39]

The patient is positioned prone. The transducer is placed over the popliteal fossa in the region of the medial head of the gastrocnemius and semimembranosus tendons to evaluate for a Baker cyst, best evaluated in the transverse plane. The needle is advanced in-plane until the tip is positioned within the cyst at the level of the neck (Fig. 9). Internal septations, if present, can be fenestrated to maximize cyst decompression. However, repeated fenestration of the cyst walls can lead to decompression of cyst contents into the surrounding soft tissues.

Platelet-rich plasma
Patellar tendon Patellar tendinopathy is a common condition in both recreational and elite athletes. Incidence has been reported as high as 45% in high-risk sports such as basketball and volleyball.[40] Cumulative repetitive microtrauma from overuse overwhelms the healing capacity of

the tendon, leading to disorganized collagen fibers, calcification, fibrosis, and neovascularization.[41,42] A systematic review of PRP in the treatment of patellar tendinopathy demonstrated significant symptomatic pain relief and improved function following PRP injection; however, there was insufficient evidence to confirm superiority over control treatments.[43]

The patient is positioned supine with the knee in 20° of flexion. The transducer is placed in the longitudinal plane over the anterior knee to visualize the patellar tendon in long axis. The patellar tendon should be assessed for tendinosis, tears, calcifications, and hyperemia (Fig. 10A). The needle is advanced in-plane from caudal to cranial, and the most tendinopathic and hyperemic regions of the tendon are targeted. Subsequently, the needle is advanced until the tip contacts the periosteum overlying the proximal patellar tendon attachment (Fig. 10B) and approximately 1 mL of PRP injected at the enthesis. The remainder of the PRP is instilled into the diseased portions of the tendon.

Foot/Ankle

Corticosteroid
Ankle (tibiotalar) joint Symptomatic arthritis in the ankle is 9 times less frequent relative to the knee and hip and is most commonly secondary to trauma or abnormal biomechanics.[44] Corticosteroid injections for treatment of ankle pain are less well studied than in the hip and knee; however, one study examining the efficacy of foot

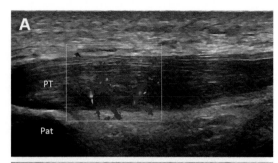

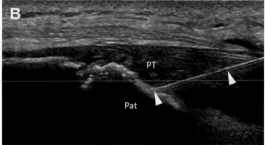

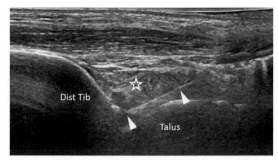

Fig. 11. Ankle injection in a 33-year-old runner with persistent left ankle pain and swelling. Longitudinal sonographic grayscale image during an intraarticular ankle injection demonstrates the needle (*arrowheads*) advanced in-plane from distal to proximal. The needle is advanced until the tip contacts the anterior lip of the distal tibia (*Dist Tib*). Injectate distends the tibiotalar joint and uplifts the overlying anterior ankle joint fat pad (*open star*).

Fig. 10. Patellar tendon PRP injection in a 20-year-old man with persistent left anterior knee pain since lateral patellar dislocation and patellar avulsion fracture. (*A*) Preprocedural longitudinal color Doppler image of the inferior pole of the patella (*Pat*) demonstrates a thickened and hyperemic patellar tendon (*PT*). (*B*) Longitudinal sonographic grayscale image during PRP instillation demonstrates the needle (*arrowheads*) advanced in-plane from caudal to cranial. The needle is advanced through the region of patellar tendinopathy, with tip positioned at the proximal patellar tendon enthesis.

and ankle corticosteroid injections found that 82% of patients with hindfoot and midfoot osteoarthritis received significant short-term benefit from intraarticular corticosteroid injections.[45]

The patient is positioned supine with the foot slightly plantarflexed. The transducer is placed in the longitudinal plane over the anterior ankle joint. The anterior ankle tendons, dorsalis pedis artery, and superficial and deep peroneal nerves lie over the anterior ankle joint and should be avoided. The needle is advanced in-plane from distal to proximal until the tip contacts the anterior lip of the distal tibia. Installation of injectate should result in uplifting of the fat pad within the anterior ankle joint recess, which is intraarticular but extrasynovial in location (**Fig. 11**).

Peroneal tendon sheath The peroneus longus and brevis tendons share a synovial sheath at the level of the distal fibula, coursing inferiorly along the lateral ankle before splitting into 2 separate tendon sheaths at the peroneal tubercle of the calcaneus. The peroneal tendons are prone to injury with

ankle plantarflexion and inversion,[46] with pathology including tenosynovitis, degeneration, tears, and subluxation or dislocation. Corticosteroid injections can provide symptomatic relief; however, they may also increase the risk of propagating preexisting tendon tears and have been reported to be associated with peroneus longus tendon rupture.[47]

The patient is placed in lateral decubitus position with the affected side up or prone. The transducer is placed in the short axis plane of the peroneal tendon sheath near the site of the patient's maximal symptoms, and the needle is advanced in-plane from posterior to anterior until the tip is positioned within the tendon sheath (**Fig. 12**). Injection with the needle tip within the tendon substance should be avoided due to the risk of inducing a tendon tear. Postprocedural images of the peroneal tendon sheath should confirm spread of injectate within the tendon sheath proximal and distal to the site of injection.

Retrocalcaneal bursa The retrocalcaneal bursa is located dorsal to the posterior superior calcaneus and deep to the Achilles tendon. Retrocalcaneal bursitis can occur with repetitive microtrauma, inflammatory conditions such as rheumatoid arthritis, or in the setting of Achilles tendinopathy.[48] A short-term follow-up study of patients with retrocalcaneal bursitis demonstrated statistically significant pain relief following corticosteroid injection.[49]

The patient is positioned prone. The transducer is placed in the transverse plane over the posterior ankle to identify the retrocalcaneal bursa deep to the Achilles tendon. Preprocedural imaging may

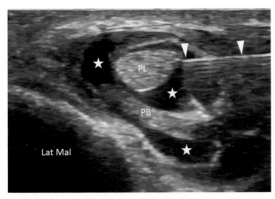

Fig. 12. Peroneal tendon sheath injection in a 16-year-old woman with 2-month history of lateral left ankle pain since ankle inversion injury. Transverse sonographic grayscale image of the lateral ankle during peroneal tendon sheath injection demonstrates the needle (*arrowheads*) advanced in-plane from posterior to anterior. The peroneus longus (*PL*) and peroneus brevis (*PB*) tendons are visualized in short axis at the level of the lateral malleolus (*Lat Mal*). The needle tip is positioned within the peroneal tendon sheath, which is distended with anechoic injectate (*stars*).

reveal Achilles tendinopathy or fluid within the retrocalcaneal bursa. The needle is advanced in-plane from lateral to medial, and the needle tip is positioned deep to the distal Achilles tendon. Instillation of injectate should result in bursal distension (**Fig. 13**).

Plantar fascia The plantar fascia is a fibrous aponeurosis, which arises from the medial calcaneal tuberosity and extends toward the metatarsal heads and toes. Plantar fasciitis is the most common cause of heel pain and occurs secondary to

repetitive microtrauma and inflammation.[50] US may be a useful adjunct when the clinical diagnosis is uncertain or the patient fails to respond to conservative therapy; a systematic review found US to be effective for diagnosis of plantar fasciitis when compared with both clinical examination and MRI.[51] Plantar fascia thickness greater than 4 mm is typically considered abnormal, and decreasing thickness following therapy is often used to assess favorable response to treatment.[52] A consensus statement by the American College of Foot and Ankle Surgeons stated that corticosteroid injections are safe and effective in the treatment of plantar fasciitis.[53]

The patient is positioned prone. The transducer is placed over the plantar heel in the longitudinal plane for visualization of the plantar fascia in long axis. The needle is advanced in-plane from proximal to distal until the needle tip is positioned immediately superficial to the region of maximal plantar fascia thickening. Care should be taken not to fenestrate the plantar fascia, which could induce a tear. Instillation of injectate should result in spread of fluid along the fascial plane deep to the subcutaneous fat and superficial to the plantar fascia (**Fig. 14**).

Platelet-rich plasma
Achilles tendon Achilles tendon overuse is a common disorder that affects both athletes and nonactive middle-aged individuals. Achilles tendinopathy is characterized by abnormal tissue repair and degeneration rather than inflammation. Conservative therapies include rest and eccentric exercises; however, these have been found to be more effective for treatment of midsubstance

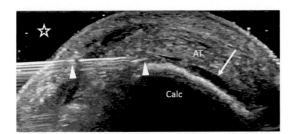

Fig. 13. Retrocalcaneal bursal injection in a 66-year-old woman with posterior left heel pain and Achilles tendinopathy. Transverse sonographic grayscale image at the level of the posterior superior calcaneus (*Calc*) during retrocalcaneal bursa injection demonstrates the needle (*arrowheads*) advanced in-plane from lateral to medial. A gel standoff pad (*open star*) optimizes visualization of the needle by enabling a trajectory parallel to the transducer. The needle tip is positioned subjacent to the distal Achilles tendon (*AT*), with anechoic injectate distending the retrocalcaneal bursa (*arrow*).

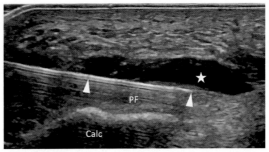

Fig. 14. Plantar fascial injection in a 38-year-old woman with left heel pain and plantar fasciopathy. Longitudinal sonographic grayscale image of the plantar calcaneus (*Calc*) during plantar fascia injection demonstrates a needle (*arrowheads*) advanced in-plane from proximal to distal. The needle tip is positioned superficial to the thickened plantar *fascia* (*PF*). Anechoic injectate (*star*) distends the fascial plane between the subcutaneous fat and plantar fascia.

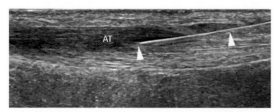

Fig. 15. Achilles tendon PRP injection in a 67-year-old woman with chronic right Achilles tendinopathy recalcitrant to conservative therapy. Longitudinal sonographic grayscale image of the distal Achilles tendon during PRP instillation demonstrates a needle (*arrowheads*) advanced in-plane from caudal to cranial. The needle tip is positioned within the hypoechoic and thickened superficial fibers of the Achilles tendon (*AT*) at the level of maximal tendinopathy.

compared with insertional Achilles tendinopathy.[54] Literature on the efficacy of PRP for Achilles tendinopathy is mixed, with one study demonstrating no statistically significant difference between PRP and sham injection with saline.[55] However, the act of fenestration and saline injection may, in itself, disrupt vascular and neural ingrowth, promote local bleeding, and lead to platelet recruitment.[56]

The patient is positioned prone with the foot slightly dorsiflexed. A large gel pad should be used for optimal visualization of the posterior ankle. The transducer is placed in the anatomic sagittal plane over the posterior ankle to obtain a long axis view of the Achilles tendon. The Achilles tendon should be assessed for tendinosis, tears, calcification, or hyperemia. The needle is advanced in-plane from caudal to cranial into the most tendinopathic and hyperemic portion of the tendon (**Fig. 15**). Postprocedural imaging should be performed to assess for resolution of hyperemia following injection.

SUMMARY

Diagnostic and therapeutic interventions of the pelvis and lower extremity are commonly performed in MSK radiology. As US-guided interventions for the management of MSK conditions become more commonplace, familiarity with these techniques is becoming increasingly important. Understanding the relevant anatomy and technical considerations of commonly performed US-guided interventions is key to ensuring patient safety and procedural accuracy.

REFERENCES

1. Björklund L. The bone and joint decade 2000-2010. Inaugural meeting 17 and 18 April 1998, Lund, Sweden. Acta Orthop Scand 1998;69:67–86.

2. Ortman JM, Velkoff VA, Hogan H. An aging nation: the older population in the United States. In: Current Population Reports. 2014. Available at: https://www.census.gov/content/dam/Census/library/publications/2014/demo/p25-1140.pdf. Accessed January 20, 2018.

3. Parker L, Nazarian LN, Carrino JA, et al. Musculoskeletal imaging: medicare use, costs, and potential for cost substitution. J Am Coll Radiol 2008;5:182–8.

4. Joines MM, Motamedi K, Seeger LL, et al. Musculoskeletal interventional ultrasound. Semin Musculoskelet Radiol 2007;11:192–8.

5. Hoeber S, Aly AR, Ashworth N, et al. Ultrasound-guided hip joint injections are more accurate than landmark-guided injections: a systematic review and meta-analysis. Br J Sports Med 2016;50:392–6.

6. Berkoff DJ, Miller LE, Block JE. Clinical utility of ultrasound guidance for intra-articular knee injections: a review. Clin Interv Aging 2012;7:89–95.

7. Heidari N, Pichler W, Grechenig S, et al. Does the anteromedial or anterolateral approach alter the rate of joint puncture in injection of the ankle? A cadaver study. J Bone Joint Surg Br 2010;92:176–8.

8. Reach JS, Easley ME, Chuckpaiwong B, et al. Accuracy of ultrasound guided injections in the foot and ankle. Foot Ankle Int 2009;30:239–42.

9. Finnoff JT, Hurdle MF, Smith J. Accuracy of ultrasound-guided versus fluoroscopically guided contrast-controlled piriformis injections: a cadaveric study. J Ultrasound Med 2008;27:1157–63.

10. Rutten MJ, Collins JM, Maresch BJ, et al. Glenohumeral joint injection: a comparative study of ultrasound and fluoroscopically guided techniques before MR arthrography. Eur Radiol 2009;19:722–30.

11. Odoom JE, Allen GM, Wilson DJ. Response to local anaesthetic injection as a predictor of successful hip surgery. Clin Radiol 1999;54:430–3.

12. Koski JM, Anttila PJ, Isomäki HA. Ultrasonography of the adult hip joint. Scand J Rheumatol 1989;18:113–7.

13. Wank R, Miller TT, Shapiro JF. Sonographically guided injection of anesthetic for iliopsoas tendinopathy after total hip arthroplasty. J Clin Ultrasound 2004;32:354–7.

14. Chandler SB. The iliopsoas bursa in man. Anat Rec 1934;58:235–40.

15. Aszmann O, Dellon E, Dellon A. Anatomical course of the lateral femoral cutaneous nerve and its susceptibility to compression and injury. Plast Reconstr Surg 1997;100:600–4.

16. Rudin D, Manestar M, Ullrich O, et al. The anatomical course of the lateral femoral cutaneous nerve with special attention to the anterior approach to the hip joint. J Bone Joint Surg Am 2016;98:561–7.

17. Shumway NK, Cole E, Fernandez KH. Neurocutaneous disease: neurocutaneous dysesthesias. J Am Acad Dermatol 2016;74:215–28.

18. Goulding K, Beaulé PE, Kim PR, et al. Incidence of lateral femoral cutaneous nerve neuropraxia after anterior approach to hip arthroplasty. Clin Orthop Relat Res 2010;468:2397–404.

19. Shbeeb MI, Matteson EL. Trochanteric bursitis (greater trochanter pain syndrome). Mayo Clin Proc 1996;71:565–9.

20. Long SS, Surrey DE, Nazarian LN. Sonography of greater trochanteric pain syndrome and the rarity of primary bursitis. AJR Am J Roentgenol 2013; 201:1083–6.

21. Blankenbaker DG, Ullrick SR, Davis KW, et al. Correlation of MRI findings with clinical findings of trochanteric pain syndrome. Skeletal Radiol 2008; 37:903–9.

22. Silva F, Adams T, Feinstein J, et al. Trochanteric bursitis: refuting the myth of inflammation. J Clin Rheumatol 2008;14:82–6.

23. Lustenberger DP, Ng VY, Best TM, et al. Efficacy of treatment of trochanteric bursitis: a systematic review. Clin J Sport Med 2011;21:447–53.

24. McEvoy JR, Lee KS, Blankenbaker DG, et al. Ultrasound-guided corticosteroid injections for treatment of greater trochanteric pain syndrome: greater trochanter bursa versus subgluteus medius bursa. AJR Am J Roentgenol 2013;201:W313–7.

25. Cho KH, Lee SM, Lee YH, et al. Non-infectious ischiogluteal bursitis: MRI findings. Korean J Radiol 2004;5:280–6.

26. Van Mieghem IM, Boets A, Sciot R, et al. Ischiogluteal bursitis: an uncommon type of bursitis. Skeletal Radiol 2004;33:413–6.

27. Kim SM, Shin MJ, Kim KS, et al. Imaging features of ischial bursitis with an emphasis on ultrasonography. Skeletal Radiol 2002;31:631–6.

28. Wisniewski SJ, Hurdle MF, Ericsson JM, et al. Ultrasound-guided ischial bursa injection: technique and positioning considerations. PM R 2014;6: 56–60.

29. Torriani M, Souto SC, Thomas BJ, et al. Ischiofemoral impingement syndrome: an entity with hip pain and abnormalities of the quadratus femoris muscle. AJR Am J Roentgenol 2009;193:186–90.

30. Taneja AK, Bredella MA, Torriana M. Ischiofemoral impingement. Magn Reson Imaging Clin N Am 2013;21:65–73.

31. Backer MW, Lee KS, Blankenbaker DG, et al. Correlation of ultrasound-guided corticosteroid injection of the quadratus femoris with MRI findings of ischiofemoral impingement. AJR Am J Roentgenol 2014; 203:589–93.

32. Wilson MD, Keene JS. Treatment of ischiofemoral impingement: results of diagnostic injections and arthroscopic resection of the lesser trochanter. J Hip Preserv Surg 2016;3:146–53.

33. Hamilton B, Tol JL, Almusa E, et al. Platelet-rich plasma does not enhance return to play in hamstring injuries: a randomised controlled trial. Br J Sports Med 2015;49:943–50.

34. Murphy L, Schwartz TA, Helmick CG, et al. Lifetime risk of symptomatic knee osteoarthritis. Arthritis Rheum 2008;59:1207–13.

35. da Costa BR, Hari R, Jüni P. Intra-articular corticosteroids for osteoarthritis of the knee. JAMA 2016; 316:2671–2.

36. McAlindon TE, LaValley MP, Harvey WF, et al. Effect of intra-articular triamcinolone vs saline on knee cartilage volume and pain in patients with knee osteoarthritis: a randomized clinical trial. JAMA 2017; 317:1967–75.

37. Rupp S, Seil R, Jochum P, et al. Popliteal cysts in adults. Prevalence, associated intra-articular lesions, and results after arthroscopic treatment. Am J Sports Med 2002;30:112–5.

38. Sanchez JE, Conkling N, Labropoulos N. Compression syndromes of the popliteal neurovascular bundle due to Baker cyst. J Vasc Surg 2011;54: 1821–9.

39. Smith MK, Lesniak B, Baraga MG, et al. Treatment of popliteal (Baker) cysts with ultrasound-guided aspiration, fenestration, and injection: long-term follow-up. Sports Health 2015;7:409–14.

40. Lian OB, Engebretsen L, Bahr R. Prevalence of jumper's knee among elite athletes from different sports: a cross-sectional study. Am J Sports Med 2005;33: 561–7.

41. van Ark M, Zwerver J, van den Akker-Scheek I. Injection treatments for patellar tendinopathy. Br J Sports Med 2011;45:1068–76.

42. Warden SJ, Brukner P. Patellar tendinopathy. Clin Sports Med 2003;22:743–59.

43. Liddle AD, Rodríguez-Merchán EC. Platelet-rich plasma in the treatment of patellar tendinopathy: a systematic review. Am J Sports Med 2015;43: 2583–90.

44. Thomas RH, Daniels TR. Ankle arthritis. J Bone Joint Surg Am 2003;85-A:923–36.

45. Grice J, Marsland D, Smith G, et al. Efficacy of foot and ankle corticosteroid injections. Foot Ankle Int 2017;38:8–13.

46. Roster B, Michelier P, Giza E. Peroneal tendon disorders. Clin Sports Med 2015;34:625–41.

47. Borland S, Jung S, Hugh IA. Complete rupture of the peroneus longus tendon secondary to injection. Foot (Edinb) 2009;19:229–31.

48. Reddy SS, Pedowitz DI, Parekh SG, et al. Surgical treatment for chronic disease and disorders of the Achilles tendon. J Am Acad Orthop Surg 2009;17: 3–14.

49. Goldberg-Stein S, Berko N, Thornhill B, et al. Fluoroscopically guided retrocalcaneal bursa steroid injection: description of the technique and pilot study of short-term patient outcomes. Skeletal Radiol 2016; 45:1107–12.

50. Goff JD, Crawford R. Diagnosis and treatment of plantar fasciitis. Am Fam Physician 2011;84:676–82.

51. Radwan A, Wyland M, Applequist L, et al. Ultrasonography, an effective tool in diagnosing plantar fasciitis: a systematic review of diagnostic trials. Int J Sports Phys Ther 2016;11:663–71.

52. Mahowald S, Legge BS, Grady JF. The correlation between plantar fascia thickness and symptoms of plantar fasciitis. J Am Podiatr Med Assoc 2011;101:385–9.

53. Schneider HP, Baca J, Carpenter B, et al. American College of Foot and Ankle Surgeons clinical consensus statement: diagnosis and treatment of adult acquired infracalcaneal heel pain. J Foot Ankle Surg 2018. https://doi.org/10.1053/j.jfas.2017.10.018.

54. Rees JD, Maffulli N, Cook J. Management of tendinopathy. Am J Sports Med 2009;37:1855–67.

55. de Vos RJ, Weir A, van Schie HT, et al. Platelet-rich plasma injection for chronic Achilles tendinopathy: a randomized controlled trial. JAMA 2010;303:144–9.

56. Rabago D, Wilson J, Zgierska A. Platelet-rich plasma for treatment of Achilles tendinopathy (letter and reply). JAMA 2010;303:1696–8.

UNITED STATES POSTAL SERVICE®
Statement of Ownership, Management, and Circulation
(All Periodicals Publications Except Requester Publications)

1. Publication Title	2. Publication Number	3. Filing Date
RADIOLOGIC CLINICS OF NORTH AMERICA	596 – 510	9/18/2018

4. Issue Frequency	5. Number of Issues Published Annually	6. Annual Subscription Price
JAN, MAR, MAY, JUL, SEP, NOV	6	$493.00

7. Complete Mailing Address of Known Office of Publication (Not printer) (Street, city, county, state, and ZIP+4®)
ELSEVIER INC.
230 Park Avenue, Suite 800
New York, NY 10169

Contact Person: STEPHEN R. BUSHING
Telephone (Include area code): 215-239-3688

8. Complete Mailing Address of Headquarters or General Business Office of Publisher (Not printer)
ELSEVIER INC.
230 Park Avenue, Suite 800
New York, NY 10169

9. Full Names and Complete Mailing Addresses of Publisher, Editor, and Managing Editor (Do not leave blank)

Publisher (Name and complete mailing address)
TAYLOR E BALL, ELSEVIER INC.
1600 JOHN F KENNEDY BLVD. SUITE 1800
PHILADELPHIA, PA 19103-2899

Editor (Name and complete mailing address)
JOHN VASSALLO, ELSEVIER INC.
1600 JOHN F KENNEDY BLVD. SUITE 1800
PHILADELPHIA, PA 19103-2899

Managing Editor (Name and complete mailing address)
PATRICK MANLEY, ELSEVIER INC.
1600 JOHN F KENNEDY BLVD. SUITE 1800
PHILADELPHIA, PA 19103-2899

10. Owner (Do not leave blank. If the publication is owned by a corporation, give the name and address of the corporation immediately followed by the names and addresses of all stockholders owning or holding 1 percent or more of the total amount of stock. If not owned by a corporation, give the names and addresses of the individual owners. If owned by a partnership or other unincorporated firm, give its name and address as well as those of each individual owner. If the publication is published by a nonprofit organization, give its name and address.)

Full Name	Complete Mailing Address
WHOLLY OWNED SUBSIDIARY OF REED/ELSEVIER, US HOLDINGS	1600 JOHN F KENNEDY BLVD, SUITE 1800 PHILADELPHIA, PA 19103-2899

11. Known Bondholders, Mortgagees, and Other Security Holders Owning or Holding 1 Percent or More of Total Amount of Bonds, Mortgages, or Other Securities. If none, check box ▶ ☐ None

Full Name	Complete Mailing Address
N/A	

12. Tax Status (For completion by nonprofit organizations authorized to mail at nonprofit rates) (Check one)
The purpose, function, and nonprofit status of this organization and the exempt status for federal income tax purposes:
☒ Has Not Changed During Preceding 12 Months
☐ Has Changed During Preceding 12 Months (Publisher must submit explanation of change with this statement)

PS Form 3526, July 2014 (Page 1 of 4 (see instructions page 4))   PSN: 7530-01-000-9931   PRIVACY NOTICE: See our privacy policy on www.usps.com

---

13. Publication Title			14. Issue Date for Circulation Data Below
RADIOLOGIC CLINICS OF NORTH AMERICA			JULY 2018

15. Extent and Nature of Circulation			Average No. Copies Each Issue During Preceding 12 Months	No. Copies of Single Issue Published Nearest to Filing Date
a. Total Number of Copies (Net press run)			867	1153
b. Paid Circulation (By Mail and Outside the Mail)	(1)	Mailed Outside-County Paid Subscriptions Stated on PS Form 3541 (Include paid distribution above nominal rate, advertiser's proof copies, and exchange copies)	566	701
	(2)	Mailed In-County Paid Subscriptions Stated on PS Form 3541 (Include paid distribution above nominal rate, advertiser's proof copies, and exchange copies)	0	0
	(3)	Paid Distribution Outside the Mails Including Sales Through Dealers and Carriers, Street Vendors, Counter Sales, and Other Paid Distribution Outside USPS®	192	313
	(4)	Paid Distribution by Other Classes of Mail Through the USPS (e.g. First-Class Mail®)	0	0
c. Total Paid Distribution (Sum of 15b (1), (2), (3) and (4))		▶	758	1014
d. Free or Nominal Rate Distribution (By Mail and Outside the Mail)	(1)	Free or Nominal Rate Outside-County Copies included on PS Form 3541	76	122
	(2)	Free or Nominal Rate In-County Copies Included on PS Form 3541	0	0
	(3)	Free or Nominal Rate Copies Mailed at Other Classes Through the USPS (e.g. First-Class Mail)	0	0
	(4)	Free or Nominal Rate Distribution Outside the Mail (Carriers or other means)	76	122
e. Total Free or Nominal Rate Distribution (Sum of 15d (1), (2), (3) and (4))		▶	76	122
f. Total Distribution (Sum of 15c and 15e)		▶	834	1136
g. Copies not Distributed (See instructions to Publishers #4 (page #3))		▶	33	17
h. Total (Sum of 15f and g)		▶	867	1153
i. Percent Paid (15c divided by 15f times 100)		▶	90.89%	89.26%

* If you are claiming electronic copies, go to line 16 on page 3. If you are not claiming electronic copies, skip to line 17 on page 3.

16. Electronic Copy Circulation	Average No. Copies Each Issue During Preceding 12 Months	No. Copies of Single Issue Published Nearest to Filing Date
a. Paid Electronic Copies ▶	0	0
b. Total Paid Print Copies (Line 15c) + Paid Electronic Copies (Line 16a) ▶	758	1014
c. Total Print Distribution (Line 15f) + Paid Electronic Copies (Line 16a) ▶	834	1136
d. Percent Paid (Both Print & Electronic Copies) (16b divided by 16c × 100) ▶	90.89%	89.26%

☒ I certify that 50% of all my distributed copies (electronic and print) are paid above a nominal price.

17. Publication of Statement of Ownership
☒ If the publication is a general publication, publication of this statement is required. Will be printed in the NOVEMBER 2018 issue of this publication.   ☐ Publication not required.

18. Signature and Title of Editor, Publisher, Business Manager, or Owner   Date: 9/18/2018
STEPHEN R. BUSHING, INVENTORY DISTRIBUTION CONTROL MANAGER

I certify that all information furnished on this form is true and complete. I understand that anyone who furnishes false or misleading information on this form or who omits material or information requested on the form may be subject to criminal sanctions (including fines and imprisonment) and/or civil sanctions (including civil penalties).

PS Form 3526, July 2014 (Page 2 of 4)   PRIVACY NOTICE: See our privacy policy on www.usps.com

Moving?

Make sure your subscription moves with you!

To notify us of your new address, find your **Clinics Account Number** (located on your mailing label above your name), and contact customer service at:

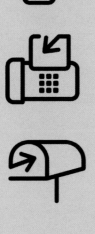

Email: journalscustomerservice-usa@elsevier.com

800-654-2452 (subscribers in the U.S. & Canada)
314-447-8871 (subscribers outside of the U.S. & Canada)

Fax number: 314-447-8029

Elsevier Health Sciences Division
Subscription Customer Service
3251 Riverport Lane
Maryland Heights, MO 63043